PSYCHIATRIC
CARE PLANNING

PSYCHIATRIC
CARE PLANNING

Susan L.W. Krupnick, RN, MSN, CARN, CCRN, CS
Psychiatric Consultation-Liaison Nurse
Hospital of the University of Pennsylvania
Adjunct Lecturer
University of Pennsylvania
Philadelphia

Andrew J. Wade, RN, MSN
Psychiatric Clinical Nurse Specialist
Inpatient Emergency Psychiatric Nursing
Thomas Jefferson University Hospital
Adjunct Lecturer
Thomas Jefferson University
Philadelphia

Springhouse Corporation
Springhouse, Pennsylvania

Staff

Executive Director, Editorial
Stanley Loeb

Director of Trade and Textbooks
Minnie B. Rose, RN, BSN, MEd

Art Director
John Hubbard

Clinical Consultant
Maryann Foley, RN, BSN

Acquisitions Assistant
Caroline Lemoine

Drug Information Editor
George J. Blake, RPh, MS

Editors
Diane Labus, Richard Stull

Copy Editors
Mary Hohenhaus Hardy, Pamela Wingrod

Designers
Stephanie Peters (associate art director),
StellarVisions, ARC Designs (cover design)

Typography
David Kosten (director), Diane Paluba (manager), Elizabeth Bergman, Joyce Rossi Biletz, Mary Madden, Phyllis Marron, Robin Mayer, Valerie Rosenberger

Manufacturing
Deborah Meiris (manager), Anna Brindisi,
T.A. Landis

Library of Congress Cataloging-in-Publication Data
Psychiatric care planning/[edited by] Susan L.W. Krupnick, Andrew J. Wade.
    p. cm.
    Includes bibliographical references and index.
    1. Psychiatric nursing.   2. Nursing care plans.
    I. Krupnick, Susan L.W. II. Wade, Andrew J.
[DNLM: 1. Patient Care Planning—nurses' instruction.
2. Psychiatric Nursing—methods. WY 160 P9717]
RC440.P7298 1993
610.73'68—dc20
DNLM/DLC   92-2365
ISBN 0-87434-399-2   CIP

Contents

Section III: Assessment Tools

Appendices

Index

Consultant and Contributors

Consultant

Jean A. Haspeslagh, RN, DNS
Associate Professor
University of Southern Mississippi
School of Nursing
Hattiesburg

Contributors

Suzanne M. Brennan, RN, MSN, CS
Private Nurse Psychotherapist and
Family Therapist
Doctoral Student
University of Pennsylvania
Philadelphia
(Attention Deficit Disorder)

Martha G. Horton, RN, MSN, CS
Clinical Nurse Specialist
Thomas Jefferson University Hospital
Philadelphia
(Organic Mental Disorders)

Lynette W. Jack, RN, PhD, CARN
Assistant Professor
University of Pittsburgh
School of Nursing
(Polysubstance Dependence)

Catherine Knox-Fischer, RN, MSN
Mental Health Clinical Nurse Specialist
Children's Hospital of Philadelphia
(Conduct Disorder)

Susan L.W. Krupnick, RN, MSN, CARN,
CCRN, CS
Psychiatric Consultation-Liaison Nurse
Hospital of the University of
Pennsylvania
Adjunct Lecturer
University of Pennsylvania
Philadelphia
(Adjustment Disorder, Anorexia
Nervosa and Bulimia Nervosa, Central
Nervous System Depressant
Dependence, Cluster A and Cluster C
Personality Disorders, General Anxiety
Disorders, Interpersonal Violence: .
Rape-Trauma Syndrome, Phobic and
Panic Disorders, Post-traumatic Stress
Disorder, Psychophysiologic Disorders,
Sleep Disorders, Vicarious
Traumatization)

Tona Leiker, RN, MN, CARN, NCAC-II
Associate Director
Chemical Dependency Services
St. Francis Regional Medical Center
Wichita, Kan.
(Hallucinogen Dependence)

Patricia Long, RN, EdD, CARN, CS
Associate Professor and Chair
Department of Family and Community
Health Nursing
School of Nursing
State University of New York at
Stonybrook;
Private Psychotherapist
(Alcoholism)

Mimi Meiselman, RN, MS, CAC
Research Associate
Alcohol Research Program
Rush–Presbyterian–St. Luke's Medical
Center
Chicago
(Stimulant Dependence)

Alfred J. Moyer, RN, MS, CS
Psychiatric Clinical Nurse Specialist
Hospital of the University of
Pennsylvania
Adjunct Clinical Lecturer
Psychiatric Mental Health Division
School of Nursing
University of Pennsylvania
Philadelphia
(Cluster B Personality Disorders)

Lisa Rubin, RN, MSN
Nurse Clinician
Bipolar Disorders Unit
Hospital of the University of
Pennsylvania
Philadelphia
(Bipolar Disorders)

Nancy Vanore-Black, RN, MSN, CS
Psychotherapist
Bryn Mawr, Pa.
(Depressive Disorders)

Andrew J. Wade, RN, MSN
Psychiatric Clinical Nurse Specialist
Thomas Jefferson University Hospital
Adjunct Lecturer
Thomas Jefferson University
Philadelphia
(Delusional [Paranoid Disorder],
Dissociative Disorders, Gender Identity
Disorder, Interpersonal Violence: Rape-
Trauma Syndrome, Miscellaneous
Psychotic Disorders, Obsessive-
Compulsive Disorder, Schizophrenic
Disorders, Sexual Disorders)

Acknowledgments

This project could not have been accomplished without enlisting the assistance and support of many individuals. We wish to acknowledge the outstanding work that each contributor provided in strengthening the fabric of this book. We also are grateful to our families for their emotional backing and nurturance throughout the course of our work and are most appreciative of our friends, colleagues, and co-workers who "covered" us many times over.

Heartfelt thanks is extended to Marlene, Vicki, and Elizabeth for their support and guidance. We also would like to express our gratitude to Eraina Cocomero and Gail Cowan for their excellence and diligence in the technical preparation of numerous drafts. Also, without Caroline Lemoine's efforts and encouragement, this project might still be an unfulfilled idea on our "Things to Do" list.

Last, we wish to applaud each other for our resilience, persistence, and consistent commitment to enhancing the mental health of individuals.

Dedication
We dedicate this book to all of the nurses, patients, and families who struggle with psychiatric-mental health and addiction disorders. We wish them continued success in their endeavors in learning to use and help improve our country's mental health system.

S.L.K.
A.W.

Preface

Psychiatric nursing has undergone tremendous growth and development as a specialty in the past 50 years. As psychiatric nurses' roles and responsibilities have expanded, so has their need for resources that address all aspects of client care. *Psychiatric Care Planning* is a comprehensive reference for psychiatric nurses in any clinical practice environment, including inpatient psychiatric units, outpatient clinics, psychiatric emergency or crisis intervention units, long-term treatment programs, or extended care facilities. Nurses practicing in medical-surgical units also will find this manual useful when caring for the client with an illness-related emotional problem or a coexisting psychiatric diagnosis.

Section I offers a multifaceted overview of psychiatric nursing. A brief history of psychiatric and mental health care in the United States provides a context for later discussions of nursing roles and functions, conceptual models appropriate to psychiatry and psychiatric nursing, treatment modalities, stress and mental illness, and the nursing process as it applies to psychiatric nursing.

Section II offers 29 comprehensive plans of care, grouped according to psychiatric diagnosis. The plans are based on the nurse's role as both an independent and interdependent (collaborative) practitioner and consequently address both levels of practice. The plans offer both the American Nurses' Association's psychiatric diagnostic categories and classifications from the American Psychiatric Association's *Diagnostic and Statistical Manual,* third edition, revised (DSM III-R). The interface between the two diagnostic classification systems is accented throughout to foster the cooperation, coordination, and collaboration among health care professionals that is so necessary to quality health care.

Each plan begins with an introduction to basic information about the disorder and its possible causes. The next two sections cover the nursing history and physical findings, and guide the nurse through the assessment process; potential complications also are listed. Appropriate nursing diagnoses (approved by the North American Nursing Diagnosis Association [NANDA]), nursing priorities, interventions, and rationales follow. Each plan concludes with lists of outcome and discharge criteria, to facilitate evaluation and documentation, and a list of selected references, to guide further reading.

Section III provides clinically based assessment tools, interview guides, and scales to enhance the nurse's ability to perform comprehensive assessments. These tools will help the nurse focus care according to individualized responses and clinically relevant information.

The appendices provide additional information of interest to the psychiatric nurse, including the DSM III-R classification categories and codes, psychiatric nursing taxonomy, and NANDA diagnostic categories arranged by Gordon's functional health patterns; laboratory tests necessary in long-term drug therapy, psychiatric drug reactions, and managing adverse drug reactions; managing acute substance abuse; and resources for clients and their families.

Psychiatric Care Planning is an up-to-date, reliable source of practical information for planning and administering care in any practice setting. Psychiatric nurses will find it an invaluable reference and indispensable care planning tool.

Section I: Overview of Psychiatric Nursing

INTRODUCTION

The Development of Psychiatric Nursing

As the specialty of psychiatry has grown and evolved, so has the specialty of psychiatric-mental health nursing. The emphasis in psychiatric-mental health nursing has expanded from primarily custodial care, to maintaining a therapeutic environment and promoting interpersonal relationships, to an expanded focus that includes community-based practice and such therapeutic interventions as individual, group, and family therapy. The nurse's role in psychiatric-mental health care has progressed from a primary emphasis on protecting society from the client and the client from the self to promoting the client's return to a productive life or, if that is not feasible, placement in the least restrictive environment possible.

In early times, mental illness was viewed as a punishment from the gods or ancestral spirits. Fear and superstition predominated; beliefs in demonology and witchcraft were widespread. According to these beliefs, human beings are powerless to help the disturbed individual; therefore, a cure is possible only if the spirits are willing. Consequently, interventions focused on physically restraining those considered violent or dangerous. Mentally ill patients were ostracized and segregated, typically confined and isolated from the community.

During the seventeenth and eighteenth centuries, scientific investigation into the causes of some mental disturbances began. During this time, Pennsylvania Hospital in Philadelphia became the first public institution in the United States to admit mentally ill clients. Institutionalization became the focus of psychiatric care in the nineteenth century. Many small psychiatric hospitals and large state institutions were established, resulting in a system of segregated, specialized care facilities for mentally ill clients.

The first school specifically designed to prepare nurses to care for these clients was established in Waverly, Massachusetts, in the late nineteenth century (Stuart and Sundeen, 1991). It prepared psychiatric nurses to assist the physician; induce the client to eat; provide hydrotherapy, such as hot and cold showers, continuous baths, and wet packs; and administer sedative drugs (such as whiskey, chloroform, or paraldehyde). Nursing care from the late nineteenth century until the 1930s did not vary much from this model. Psychiatric nursing's primary goal was to meet the client's physical needs through custodial care. Therapeutic measures were largely limited to exhibiting tolerant, humane behavior.

The first psychiatric nurses faced three major stumbling blocks to delivering care to mentally ill clients. First, individualized care was difficult because of the large number of hospitalized clients and the limited number of professional staff. Second, the chronic nature of psychiatric illness made intervention difficult. Third, psychotic behavior compounded the difficulties in caring for mentally ill clients.

Two factors in the early twentieth century greatly influenced psychiatric care. The first was the development of the National Mental Hygiene Movement, which promoted a focus on mental health rather than on mental illness. Proponents examined the conditions in the community in which the mental illness developed and then postulated how the community contributed to the illness. Proponents believed they could use this knowledge to balance mental health care, promoting prevention along with treatment. The second factor was a growing support for Sigmund Freud's school of psychodynamic psychiatry. Freud believed that mental disorders were a maladaptive response arising from unresolved conflicts between instinctual forces and family and societal expectations. Psychoanalysis, Freud's technique for examining and treating maladaptive responses, became the dominant treatment for mental illness.

Freud's psychoanalytic model paved the way for later models, including Carl Rogers's person-centered therapy, Fredrick Perls's gestalt therapy, Albert Ellis's rational emotive therapy, and Aaron Beck's cognitive behavioral therapy. As research in the fields of psychiatry and psychology increased, numerous theorists attempted to explain the cause of psychiatric conditions.

Despite the impact of the National Mental Hygiene Movement and psychoanalysis on psychiatric care, the psychiatric nurse's role remained largely unchanged. Only nurses employed in private clinics and hospitals, where the staff numbers were adequate for the clients, were able to become more involved in treatment. The emergence in the 1930s of new somatic therapies—including insulin shock therapy, electroshock (electroconvulsive) therapy, and psychosurgery—was of greater significance to psychiatric nursing. As these therapies gained acceptance, the nurses with technical ability, medical-surgical expertise, and interpersonal skills could take a more active role in psychiatric care.

As the economic depression of the 1930s receded, the federal government's involvement in the health care system began to increase. During World War II, American and English psychiatrists working in military installations established community support systems for mentally disabled soldiers. In 1946, the U.S. National Mental Health Act was signed. Three years later, the National Institute for Mental Health (NIMH) was established to examine the causes and promote treatment of mental disorders. The NIMH also provided federal funds for training health care professionals.

After World War II, psychiatric nursing came into its own. Nurse educators recognized the need for a theoretical foundation for nursing practice. Three theoretical models emerged at that time: psychoanalytic theory, interpersonal theory, and communications theory. Hildegard Peplau developed her interpersonal theory. Early in the 1950s, education for psychiatric nursing as a clinical specialty became available at the graduate level. In the late 1950s and early 1960s, psychiatric nursing education changed its focus from somatic therapies to one in which nurses worked with clients in individual and group psychotherapy.

Also during the 1950s, psychopharmacology emerged as an important treatment modality and led to revolutionary changes in the care of mentally ill clients. New medications made possible the control of such symptoms as anxiety, agitation, and aggression without using physical restraints. By reducing these symptoms, psychotherapeutic drugs made clients more open to nursing interventions and enabled them to participate actively in their therapies. Although the nurse's initial role was drug administration and monitoring, the steady increase in the number of psychoactive drugs required psychiatric nurses to understand increasing details of pharmacology.

In 1953, Maxwell Jones introduced a new therapeutic method, known as the therapeutic community, in which the psychiatric nurse held an important and expanded role as part of a multidisciplinary team. Maxwell's method used the treatment environment to reinforce and enhance what the client learned in therapy. Once considered passive, the client was expected to participate actively in care and become an active member of the team. D. Gregg, in a 1954 nursing article, said that the role of the psychiatric nurse was to help create an environment in which the client could develop new and different behavior patterns that would facilitate a more mature adjustment to life. By this time, the foundation for multiple treatment approaches, including milieu therapy, was being laid. Psychiatric hospitals were becoming places for aggressive psychological and biological care, rather than custodial warehouses for mentally ill clients.

The delivery of care changed further in the 1960s. The Community Mental Health Act, passed in 1963, provided financial support for construction and staffing of community-based mental health centers throughout the United States. These community centers were to provide full service to all persons living within a geographic area, called a catchment area. Federal legislation required that community mental health programs include 24-hour emergency care, short-term inpatient care, partial hospitalization (including day and night treatment centers), follow-up outpatient care for clients living at home, and community consultation and education.

The Community Mental Health Act moved the focus of psychiatric treatment from inpatient care to outpatient treatment and moved many chronically mentally ill clients from institutions to the community. Their treatment and follow-up care were to be provided by community-based mental health centers. Although the intention of this was to place clients in the least restrictive environment possible, its enforcement caused problems related to client preparation for a return to the community, client financial support, and the ability of the mental health system to meet the liberated client's needs. Changing politics and erratic funding further worsened the problems.

With the passage of the Community Mental Health Act, the role of the psychiatric-mental health nurse was no longer limited to traditional models of inpatient therapy but expanded to include prevention, education, community assessment, diagnosis, intervention, and evaluation. With outpatient care, the psychiatric-mental health nurse needed an increased awareness of the role sociocultural factors can play in the development of and recovery from mental illness.

Throughout the 1960s, the psychiatric nursing community prepared advanced practitioners to meet the needs of deinstitutionalized clients and their families. The role of this clinical specialist included six components: those of teacher, therapist, consultant, practitioner, researcher, and change agent. These nurses were expected to function as therapists, base their practice on theory, and practice in whatever setting they found their clients (Wilson, 1988). In addition, two professional psychiatric nursing journals, *Perspectives in Psychiatric Care* and the *Journal of Psychiatric Nursing and Mental Health Services,* were first published during the 1960s, beginning the process of sharing and exchanging expert psychiatric nursing practice among colleagues. These journals provided early evidence that psychiatric nurses could apply their special knowledge and skills to the general hospital setting, laying the foundation for psychiatric consultation-liaison nursing.

The 1970s and 1980s saw numerous advances in the understanding and treatment of psychiatric illness, particularly in biological psychiatry. Interest in psychobiology — the study of the relationships among thought, mood, emotion, affect, and behavior — developed with the discovery of the therapeutic potential of psychoactive drugs. Psychobiological research has offered practitioners a fuller understanding of how the brain works.

During the 1970s, several significant events furthered the professional growth of psychiatric nursing. The American Nurses' Association (ANA) published *Standards of Adult Psychiatric Mental Health Nursing* (revised in 1982). The ANA also administered the first certification exam for psychiatric-mental health nurse generalists and for psychiatric clinical nurse specialists. Another journal, *Issues in Mental Health Nursing,* began publication in 1979.

In 1980, Congress passed the Mental Health Systems Act, restating the need for the federal government's involvement in mental health care. The Act identified specific psychiatric concerns for young, elderly, minority, and chronically ill clients. However, most of the provisions of this Act were ignored because of budget reductions. In 1985, the ANA published *Standards of Child and Adolescent Psychiatric and Mental Health Nursing Practice,* and in 1987, *The Journal of Psychiatric Nursing* began publication.

Although research has improved understanding about mental health, mental illness, and human behavior, many problems remain unexplained or unexplored. Researchers and clinicians will need to work collaboratively and aggressively if psychobiology is to be accepted in the psychiatric communities where strong allegiances continue to the psychoanalytic, psychodynamic, cognitive, and family systems models of treatment. However, many clinicians believe that the psychobiological model can be synthesized into an integrated model of care. Further exploration of this model will include the subspecialties of psychoendocrinology and psychoneuroimmunology. Psychoendocrinology studies the interaction between the brain and endocrine system, investigating the relationship between behavior and endocrine function and how hormones influence neurotransmission and neuroregulation to create ordered brain function. Psychoneuroimmunology investigates the relationship between the nervous and immune systems. Psychobiological research may answer some of the complex questions about how the brain interacts with environmental, psychological, and sociocultural factors to produce behavioral responses.

Selected references

Ader, R., Felten, K.L., and Cohen, N. (1991). *Psychoneuroimmunology* (2nd ed.). New York: Academic Press.

Burgess, A. (1990). *Psychiatric nursing in the hospital and the community.* Norwalk, CT: Appleton & Lange.

Gregg, D. (1954). The psychiatric nurse's role. *American Journal of Nursing.* 45, 848.

Jones, M. (1953). *The therapeutic community.* New York: Basic Books.

Murphy, S.A., and Hoeffer, B. (1987). The evolution of subspecialities in psychiatric and mental health nursing. *Archives of Psychiatric Nursing,* 1(3), 145-54.

Stuart, G.W., and Sundeen, S.J. (1991). *Principles and practice of psychiatric nursing* (4th ed.). St. Louis: Mosby-Year Book.

Wilson, H.S. (1988). *Psychiatric nursing* (3rd ed.). Menlo Park, CA: Addison-Wesley.

INTRODUCTION
Today's Psychiatric Nursing Roles

Psychiatric nursing uses an interpersonal process to promote, maintain, restore, or rehabilitate an individual's mental health. Psychiatric nurses accept individuals, families, groups, and communities as clients, using skills that draw on the psychosocial and biophysical sciences and on theories of personality and human behavior. The American Nurses' Association (ANA) considers psychiatric nursing a specialized area of nursing practice that employs the theories of human behavior as its science and "powerful use of self" as its art; the National Institute of Mental Health recognizes it as a core mental health discipline.

Psychiatric nurses practice in numerous settings, including psychiatric hospitals, community mental health centers, general hospitals, community health agencies, outpatient clinics, homes, schools, prisons, health maintenance organizations, private practice, crisis units, and industrial centers. In those settings, a psychiatric nurse can assume the role of staff nurse, administrator, consultant, in-service educator, clinical practitioner, researcher, program evaluator, primary care provider, and liaison between the client and other members of the health care delivery system.

Various factors determine the level at which a psychiatric nurse practices, including state nurse practice acts, education and experience, certification, practice setting, personal initiative, and professional standards.

Nurse practice acts. Nurse practice acts regulate entry into the profession and define the legal limits of nursing practice. Some state nurse practice acts also address advanced practice.

Education and experience. Education and experience determine whether a psychiatric nurse practices as a generalist or a specialist. The *psychiatric nurse generalist* has received basic nursing preparation, typically a baccalaureate degree, and meets the profession's standards of knowledge, experience, and quality of care. This nurse provides most of the nursing care to patients in inpatient settings, offering direct and indirect care through the nurse-client relationship. However, the psychiatric nurse generalist is not prepared to conduct psychotherapy. The *psychiatric clinical nurse specialist* is a graduate of a master's degree program and has had supervised clinical experience. The specialist has in-depth knowledge, competence, and skill in psychiatric nursing practice and may also be certified by a professional nursing organization. The specialist also can provide individual, family, and group psychotherapy in inpatient, outpatient, and community health settings and in private practice. The specialist can also provide indirect services, teaching, consultation, and administration; the psychiatric liaison nurse provides these services in a general hospital setting.

Certification. Psychiatric nurses may be certified by professional organizations. ANA certification requires a formal review, including a written test. Certification provides credentials for clinical practice as a generalist or specialist.

Practice setting. A health care organization's philosophy of mental health and mental illness and approach toward treatment shape the nurse's and client's expectations. Administrative policies will either foster or limit the full use of the psychiatric nurse's services.

Personal initiative. The willingness to act as a change agent, knowledge of personal strengths and weaknesses, and realization of clinical competence will influence the level at which the psychiatric nurse performs.

Professional standards. Professional standards define nursing practice and performance. The ANA first developed standards for adult psychiatric and mental health nursing in 1973 and revised them in 1982. Standards for child and adolescent psychiatric and mental health nursing were established in 1985; standards for psychiatric consultation-liaison nursing were established in 1990. (See *Selected practice standards,* pages 6 and 7.)

Psychiatric nursing functions involve direct and indirect care. The ANA defines psychiatric nursing functions to include:
- maintaining a therapeutic milieu
- working to solve the client's current problems
- fulfilling a surrogate parent role
- using somatic therapies to alleviate the client's health problems
- educating consumers about factors that influence mental health
- promoting change to improve socioeconomic conditions
- providing leadership and clinical supervision to colleagues
- conducting psychotherapy
- engaging in social and community mental health efforts.

In addition, the psychiatric nurse participates in in-service and continuing education, participates in nursing administration, and engages in consultation and research.

Nursing functions occur on three levels of prevention: primary, secondary, and tertiary. When the psychiatric nurse is involved in *primary prevention,* the functions include conducting health education, improving socioeconomic conditions, offering consumer education about normal growth and development, providing referrals before symptoms develop, supporting family members, and engaging in community and political activities. In *secondary prevention,* the functions include

(Text continues on page 8.)

SELECTED PRACTICE STANDARDS

This chart outlines the American Nurses' Association (ANA) standards for general psychiatric, psychiatric consultation-liaison, and child and adolescent psychiatric nursing.

ANA Standards of Psychiatric and Mental Health Nursing Practice

PROFESSIONAL PRACTICE STANDARDS

Standard I. Theory
The nurse applies appropriate theory that is scientifically sound as a basis for decisions regarding nursing practice.

Standard II. Data Collection
The nurse continuously collects data that are comprehensive, accurate, and systematic.

Standard III. Diagnosis
The nurse utilizes nursing diagnoses and/or standard classification of mental disorders to express conclusions supported by recorded assessment data and current scientific premises.

Standard IV. Planning
The nurse develops a nursing care plan with specific goals and interventions delineating nursing actions unique to each client's needs.

Standard V. Intervention
The nurse intervenes as guided by the nursing care plan to implement nursing actions that promote, maintain, or restore physical and mental health; prevent illness; and effect rehabilitation.

Standard V-A. Intervention: Psychotherapeutic Interventions
The nurses uses psychotherapeutic interventions to assist clients in regaining or improving their previous coping abilities and to prevent further disability.

Standard V-B. Intervention: Health Teaching
The nurse assists clients, families, and groups to achieve satisfying and productive patterns of living through health teaching.

Standard V-C. Intervention: Activities of Daily Living
The nurse uses the activities of daily living in a goal-directed way to foster adequate self-care and physical and mental well-being of clients.

Standard V-D. Intervention: Somatic Therapies
The nurse uses knowledge of somatic therapies and applies related clinical skills in working with clients.

Standard V-E. Intervention: Therapeutic Environment
The nurse provides, structures, and maintains a therapeutic environment in collaboration with the client and other health care providers.

Standard V-F. Intervention: Psychotherapy*
The nurse utilizes advanced clinical expertise in individual, group, and family psychotherapy; child psychotherapy, and other treatment modalities to function as a psychotherapist and recognizes professional accountability for nursing practice.

Standard VI. Evaluation
The nurse evaluates client responses to nursing actions in order to revise the data base, nursing diagnoses, and nursing care plan.

PROFESSIONAL PERFORMANCE STANDARDS

Standard VII. Peer Review
The nurse participates in peer review and other means of evaluation to assure quality of nursing care provided for clients.

Standard VIII. Continuing Education
The nurse assumes responsibility for continuing education and professional development and contributes to the professional growth of others.

Standard IX. Interdisciplinary Collaboration
The nurse collaborates with other health care providers in assessing, planning, implementing, and evaluating programs and other mental health activities.

Standard X. Utilization of Community Health Systems*
The nurse participates with other members of the community in assessing, planning, implementing, and evaluating mental health services and community systems that include the promotion of the broad continuum of primary, secondary, and tertiary prevention of mental illness.

Standard XI. Research
The nurse contributes to nursing and the mental health field through innovations in theory and practice and participation in research.

* Specific to clinical specialists with a master's degree in psychiatric or mental health nursing.

From *Standards of Psychiatric and Mental Health Nursing Practice.* Kansas City: American Nurses' Association, 1982. Used with permission.

ANA Standards of Psychiatric Consultation-Liaison Nursing Practice

PROFESSIONAL PRACTICE STANDARDS

Standard I. Theory
The psychiatric consultation-liaison nurse specialist (PCLNS) applies appropriate, scientifically sound theory as a basis for decisions regarding nursing practice.

Standard II. Assessment
The PCLNS systematically collects, records, and analyzes data that are comprehensive and accurate.

Standard III. Diagnosis
The PCLNS utilizes nursing diagnoses and/or standard classification of mental disorders and systems diagnoses to express conclusions supported by assessment data and current scientific premises.

Standard IV. Planning
The PCLNS collaborates with consultees to develop a plan with specific goals and interventions related to both client, family, and systems needs.

Standard V-A. Intervention: Direct Care—Psychotherapeutic Interventions
The PCLNS uses psychotherapeutic interventions to assist clients and families in developing, improving, or regaining their adaptive functioning; promote health; prevent illness; and facilitate rehabilitation.

Standard V-B. Intervention: Direct Care—Health Teaching and Anticipatory Guidance
The PCLNS assists clients, families, and groups to achieve more satisfying and productive patterns of living through health teaching and anticipatory guidance.

SELECTED PRACTICE STANDARDS *(continued)*

Standard V-C. Intervention: Direct Care—Somatic Therapies
The PCLNS uses knowledge of somatic therapies and applies related clinical skills in working with clients, families, and consultees.

Standard V-D. Intervention: Direct Care—Psychotherapies
The PCLNS uses advanced clinical expertise in individual, group, and family psychotherapy and other treatment modalities to function as a psychotherapist, and recognizes and accepts professional accountability for nursing practice.

Standard VI-A. Intervention: Indirect Care—Consultation
The PCLNS uses consultation as a modality to effect appropriate psychiatric and psychosocial care for clients and families and enhance the abilities of nonpsychiatric health care providers to provide such care.

Standard VI-B. Intervention: Indirect Care—Education
The PCLNS participates in the professional growth and development of other health care providers through formal and informal educational activities.

Standard VI-C. Intervention: Indirect Care—Therapeutic Environment
The PCLNS consults and collaborates with other health care providers to provide, structure, and maintain a therapeutic environment.

Standard VI-D. Intervention: Indirect Care—Systems
The PCLNS applies expertise in systems theory and organizational dynamics to plan programs, develop policy, and facilitate communication networks in order to provide an optimal climate for quality client and family care.

Standard VII. Evaluation
The PCLNS collaborates with the consultee to evaluate responses of the client and family to nursing actions, in order to revise the data base, nursing diagnosis, and nursing care plan.

PROFESSIONAL PERFORMANCE STANDARDS

Standard VIII. Quality Assurance
The PCLNS participates in peer review and/or other means of evaluation to assure the quality of the PCLNS role and the quality of client care.

Standard IX. Professional Development
The PCLNS assumes responsibility for continuing education and professional development.

Standard X. Multidisciplinary Collaboration
The PCLNS collaborates with other health care providers in assessing needs; planning, implementing, and evaluating interventions; and other activities related to psychiatric consultation-liaison nursing.

Standard XI. Utilization of Community Health Systems
The PCLNS participates with other members of the community in assessing, planning, implementing, and evaluating psychiatric-mental health services and community systems that include promotion of the broad continuum of primary, secondary, and tertiary preventions of mental illness.

Standard XII. Research
The PCLNS contributes to nursing and the psychiatric-mental health field through innovations in theory and practice, utilization of and participation in research, and communication about these contributions.

From *Standards of Psychiatric Consultation-Liaison Nursing Practice.* Kansas City: American Nurses' Association, 1990. Used with permission.

ANA Standards of Child and Adolescent Psychiatric and Mental Health Nursing Practice

Standard I. Theory
The nurse applies appropriate, scientifically sound theory as a basis for nursing practice decision.

Standard II. Assessment
The nurse systematically collects, records, and analyzes data that are comprehensive and accurate.

Standard III. Diagnosis
The nurse in expressing conclusions supported by recorded assessment data and current scientific premises, uses nursing diagnoses and/or standard classifications of mental disorders for childhood and adolescence.

Standard IV. Planning
The nurse develops a nursing care plan with specific goals and interventions delineating nursing actions unique to the needs of each child or adolescent, as well as those of the family and other relevant interactive social systems.

Standard V. Intervention
The nurse intervenes as guided by the nursing care plan to implement nursing actions that promote, maintain, or restore physical and mental health, prevent illness, effect rehabilitation in childhood and adolescence, and restore developmental progression.

Standard V-A. Intervention: Therapeutic Environment
The nurse provides, structures, and maintains a therapeutic environment in collaboration with the child or adolescent, the family, and other health care providers.

Standard V-B. Intervention: Activities of Daily Living
The nurse uses the activities of daily living in a goal-directed way to foster the physical and mental well-being of the child or adolescent and family.

Standard V-C. Intervention: Psychotherapeutic Interventions
The nurse uses psychotherapeutic interventions to assist children or adolescents and families to develop, improve, or regain their adaptive functioning to promote health, prevent illness, and facilitate rehabilitation.

Standard V-D. Intervention: Psychotherapy
The child and adolescent psychiatric and mental health specialist uses advanced clinical expertise to function as a psychotherapist for the child or adolescent and family and accepts professional accountability for nursing practice.

Standard V-E. Intervention: Health Teaching and Anticipatory Guidance
The nurse assists the child or adolescent and family to achieve more satisfying and productive patterns of living through health teaching and anticipatory guidance.

Standard V-F. Intervention: Somatic Therapies
The nurse uses knowledge of somatic therapies with the child or adolescent and family to enhance therapeutic interventions.

Standard VI. Evaluation
The nurse evaluates the response of the child or adolescent and family to nursing actions in order to revise the data base, nursing diagnoses, and nursing care plan.

From *Standards of Child and Adolescent Psychiatric and Mental Health Nursing Practice.* Kansas City: American Nurses' Association, 1985. Used with permission.

screening and evaluating clients promptly; providing emergency treatment, crisis intervention, and a therapeutic milieu; supervising medication administration; preventing suicide; counseling on a time-limited basis; conducting psychotherapy; and initiating community and organization interventions, such as helping to set up shelters for the homeless. In *tertiary prevention*, nursing functions include establishing vocational training, rehabilitation programs, and after care, and participating in partial hospitalization if necessary.

Legal issues also shape psychiatric nursing roles. Psychiatric nurses are held to the same standards of reasonable and prudent behavior expected of other professionals with the same education in similar circumstances and must provide care that meets with professional standards established by the ANA. Psychiatric nurses must know and abide by statutory provisions concerning client admissions into psychiatric care. Obtaining informed consent is the physician's responsibility, but the nurse should supply the client with relevant information about consent and document whether or not the consent was valid. A nurse who must violate a client's rights, for whatever reason, should carefully document all signs and symptoms, treatments, and treatment effects as a precaution against litigation. A nurse can legally use restraints or seclusion if clinically necessary to protect a client's safety; indeed, the nurse has an obligation to protect a client from self-harm, even against the client's wishes.

Selected references

American Nurses' Association (1982). *Standards of psychiatric and mental health nursing practice.* Kansas City, MO: American Nurses' Association.

American Nurses' Association (1985). *Standards of child and adolescent psychiatric and mental health nursing practice.* Kansas City, MO: American Nurses' Association.

American Nurses' Association (1990). *Standards of psychiatric consultation-liaison nursing practice.* Kansas City, MO: American Nurses' Association.

Burgess, A. (1990). *Psychiatric nursing in the hospital and the community.* Norwalk, CT: Appleton & Lange.

Murphy, S.A., and Hoeffer, B. (1987). The evolution of subspecialities in psychiatric and mental health nursing. *Archives of Psychiatric Nursing, 1*(3), 145-54.

Northrop, C.E., and Kelly, M.E. (1988). *Legal issues in nursing.* St. Louis: Mosby.

Stuart, G.W., and Sundeen, S.J. (1991). *Principles and practice of psychiatric nursing* (4th ed.). St. Louis: Mosby-Year Book.

Wilson, H.S. (1988). *Psychiatric nursing* (3rd ed.). Menlo Park, CA: Addison-Wesley.

INTRODUCTION
Conceptual and Nursing Models

Most psychiatric and mental health professionals practice within the framework of a model. A model is a means of organizing a complex body of knowledge, such as concepts and beliefs about human behavior. A model suggests appropriate tasks and activities for fulfilling therapeutic role requirements, and provides criteria for evaluating personal effectiveness in that role. Because scientific knowledge about human behavior is limited, no one model or its parts is correct or incorrect. The important issue is a model's usefulness — whether it helps the user provide effective care.

Conceptual models
Current conceptual models include the psychoanalytical, the behavioral, the existential, the interpersonal, the biogenic, the social, and the medical.

Psychoanalytical model
Based on the work of Sigmund Freud, this model was developed and refined in the late nineteenth and early twentieth centuries. Freud developed his psychoanalytic theory from his study of neurotic behavior; many of his ideas were controversial for the Victorian era because they centered on sexuality.

According to the psychoanalytical model, all human behavior has a cause and can be explained. The individual has psychic energy, known as libido, derived from instincts and desires. The libido reduces tension through pleasure. Five stages of personality development (oral, anal, phallic, latent, and genital) determine how a person seeks pleasure. Freud also identified three structures of the personality — the id, ego, and superego — and maintained that the human personality functions on preconscious, conscious, or unconscious levels. According to Freud, early life events determine the individual's later behavior. This means disruptive behavior in adults originates in early developmental stages.

The psychoanalytic model uses psychoanalysis — a form of therapy in which the therapist uses such techniques as free association, dream analysis, hypnosis, and interpretation — to help the client identify repressed feelings associated with conflict and release them. The therapist plays a passive role to create an environment devoid of approval or disapproval. The goal of psychoanalysis is to create a permissive yet safe situation where the client can recall past trauma and work through residual conflicts and emotions that have delayed or stopped personal growth. The patient is motivated to work in therapy by transferring the repressed conflict onto the therapist, a technique known as transference.

Behavioral model
Rooted in psychology and neurophysiology, the behavioral model is associated with Ivan Pavlov, B.F. Skinner, and J. Wolpe. The behavioral model is concerned only with observable behavior (behavior is a response to an environmental stimulus), which defines an individual's "self." Key to the behavioral model is the idea that humans are complex animals, and that all behavior is learned. Deviations occur when undesirable behavior is reinforced.

The therapist's goal, therefore, is to determine which patient behaviors should be changed and how. The therapist helps change undesirable behaviors through desensitization, operant conditioning, counterconditioning, aversion therapy, and token economy systems. As a learner, the patient must practice uncomfortable behaviors.

Existential model
The existential model was influenced by Sartre, Heidegger, and Kierkegaard. Recent existentialists include Frederick Perls, William Glasser, Albert Ellis, Carl Rogers, and R.D. Laing. This model focuses on the individual's recent experiences, with little emphasis on the past. According to this model, humans possess the freedom to realize their potential. Social interaction modifies self-awareness, which mediates behavior. A lack of self-awareness prevents the person's participation in authentic relationships. Deviations result when the individual is alienated from the self or the environment.

Using this model, the therapist attempts to further the client's self-awareness through gestalt, rational-emotive, reality, and encounter-group therapies. The therapist acts as a guide, but discourages the client's dependence.

Interpersonal model
Most commonly associated with Harry Stack Sullivan, the interpersonal model focuses on the interactive aspects of behavior and development. Sullivan identified six phases of interpersonal development of the self-system: infancy, childhood, juvenile, preadolescence, early adolescence, and late adolescence. The self-system resists change and consists of the "good me," "bad me," and "not me."

Behavior is produced by situations and interpersonal relationships, and the drives for satisfaction and security. Personality is an enduring pattern of interpersonal relationships. Selective inattention defends against interpersonal anxiety.

In this model, therapy involves reeducation. The therapist and client review the client's life to explore progress through developmental phases. Playing the role of the participant-observer, the therapist encourages the client to learn more successful styles of relating. Successful treatment depends on a healthy client-therapist relationship: experiencing a healthy relationship with the therapist teaches the client how to have more satisfying interpersonal relationships in general.

Social model
Associated with Gerald Caplan and Thomas Szasz, the social model considers the social environment's impact on the individual. Social conditions are held largely responsible for deviant behavior.

According to this model, the self emerges through social interaction. An individual takes responsibility for behavior by deciding whether or not to conform to social expectations. Deviance is culturally defined; it is not an illness. Instead, society labels "undesirables" as mentally ill and uses diagnosis and institutionalization to exert control over deviants. Social conditions, such as poverty or inadequate education, can predispose an individual to deviant behavior.

Therapy promotes freedom of choice and community mental health. The client defines the problem, initiates therapy, and approves or disapproves of the recommended therapeutic intervention. The therapist collaborates with the client to promote change. Therapy is successful when the client is satisfied with the changes in life-style.

Medical model
Based on the physician-client relationship, the medical model focuses on the diagnosis of mental illness; the physician's diagnosis defines the treatment to be used. Treatments include pharmacotherapy, electroconvulsive therapy, and, occasionally, psychosurgery.

According to this model, deviant behavior reflects a central nervous system disorder. Several circumstances can lead to deviant behavior, including loss of nerve cells, excesses or deficits in chemical transmission, and problems with brain circuitry, control centers, or impulse transmission. Environmental and social factors that might cause mental illness, or predispose a person to it, also are considered.

Using the medical model, the physician examines the client, diagnoses the illness, and then records and classifies the diagnosis according to the American Psychiatric Association's *Diagnostic and Statistical Manual of Mental Disorders, Third Edition, Revised (DSM III-R)*. The physician then prescribes treatment based on the diagnosis. Therapy focuses on promoting the client's trust, which fosters compliance with treatment. The physician acts as the healer; the client assumes the sick role and must work to get well. The client's self-assessment and the physician's objective assessment determine treatment success.

Biogenic model
Influenced by scientific investigations into the brain's neuroanatomy and physiology, this model examines biological and chemical factors that can influence behavior, including body types, genetics, chemistry, and biological rhythms.

Maladaptive behavior results from organic illness, structural or genetic defects, or biological imbalances affecting the central nervous system. The behavior can be cured or controlled with medical or surgical treatments. Interpersonal processes play little if any role in the development of maladaptive behavior.

Certain body types predispose clients to personality traits and susceptibility to mental disorders. For example, an ectomorphic body type (light build with little muscle) has been associated with schizophrenia; an endomorphic body type (heavy build) has been linked with bipolar disorders. Research also suggests an interaction of heredity with the environment can predispose individuals to mental disorders. Chemical imbalances may be related to mental disorders. For example, schizophrenia has been associated with the defective transmethylation of catecholamines, depression has been linked with deficient norepinephrine, and mania has been related to excess norepinephrine. Biological rhythms may affect physical and psychological well-being, possibly explaining the cause of episodic or cyclic mental disorders.

In the biogenic model, therapy is similar to that of the medical model, including psychosurgery, electroconvulsive therapy, and pharmacotherapy.

Nursing models and theories
Every profession is founded on a specialized body of knowledge. In the past, the nursing profession relied on theories from the disciplines of medicine, psychology, and sociology as a basis for practice. To define nursing and nursing practice, nurses can now describe their knowledge in terms of conceptual models and theories that provide information about nursing practice, the principles that form the basis for practice, and the goals and functions of nursing.

No universally accepted model or theory exists. All incorporate a holistic approach focusing on the individual's biological, psychological, and sociocultural needs and on the nurse's caring functions. This holistic approach is expressed through the nursing metaparadigm—person, environment, health, and nursing (for a summary, see *Selected nursing models and theories and the nursing metaparadigm*, pages 11 and 12). The individual's response to actual or potential health problems is of primary importance: the client's health is viewed on a continuum and the client's behavior is seen as a result of predisposing factors and precipitating stressors.

In any nursing theory or model, the nurse-client relationship must focus on the client's needs. The nurse and client collaborate, with the nurse acting as the client's advocate. The nurse uses the nursing pro-

SELECTED NURSING MODELS AND THEORIES AND THE NURSING METAPARADIGM

The nursing metaparadigm comprises four concepts: person, environment, health, and nursing. *Person* refers to the recipient of nursing care, including physical, spiritual, psychological, and sociocultural components. *Environment* refers to all the internal and external conditions, circumstances, and influences affecting the person. *Health* refers to the degree of wellness or illness experienced by the person. *Nursing* refers to the actions, characteristics, and attributes of the individual providing the nursing care.

Theorist	Person	Environment	Health	Nursing
Peplau	• Defined as an individual • Described as a developing organism striving to reduce anxiety caused by needs • Lives in an unstable environment	• Is not specifically defined	• Implies forward movement of personality and other ongoing human processes toward creative, constructive, productive, personal, and community living • Consists of interacting physiologic and interpersonal conditions	• Is a significant, therapeutic, interpersonal process that functions cooperatively with other human processes and makes health possible • Is a human relationship between an individual who is sick or has a felt need and a nurse who is educated to recognize and respond to the need for help • Promotes the client's development of skills to deal with problems; a mutual and collaborative process
Orem	• Defined as the patient (client receiving nursing care) • Functions biologically, symbolically, and socially with the potential for learning and development • Is subject to the forces of nature and can learn to meet self-care requisites	• Consists of factors, elements, conditions, and development	• Is characterized by soundness or wholeness of bodily structure and function • Consists of physical, psychological, interpersonal, and social aspects that are inseparable • Includes promotion and maintenance of health, treatment of illness, and prevention of complications	• Viewed as a service geared toward helping the self and others • Is required when therapeutic self-care demands exceed a client's self-care agency
Roy	• Is the recipient of nursing care; plays an active role • Is a biopsychosocial being who interacts with a changing environment • Is an adaptive system who uses innate and acquired coping mechanisms to deal with stressors	• Defined as all conditions, circumstances, and influences surrounding and affecting the development and behavior of persons and groups • Is always changing and interacting with the person	• Defined as a process of being and becoming an integrated and whole person • Is the goal of the person's behavior	• Is required when a person expends increased energy on coping, thereby leaving less energy available for growth, reproduction, mastery, and survival • Uses four adaptive modes to increase a person's adaptation level
Levine	• Viewed as a holistic individual or open system • Is an everchanging organism in constant interaction with the environment and striving to maintain integrity • Experiences orderly, sequential change through adaptation; health and illness are patterns of adaptive change • Survives by using one of four organismic responses	• Is internal (such as the body's response to bacteria) • Is external and includes the perceptual environment (responded to through the five senses), the operational environment (responded to physically), and the conceptual environment (responded to through traditions, beliefs, or values)	• Described as a pattern of adaptation or change, viewed as a continuum • Involves adapting by degrees • Maintains personal unity and integrity	• Is based on the dependence of people and their relationships with others • Involves human interaction to promote the wholeness of a dependent person and to assist the person in adapting to a state of health • Uses the conservation principles to identify areas of intervention

continued

SELECTED NURSING MODELS AND THEORIES AND THE NURSING METAPARADIGM *(continued)*

Theorist	Person	Environment	Health	Nursing
King	• Is a social, sentient, rational, perceiving, controlling, purposeful, action-oriented, time-oriented being • Has a right to self-knowledge, participation in decisions that affect life and health, and acceptance or rejection of health care	• Is not specifically defined	• Described as a dynamic state in the life cycle • Implies continuous adjustment to stress in the internal and external environments, using personal resources to achieve optimal daily living	• Refers to observable nurse-client interaction, focusing on helping the individual to maintain health and function appropriately • Is an interpersonal process of action, reaction, interaction, and transaction
Rogers	• Described as an organized energy field with a unique pattern • Is a unified whole possessing integrity and manifesting characteristics more than and different from the sum of the parts • Continuously exchanges matter and energy with environmental fields, resulting in life-process changes	• Described as an irreducible four-dimensional energy field identified by pattern and having characteristics different from those of its parts • Is infinite and identified by continuously changing wave patterns	• Is not clearly defined	• Is an art and science that seeks to study the nature and direction of unitary human development in constant interaction with the environment • Seeks to promote harmonic interaction between the environment and the person to strengthen the coherence and integrity of humans • Attempts to direct and redirect patterns of interaction between the person and the environment to realize maximum health potential

Adapted from Wesley, R. (1992). *Nursing theories and models.* Springhouse, PA: Springhouse Corp.

cess to intervene at any point along the health-illness continuum. Nursing functions include coordinating health care, applying comfort measures to ease pain, and helping the client maximize capabilities. Nursing theories and models appropriate to psychiatric-mental health nursing include the interpersonal relations model, the general theory of nursing (theory of self-care), the adaptation model, the conservation model, the goal attainment theory, and the unitary human model.

Interpersonal relations model (1952)

In her publication *Interpersonal Relations in Nursing,* Hildegard Peplau challenged nurses to use interpersonal relationships as a therapeutic tool. Peplau's ideas about interpersonal techniques became the cornerstone of psychiatric nursing. In forming her model, she drew from psychoanalytical, social learning, human motivational, and personality development theories.

Peplau defined psychodynamic nursing as a significant interpersonal process and identified numerous skills, activities, and roles for the psychiatric nurse. Psychodynamic nursing applies the principles of human relations to problems arising at all levels of human experience. The nurse uses an understanding of personal behavior to help the client identify difficulties. The

nurse-client relationship has four stages of personal interactions, during which the nurse assumes the roles of teacher, resource, counselor, leader, technical expert, and surrogate.

General theory of nursing (1959)

Dorothea Orem's theory consists of three related theories—self-care theory, self-care deficit theory, and nursing systems theory.

Orem's self-care theory describes and explains those activities that the client performs independently to promote and maintain personal well-being. Self-care theory uses the concepts of self-care agency (the ability to perform self-care), self-care requisites (actions or measures used to provide self-care), and therapeutic self-care demand (activities used to meet the self-care requisites) to promote the goal of client self-care.

Central to Orem's general theory of nursing is her self-care deficit theory. The nurse can help the client who cannot meet self-care requisites in five ways: by acting or doing for, guiding, teaching, supporting, and providing an environment that promotes the client's ability to meet current or future demands.

Nursing systems theory describes the system—wholly compensatory, partly compensatory, or supportive-educative—that a nurse uses to meet a client's self-care requisites. Each system describes nursing responsibilities, the nurse's and client's role, rationales for the nurse-client relationship, and the actions needed for the client's self-care needs.

Adaptation model (1964)

Developed by Sister Callista Roy, the adaptation model is based in systems theory with a strong analysis of interactions. The model contains five essential elements: patiency (the person receiving nursing care), goal of nursing (adapting to change), health, environment, and direction of nursing activities (facilitating adaptation).

Roy's model employs a feedback cycle of input, throughput, and output. Input is the stimuli from the environment or from within the client. Throughput uses the client's processes (mechanisms for adaptation) and effectors (categories of adaptable behavior, such as physiologic function, self-concept, role function, and interdependence). Output is the client's behavior, which is either adaptive (promoting the person's integrity) or ineffective (failing to promote goal achievement).

Roy identifies two types of coping mechanisms (behavior patterns) used for self-control: the regulator and the cognator. The regulator controls internal processes related to physiologic needs; the cognator controls internal processes related to higher brain functions, such as perception, information processing, experiential learning, judgment, and emotion.

Conservation model (1966)

Myra Levine's conservation model addresses total patient care and has two components—conservation principles and the organismic response. The conservation model is limited to persons in an illness state and focuses on nursing intervention as a conservation activity aimed at restoring wholeness, integrity, and well being.

Levine uses four principles to explain nursing interventions: conservation of energy (need for a balance of energy and a constant renewal of energy resources); conservation of structural integrity (need for healing); conservation of personal integrity (need to maintain and restore self-identity and self-worth); and conservation of social integrity (need for interaction with others). According to Levine, health is socially determined and individual coping patterns determine social acceptance.

The conservation model states that a person must adapt to the environment to survive; the methods of adaptation are called redundancy. These redundant choices are part of the organismic response, which can be immediate or long-term. The four levels of organismic response include fight or flight response, inflammatory response, response to stress, and sensory response.

Goal attainment theory (1971)

Developed by Imogene King, goal attainment theory centers on an open systems framework, which assumes that humans are open systems in constant interaction with their environment. This framework consists of three interacting systems: personal, interpersonal, and social. The personal system consists solely of the individual and includes perception, self, growth and development, body image, space, and time. The interpersonal system exists when humans socialize and includes interaction, communication, transaction, role, stress, and coping. The social system exists when interpersonal systems come together to form larger systems, such as families, religious groups, schools, workplaces, and peer groups. The social system includes the social roles, behaviors, and practices—such as organization, authority, power, status, and decision making—developed to maintain values.

King's goal attainment theory incorporates the relationship between the nurse and the client as they work together to communicate, establish goals, and take action to attain goals. In this relationship, two people, usually strangers, come together in a health care organization to help or be helped to maintain a state of health. The nurse-client relationship is based on the personal and interpersonal systems, including interaction, perception, communication, transaction, role, stress, growth and development, time, and space.

Unitary human model (1983)

Martha Rogers's unitary human model is closely related to general systems theory. This model draws heavily from the liberal arts and sciences, including anthropology, psychology, sociology, astronomy, religion, philosophy, history, biology, physics, mathematics, and literature.

Rogers's model is based on her assumptions about the person and interaction with the environment and uses four building blocks: energy fields, universe of open systems, pattern, and four dimensionality. These four building blocks are the basis of the principles of homeodynamics.

Rogers views homeodynamics as a means of understanding life and the mechanisms that affect it. Homeodynamics can provide a nurse with knowledge of how to intervene to redirect a client in a desired direction. Her current model identifies three principles: integrality (continuous and mutual interaction between human and environmental fields, indicating that life processes occur as continuous revisions), resonancy (continuous change from lower frequency to higher frequency wave patterns, indicating increasing complexity), and helicy (continuous, increasing diversity of the human and environmental fields, indicating that life processes are irreversible).

Selected references

Erikson, E. (1964). *Childhood and society* (2nd ed.). New York: Norton.

Freud, S. (1932). *The complete psychological works of Sigmund Freud.* Hogarth Press: London.

Jung, C.G. (1933). *Modern man in search of a soul.* New York: Harcourt Brace.

King, I. (1971). *Toward a theory for nursing: General concepts of human behavior.* New York: John Wiley & Sons.

King, I. (1981). *A theory for nursing: Systems, concepts, and process.* New York: Delmar.

Levine, M.E. (1973). Adaptation and assessment: A rationale for nursing intervention. In Hardy, M.E. (ed.) *Theoretical foundations for nursing.* New York: Irvington.

Levine, M.E. (1988). The four conservation priniciples: Twenty years later. In Riehl-Sisca, J. (ed.) *Conceptual models for nursing practice,* (3rd ed.). East Norwalk, CT: Appleton & Lange.

Orem, D.E., ed. (1959). *Guides for developing curricula for the education of practical nurses.* Vocational Division #274, Trade and Industrial Education #68. Washington, DC: U.S. Department of Health, Education, and Welfare.

Peplau, H.E. (1952). *Interpersonal relations in nursing.* Putnam: New York.

Peplau, H.E. (1962). Interpersonal techniques: The crux of psychiatric nursing. *American Journal of Nursing.* 62, 50-54.

Rogers, M.E. (1970). *An introduction to the theoretical basis of nursing.* Philadelphia: Davis.

Rogers, M.E. (1983). Science of unitary human beings: A paradigm for nursing. In *Family health: A theoretical approach to nursing care,* edited by Chaska, N.L. New York: McGraw-Hill.

Roy, C., and Riehl, J.P. (eds.) (1980). *Conceptual models for nursing practice,* 2nd ed. Englewood Cliffs, NJ: Prentice-Hall.

Roy, C., and Roberts, S. (1981). *Theory construction in nursing: An adaptation model.* Englewood Cliffs, NJ: Prentice-Hall.

Roy, C. (1984). Introduction to nursing: An adaptation model, 2nd ed. East Norwalk, CT: Appleton & Lange.

Roy, C., and Andrews, H. (1986). *Essentials of the Roy adaptation model.* East Norwalk, CT: Appleton-Century-Crofts.

Roy, C., and Andrews, H. (1991). *The Roy adaptation model: The definitive statement.* East Norwalk, CT: Appleton & Lange.

Treatment Modalities

Various treatment modalities, including psychotherapy, crisis intervention, group therapy, family therapy, milieu therapy, behavioral therapy, biological therapies, and psychopharmacology, are used with psychiatric and mental health clients. Each treatment can be used alone or in combination with another modality.

Psychotherapy

This treatment facilitates change in a person's feelings, attitudes, and beliefs through interpersonal relationships. The therapist communicates verbally and nonverbally to build a relationship with the client in an attempt to achieve understanding and relieve emotional pain. The client usually is anxious and expresses a symptomatic need for help. Traditionally, psychotherapy has emphasized the client's memories of childhood relationships and events. Today, psychotherapy tends to concentrate more on the client's behavior in current relationships. However, both approaches focus on the client's interpersonal relationships.

Psychotherapy may be the method of choice for treating certain emotional disorders, helping people who are not emotionally ill deal with problems or gain insight and self-knowledge, and training persons in the helping professions. It also can be used for stress reduction and as an adjunct treatment for medical problems.

Psychotherapy can be supportive, re-educative, or reconstructive. In supportive psychotherapy, the therapist encourages the client to express feelings, explore choices, and make decisions in a safe, caring relationship. Existing coping mechanisms are reinforced and no new means of coping are introduced. Re-educative therapy introduces the client to new ways of perceiving and behaving. These alternatives are examined in a planned, systematic manner that takes somewhat longer than supportive psychotherapy. The client enters into a contract that identifies the desired behavior change. Changing specific behaviors may change the client's self-perception. Reconstructive therapy, a long-term interaction that explores all aspects of the client's life, involves both the cognitive and emotional levels. Ultimately, the client increases understanding of the self and others, emotional freedom, the potential for new abilities, and capacity for love and work.

Psychotherapy evolves through three stages. In the introductory stage, the client and therapist begin to work together. The client's background and problems, including any factors or events that caused the client to seek help, are explored. The client discusses personal perceptions of problems and needs and identifies expectations of therapy, and the therapist forms some preliminary ideas about the client's needs. Together, they discuss specific issues, such as duration of ther-

apy, cost, goals, and meeting times. This stage may last from a few weeks to years. The therapist's goal is to develop trust so that the client will set aside defense mechanisms and reveal the self.

In the working stage, the client begins self-exploration. The client and therapist examine thoughts, feelings, and behaviors that have caused pain or problems. During the sessions, the client relates to the therapist as to other people. Patterns of client behavior become apparent as therapy continues. With greater recall, insight, and self-expression, the client develops greater understanding of personal behavior.

In the working through stage, the client uses increased self-understanding to experiment with new ways of thinking, feeling, and behaving. The client becomes more autonomous and functions more effectively.

Crisis intervention

During a crisis, stress overwhelms an individual's coping mechanisms. Predisposing factors include a disastrous event, threatened loss of a basic gratification, failure to cope with stress, or a perceived absence of support. Confronting a problem or threat (real or perceived), the individual uses strategies that have worked previously. When these methods fail, disorganization and disequilibrium result, with an increase in general anxiety. A state of emergency occurs and may lead to the client's breaking point. A crisis is typically self-limiting, resolving within 6 weeks.

Crisis intervention attempts to resolve the emergency positively. Interventions offer immediate help by reestablishing equilibrium. The goal is to restore the client to precrisis functioning by teaching new ways of problem solving.

Crisis intervention involves a step-wise approach. First, the therapist assesses the nature of the crisis, its effect on the client, and the client's coping mechanisms and support systems. Then the therapist plans a step-by-step solution. Next, interventions (environmental manipulation) provide direct support or remove stress and reassure the client that the therapist understands and will help (general support measures). The therapist can use a generic approach, using standard interventions for a given crisis, or an individual approach, tailoring interventions to a particular client. Finally, evaluation determines whether the crisis has been resolved.

Techniques of crisis intervention include taking an active role in exploring the client's problem; maintaining the client's orientation; encouraging expression of feelings and an awareness of the relationships among events, current feelings, and behavior; persuading the client to view the therapist as a helper; promoting and reinforcing adaptive behavior; supporting the client's defenses; increasing the client's self-esteem; and exploring solutions to the cause of the crisis.

Group therapy

A group is a gathering of three or more individuals who share similar goals. Because humans are social and desire interaction with others, groups can offer a safe environment for sharing emotional experiences. Many forces can influence the group's goals, including intrapersonal and interpersonal characteristics, needs, the physical environment, and the unique interaction of the group.

Group therapy can alleviate emotional distress or modify personality traits. Group dynamics can help modify behavior, focusing on interpersonal, cognitive, or behavioral changes. A group proceeds through three stages of development; in each stage, conflicts may arise, but these can further emotional bonding within the group. In the initial stage, the conflict issues are dependency and authority. This stage involves superficial communication, where the members become acquainted and search for personal similarities. Norms of behavior, roles, and responsibilities may be established during this time. In the middle or working stage, the conflict issues are intimacy, cooperation, and productivity. The group approaches problems and possible solutions and makes decisions through sharing and discussion. In the final or termination stage, the conflict issues are disengagement and dissolution. The group evaluates the experience and explores the members' feelings about the experience and impending separation.

For group therapy to be effective, the leader must adopt a style that is most effective for that group. Generally, the leader adopts one of three styles: autocratic (maintains control over decision making), democratic (encourages all members to participate in decision making), or laissez-faire (relinquishes control over decision making and provides little, if any, guidance or support). The effective group leader is skilled in techniques and interventions that foster interaction and shape behavior.

A group may be one of several types, including growth groups (such as self-help groups), psychoanalytic groups, psychodrama groups, marathon groups, encounter groups, T-groups, and community support groups. Methods of group therapy include transactional analysis, rational-emotive therapy, Rogerian group therapy, gestalt therapy, interpersonal group therapy, and the bion method.

Family therapy

Family therapy identifies a problem within a context, explores how family members relate to the problem, and focuses on how family interaction perpetuates the problem. The entire family is viewed as the client; the goal of therapy is to enable each member to function independently.

Family therapy may be structural or strategic. Structural therapy examines the individual within the family's social context. According to this model, behavior results from the family's organization and the interactions among members. It explores the family as a social system that undergoes predictable stages of development and requires adaptive restructuring. The structural model also explores the issues of power, influence, relationships, and boundaries within the family. The goal of structural therapy is not to change behavior but to change the family's organization so that dysfunctional behaviors are not supported. Change in the family's organization and feedback mechanisms forces members to change individually and as part of the group. The therapist becomes a temporary part of the context.

Strategic therapy, also known as problem-solving or brief family therapy, has its roots in communication theory. This model explores a behavior's function rather than its meaning. Consequently, treatment focuses on the presenting problem and the behaviors that maintain it, not on the problem's history or the motivation behind it. The therapist is an active and deliberate change agent who assumes responsibility for a successful outcome.

Milieu therapy

This group therapy approach uses a total living experience to achieve its therapeutic objectives; it draws on recreational, occupational, psychosocial, psychiatric, nursing, medical, and mental health therapies. It focuses on the client's interaction with the environment, creating a secure atmosphere in which the client can develop appropriate responses to people and situations. It is deliberately planned and structured to modify maladaptive behaviors and to promote positive insights and coping skills.

In milieu therapy, communication is encouraged, developed, and maintained between the treatment team and the client. Limits and external controls are set on unacceptable behavior. A homelike atmosphere encourages the client to use psychosocial skills. Milieu therapy focuses on client action and problem solving, on how the client and family relate to the community, on effective relationships among team members, and on a humanistic approach to treatment.

Behavioral therapy

Also called behavior modification, behavioral therapy deals with maladaptive behavior. Assuming that most behaviors are learned, behavioral therapy teaches the client to substitute adapative behaviors for maladaptive ones. Techniques used include generalization, discrimination, extinction, prompting and fading, shaping, modeling, imagery, and progressive muscle relaxation.

Behavioral therapy relies on classical conditioning and operant conditioning. In classical conditioning, an unconditioned stimulus elicits an unconditioned response. When a conditioned stimulus is paired with an unconditioned stimulus, a conditioned response may result. The original unconditioned response, whether positive or negative, reinforces the conditioned stimulus and response.

Operant conditioning, also called operant reinforcement therapy, uses reinforcement to increase the probability of a desired response. The unconditioned stimulus is paired with a conditioned stimulus, and the combination acts as a reinforcer. The reinforcer must meet a need and be goal directed. A positive reinforcer strengthens desired behavior; a negative reinforcer encourages avoidance of undesirable behavior.

Biological therapies

Biological therapies follow the medical model, viewing psychiatric problems as illness, and focus on symptoms, diagnosis, and prognosis. Biological therapies include psychoactive medications (see below for more information), electroconvulsive therapy, psychosurgery, insulin coma, hydrotherapy, nonconvulsive electrical stimulation therapy, and hemodialysis.

Psychopharmacology

Drug treatment for psychiatric disorders is relatively new — chlorpromazine's value in treating schizophrenia did not occur until the 1950s — but has dramatically improved the client's prognosis. Schizophrenics, for example, may leave inpatient care sooner, live in the community, and take part in other therapies previously unavailable to them.

In the past 40 years, additional drugs have become available to treat psychiatric disorders. Antianxiety agents, such as diazepam, and antidepressants, such as amitriptyline, are prescribed commonly. (For more information, refer to *Selected psychotropic drugs*, pages 18 to 29). Although medications may be used alone, they are usually used in conjunction with other therapeutic modalities, such as psychotherapy.

Drugs that alter behavior or promote sleep are likely to be prescribed for long-term therapy. Consequently, the client should be monitored closely for adverse reactions and signs of noncompliance, such as return of the original symptoms. Because some psychoactive drugs are addictive, the health care professional must watch for signs of dependence and, when the drug is discontinued, withdrawal.

Antianxiety agents

Also called anxiolytics, antianxiety agents include some of the most commonly prescribed drugs in the United States. They are used primarily to treat anxiety disorders. Benzodiazepines have replaced barbiturates for treating anxiety because they interact with fewer drugs and cause fewer adverse reaction. Benzodiazepines do interact with other CNS depressants, causing additive effects. The most common adverse reactions affect the CNS, producing drowsiness, motor incoordination, and increased reaction time. Meprobam-

ate appears to be less effective than other antianxiety agents and is used rarely to treat anxiety.

Buspirone (BuSpar) is one of the newest antianxiety agents. Preliminary data indicate that it interacts only with MAO inhibitors. Buspirone appears to have no abuse potential, causes almost no sedation, and produces only minor adverse reactions, such as dizziness and headache. Nevertheless, a client receiving this agent must be monitored closely until more is known about its long-term effects.

Antidepressant and antimanic agents

Affective disorders respond to antidepressant and antimanic agents. These include monoamine oxidase (MAO) inhibitors, tricyclic antidepressants, second generation antidepressants, and lithium.

MAO inhibitors are the treatment of choice for atypical depression. They also may be used in treatment-resistant depression or when other therapies are contraindicated. However, MAO inhibitors interact with many drugs and foods.

The tricyclic antidepressants are preferred for treating major depressive episodes. Like MAO inhibitors, they can interact with many other agents. The second-generation antidepressants also are used to treat major depression, although they are less effective than the tricyclic antidepressants. They cause fewer adverse reactions than tricyclic antidepressants and MAO inhibitors.

Lithium effectively treats manic episodes and prevents relapses of bipolar disorders (disorders characterized by alternating periods of manic behavior and clinical depression). Because this drug has a narrow therapeutic range and a high incidence of adverse effects, close monitoring is crucial.

Antipsychotic agents

Antipsychotic agents control psychotic symptoms, such as delusions, hallucinations, and thought disorders, that can occur with schizophrenia, mania, and other psychoses. They can help treat organic psychiatric disorders, such as dementia, delirium, and stimulant-induced psychoses, and can sedate agitated clients. Antipsychotic agents are also called major tranquilizers, because they can reduce agitation, or neuroleptics, because of their neurologic effects. All antipsychotic agents may be classified as phenothiazines or nonphenothiazines.

Serious adverse reactions to antipsychotic agents include extrapyramidal symptoms and tardive dyskinesia (abnormal muscle movement). Other adverse reactions include hypotension, seizures, anticholinergic effects, photosensitivity, blood dyscrasias, and jaundice.

Clozapine (Clozaril), one of the newest nonphenothiazines, can cause severe neutropenia and agranulocytosis. Consequently, clozapine is reserved for clients who do not respond to standard antipsychotic agents or who experience tardive dyskinesia. Regardless of

(Text continues on page 29.)

SELECTED PSYCHOTROPIC DRUGS

This chart summarizes the most common antianxiety, antidepressant and antimanic, antipsychotic, and sedative and hypnotic agents currently in clinical use.

Drug	Major indications	Usual adult dosages	Contraindications and precautions
Antianxiety agents			
Barbiturates			
pentobarbital (Nembutal)	Anxiety, sedation	20 mg P.O. t.i.d. or q.i.d.	• Know that pentobarbital is contraindicated in a pregnant client or one with porphyria or known hypersensitivity to the drug. • Administer with caution to a lactating client or one with depression, suicidal tendencies, hepatic damage, or a history of drug abuse.
phenobarbital (Barbita)	Anxiety	30 to 120 mg P.O. daily in two or three divided doses	• Know that phenobarbital is contraindicated in a pregnant client or one with porphyria, nephritis, renal insufficiency, or known hypersensitivity to the drug. • Administer with caution to a lactating client or one with depression, suicidal tendencies, hepatic damage, or a history of drug abuse.
Benzodiazepines			
alprazolam (Xanax)	Anxiety associated with depression	0.025 to 0.5 mg P.O. t.i.d. increased as tolerated to a maximum of 4 mg/day in divided doses	• Know that alprazolam is contraindicated in a pregnant or lactating client or one with acute narrow-angle glaucoma or known hypersensitivity to the drug. • Administer with caution to an elderly or debilitated client, a client receiving another psychotropic agent, or one with impaired renal or hepatic function or a history of drug dependence.
chlorazepate (Tranxene)	Anxiety	15 to 60 mg P.O. daily	• Know that chlorazepate is contraindicated in clients with known hypersensitivity and in those with acute narrow-angle glaucoma or untreated open-angle glaucoma, shock or coma, acute alcohol intoxication, or suicidal ideation. • Administer with caution to clients with psychoses, myasthenia gravis or Parkinson's disease, or impaired renal or hepatic function. • Administer with caution to elderly or debilitated clients and those prone to addiction or drug abuse.
chlordiazepoxide hydrochloride (Librium)	Anxiety	5 to 25 mg P.O. t.i.d. or q.i.d. daily	• Know that chlordiazepoxide is contraindicated in clients with known hypersensitivity and in those with acute narrow-angle glaucoma or untreated open-angle glaucoma, shock, coma, or acute alcohol intoxication. • Administer with caution to clients with psychoses, myasthenia gravis or Parkinson's disease, or impaired renal or hepatic function. • Administer with caution to elderly or debilitated clients and those prone to addiction or drug abuse.
	Severe alcohol withdrawal	50 to 100 mg P.O., I.M., or I.V. to a maximum dosage of 300 mg daily	

SELECTED PSYCHOTROPIC DRUGS *(continued)*

Drug	Major indications	Usual adult dosages	Contraindications and precautions
Antianxiety agents *(continued)*			
clonazepam (Klonopin)	Anxiety	1.5 to 10 mg daily	• Know that clonazepam is contraindicated in clients with known hypersensitivity and in those with significant hepatic disease, chronic respiratory disease, or untreated open-angle glaucoma or narrow-angle glaucoma.
	Seizures	1.5 mg P.O. daily in divided doses	• Administer with caution to clients with decreased renal function.
diazepam (Valium)	Anxiety	2 to 10 mg P.O. b.i.d. to q.i.d.	• Know that diazepam is contraindicated in a pregnant client or one with acute narrow-angle glaucoma or known hypersensitivity to the drug.
	Alcohol withdrawal	10 mg P.O. t.i.d. or q.i.d. for 24 hours, decreased to 5 mg t.i.d. or q.i.d.	• Administer with caution to a client with severe or latent depression, impaired renal or hepatic function, or a history of drug dependence.
	Skeletal muscle spasms	2 to 10 mg P.O. t.i.d. or q.i.d.	
	Status epilepticus	5 to 10 mg slow I.V. push repeated every 10 to 15 minutes to a maximum of 30 mg	
halazepam (Paxipam)	Anxiety	20 to 40 mg P.O. t.i.d. or q.i.d.; optimal daily dose of 80 to 160 mg	• Halazepam is contraindicated in clients with known hypersensitivity and in those with acute narrow-angle glaucoma or untreated open-angle glaucoma, shock or coma, or acute alcohol intoxication. • Administer with caution to clients with psychoses, myasthenia gravis or Parkinson's disease, or impaired renal or hepatic function. • Administer with caution to elderly or debilitated clients and those prone to addiction or drug abuse.
oxazepam (Serax)	Anxiety	10 to 30 mg P.O. t.i.d. or q.i.d.	• Know that oxazepam is contraindicated in clients with known hypersensitivity and in those with acute narrow-angle glaucoma or untreated open-angle glaucoma, coma, acute alcohol intoxication, or tartrazine allergy. • Administer with caution to clients with psychoses, myasthenia gravis or Parkinson's disease, or impaired hepatic or renal function. • Administer with caution to elderly or debilitated clients and those prone to addiction or drug abuse.

continued

SELECTED PSYCHOTROPIC DRUGS *(continued)*

Drug	Major indications	Usual adult dosages	Contraindications and precautions

Antianxiety agents (continued)

Benzodiazepines *(continued)*

Drug	Major indications	Usual adult dosages	Contraindications and precautions
prazepam (Centrax)	Anxiety	30 mg P.O. daily in divided doses	• Know that prazepam is contraindicated in clients with known hypersensitivity and in those with acute narrow-angle glaucoma or untreated open-angle glaucoma, coma, or acute alcohol intoxication. • Administer with caution to clients with psychoses, myasthenia gravis or Parkinson's disease, or impaired hepatic or renal function. • Administer with caution to elderly or debilitated clients and those prone to addiction or drug abuse.

Buspirone

Drug	Major indications	Usual adult dosages	Contraindications and precautions
buspirone (BuSpar)	Anxiety	5 mg P.O. t.i.d., increased by 5 mg q 2 to 3 days, as needed, to a maximum of 60 mg/day	• Know that buspirone is contraindicated in a lactating client, one with impaired renal or hepatic function or known hypersensitivity to the drug, or one who uses monoamine oxidase inhibitors concomitantly. • Administer with caution to a pregnant client.

Antidepressant and antimanic agents

Atypical antidepressants

Drug	Major indications	Usual adult dosages	Contraindications and precautions
bupropion (Wellbutrin)	Depression	100 mg b.i.d., up to 150 mg t.i.d.	• Know that bupropion is contraindicated in clients with known allergy, those who have taken MAO inhibitors within the past 14 days, and those with seizure disorders or history of bulimia nervosa or anorexia nervosa. • Administer with caution to clients with psychosis or hepatic, renal, or cardiac disease. • Administer with caution to suicidal, elderly, or debilitated clients.
fluoxetine (Prozac)	Endogenous depression, major depressive episode	20 mg P.O. daily increased to 40 mg daily (not to exceed 80 mg daily)	• Know that fluoxetine is contraindicated in clients with known hypersensitivity. • Be aware that clients taking fluoxetine may experience anxiety, nervousness, and insomnia; administer early in the day to avoid sleep disturbance. • Administer with caution to underweight clients.

Lithium

Drug	Major indications	Usual adult dosages	Contraindications and precautions
lithium (Eskalith)	Mania and bipolar disorder relapse	300 to 600 mg P.O. up to q.i.d., adjusted to achieve lithium blood level of 1 to 1.5 mEq/liter for acute mania, 0.6 to 1.2 mEq/liter to prevent bipolar disorder relapses, and 2 mEq/liter as a maximum dose	• Know that lithium is contraindicated in a pregnant, lactating, elderly, or debilitated client; a client who cannot be monitored closely; or one with epilepsy, renal or cardiovascular disease, brain damage, severe dehydration, or sodium depletion. • Administer with caution to a client with a thyroid disorder.

SELECTED PSYCHOTROPIC DRUGS *(continued)*

Drug	Major indications	Usual adult dosages	Contraindications and precautions

Antidepressant and antimanic agents (continued)

MAO inhibitors

Drug	Major indications	Usual adult dosages	Contraindications and precautions
isocarboxazid (Marplan)	Atypical depression	30 mg P.O. daily in a single dose or divided doses, reduced to 10 to 20 mg/day when condition improves	• Know that isocarboxazid is contraindicated in an elderly or debilitated client and in a client with severe hepatic or renal impairment; congestive heart failure; pheochromocytoma; hypertensive, cardiovascular, or cerebrovascular disease; severe or frequent headaches; or known hypersensitivity to the drug. It also is contraindicated within 10 days of elective surgery requiring general anesthesia, a local anesthetic containing sympathomimetic vasoconstrictors, or cocaine; and with concurrent use of other MAO inhibitors, dibenzazepines, buspirone, clomipramine, central nervous system depressants, sympathomimetic drugs, high-tryptophan foods, high-tyramine foods, or excessive amounts of caffeine. • Administer with caution to a hyperactive, agitated, schizophrenic, or suicidal client and to a client with diabetes or epilepsy or one taking antihypertensive drugs including thiazide diuretics. Also administer with caution to a pregnant or lactating client.
phenelzine (Nardil)	Severe depression, depression accompanied by anxiety	15 mg P.O. t.i.d. daily up to a maximum dose of 90 mg	• Know that phenelzine is contraindicated in clients with uncontrolled hypertension and seizure disorders. • Administer with caution to clients with angina pectoris and other cardiovascular disease, Type I and Type II diabetes, Parkinson's disease and other motor disorders, hyperthyroidism, pheochromocytoma, renal or hepatic insufficiency, or bipolar disorder.
tranylcypromine (Parnate)	Atypical depression	10 mg P.O. b.i.d., increased to a maximum of 30 mg/day after 2 to 3 weeks, if necessary	• Know that tranylcypromine is contraindicated in a client with cerebrovascular defects, cardiovascular disorders, pheochromocytoma, liver disease, known hypersensitivity to the drug, or with concurrent use of MAO inhibitors, dibenzazepines, fluoxetine, buspirone, sympathomimetics, meperidine, dextromethorphan, or high-tyramine foods. It also is contraindicated in a client undergoing elective surgery or one who uses narcotics, alcohol, hypotensive agents, or excessive amounts of caffeine. • Administer with caution to a pregnant or lactating client; one with impaired renal function, epilepsy, diabetes, or hyperthyroidism; or one who is receiving antiparkinsonian agents or disulfiram (Antabuse).

continued

SELECTED PSYCHOTROPIC DRUGS   *(continued)*

Drug	Major indications	Usual adult dosages	Contraindications and precautions

Antidepressant and antimanic agents *(continued)*

Second-generation antidepressants

Drug	Major indications	Usual adult dosages	Contraindications and precautions
trazodone (Desyrel)	Depression	150 mg P.O. daily in divided doses, increased by 50 mg/day every 3 to 4 days up to a maximum of 400 mg/day (600 mg/day for a severely ill client)	• Know that trazodone is contraindicated in a client with known hypersensitivity to the drug. • Administer with caution to a pregnant or lactating client or one with cardiac disease.

Tricyclic antidepressants

Drug	Major indications	Usual adult dosages	Contraindications and precautions
amitriptyline (Elavil)	Depression	50 to 75 mg P.O. increased to 200 mg/day, then to a maximum of 300 mg daily, if needed; or 20 to 30 mg I.M. q.i.d. or as a single dose h.s.	• Know that amitriptyline is contraindicated in a client with a known hypersensitivity to the drug or during the acute recovery phase of myocardial infarction. • Administer with caution to a pregnant or lactating client, a client receiving electroconvulsive therapy or undergoing elective surgery, or one with seizures, suicidal tendencies, urine retention, narrow-angle glaucoma, increased intraocular pressure, cardiovascular disease, hyperthyroidism, or impaired hepatic function.
amoxapine (Asendin)	Depression associated with melancholia or psychotic symptoms, depressive phase of bipolar disorder, depression associated with organic disease or alcoholism, psychoneurotic anxiety, mixed symptoms of anxiety or depression	Initial dosage of 50 mg t.i.d.; may increase to 100 mg t.i.d. on third day of treatment; maximum dosage of 600 mg in hospitalized clients	• Know that amoxapine is contraindicated in clients with known hypersensitivity and in those in the acute recovery phase of a myocardial infarction, in coma or severe respiratory depression, and during or within 14 days of MAO therapy. • Administer with caution to clients with other cardiac diseases (arrhythmias, congestive heart disease, angina, valvular disease, or heart block), respiratory disorders, seizure disorders, bipolar disease, glaucoma, hyperthyroidism (or taking thyroid hormone replacement), Type I and Type II diabetes, prostatic hypertrophy, paralytic ileus or urine retention, hepatic or renal dysfunction, Parkinson's disease, or tardive dyskinesis. • Administer with caution to clients undergoing surgery with general anesthesia or scheduled for electroconvulsive therapy.
clomipramine (Anafranil)	Obsessive-compulsive disorder	25 mg P.O. daily, gradually increasing to 100 mg P.O. daily in divided doses during the first two weeks with a maximum dosage of 250 mg	• Know that clomipramine is contraindicated in clients with a history of hypersensitivity, during or within 14 days of MAO therapy, and during the acute recovery period after a myocardial infarction. • Administer with caution to clients with history of seizure disorders, or brain damage, or those receiving other seizure-threshold lowering drugs; in clients with hyperthyroidism (or receiving thyroid hormone replacement therapy), urine retention, narrow-angle glaucoma or increased intraocular pressure, cardiovascular disease, impaired hepatic or renal function, tumors of the adrenal medulla, or acute intermittent porphyria.

SELECTED PSYCHOTROPIC DRUGS (continued)

Drug	Major indications	Usual adult dosages	Contraindications and precautions

Antidepressant and antimanic agents (continued)

Drug	Major indications	Usual adult dosages	Contraindications and precautions
clomipramine (Anafranil) (continued)			• Administer with caution to elderly or debilitated clients or those receiving electroconvulsive therapy or electrocautery. • Remember that safe use in pregnancy and lactation has not been established.
desipramine (Norpramin)	Endogenous depression; major depression with melancholia or psychotic symptoms; depression associated with organic disease, alcoholism, schizophrenia, mental retardation or depressive phase of bipolar disorder	75 to 150 mg daily in divided doses increasing to a maximum of 300 mg daily	• Know that desipramine is contraindicated in clients with known hypersensitivity and in the acute recovery phase of a myocardial infarction, in coma or severe respiratory depression, and during or within 14 days of MAO therapy. • Administer with caution to clients with other cardiac diseases (arrhythmias, congestive heart failure, angina, valvular disease, or heart block), respiratory disorders, seizure disorders, bipolar disease, glaucoma, hyperthyroidism (or taking thyroid hormone replacement), Type I and Type II diabetes, prostatic hypertrophy, paralytic ileus or urine retention, hepatic or renal dysfunction, or Parkinson's disease. • Administer with caution to clients undergoing surgery with general anesthesia or scheduled for electroconvulsive therapy.
doxepin (Sinequan)	Depression	25 to 50 mg P.O. daily initially, increased to a maximum of 300 mg daily, if necessary	• Know that doxepin is contraindicated in a client with urine retention, narrow-angle glaucoma, or known hypersensitivity to the drug. • Administer with caution to a pregnant or lactating client or one with suicidal tendencies.
imipramine (Tofranil)	Depression	75 to 100 mg P.O. daily in divided doses, with 25- to 50-mg increments up to 200 mg for outpatients and 300 mg daily for hospitalized clients	• Know that imipramine is contraindicated in clients with known hypersensitivity and in those in the acute recovery phase of a myocardial infarction, in coma or severe respiratory depression, and during or within 14 days of MAO therapy. • Administer with caution to clients with other cardiac diseases (arrhythmias, CHF, angina, valvular disease or heart block), respiratory disorders, seizure disorders, bipolar disease, glaucoma, hyperthyroidism (or taking thyroid hormone replacement), Type I and Type II diabetes, prostatic hypertrophy, paralytic ileus or urine retention, hepatic or renal dysfunction, or Parkinson's disease. • Administer with caution to clients undergoing surgery with general anesthesia or scheduled for electroconvulsive therapy.

continued

SELECTED PSYCHOTROPIC DRUGS *(continued)*

Drug	Major indications	Usual adult dosages	Contraindications and precautions
Antidepressant and antimanic agents *(continued)*			
Tricyclic antidepressants *(continued)* trimipramine (Surmontil)	Major depression, depression with melancholia or psychotic symptoms	75 mg daily in divided doses, increased to 200 mg daily	• Know that trimipramine is contraindicated in clients with known hypersensitivity and in those in the acute recovery phase of a myocardial infarction, in coma or severe respiratory depression, and during or within 14 days of MAO therapy. • Administer with caution to clients with other cardiac diseases (arrhythmias, congestive heart failure, angina, valvular disease or heart block), respiratory disorders, seizure disorders, bipolar disease, glaucoma, hyperthyroidism (or taking thyroid hormone replacement), Type I and Type II diabetes, prostatic hypertrophy, paralytic ileus or urine retention, hepatic or renal dysfunction, and in those undergoing surgery with general anesthesia.
Antipsychotic agents			
Butyrophenone haloperidol, haloperidol decanoate (Haldol, Haldol Decanoate)	Symptomatic relief of psychoses, relief of dyskinesia in Gilles de la Tourette's syndrome	0.5 to 5 mg P.O. b.i.d. or t.i.d., increased as needed up to 100 mg/day	• Know that haloperidol and haloperidol decanoate are contraindicated in a pregnant or lactating client or one with toxic CNS depression, coma, Parkinson's disease, or known hypersensitivity. • Administer with caution to a client with severe cardiovascular disease or known allergies, or to a client who also receives an anticonvulsant or anticoagulant.
Dibenzodiazepine (atypical) clozapine (Clozaril)	Schizophrenia unresponsive to other therapies	25 mg P.O. daily or b.i.d., increased to a daily dosage of 300 to 450 mg daily (may increase to 300 to 600 mg daily, but not to exceed 900 mg daily)	• Know that clozapine is contraindicated in clients with a history of clozapine-induced agranulocytosis or severe granulocytopenia, severe CNS depression or coma, or in bone marrow suppression. • Administer with caution to clients with prostatic hypertrophy, glaucoma, or seizure disorders.
Phenothiazines chlorpromazine (Thorazine)	Symptomatic relief of psychoses	200 to 600 mg P.O. daily in divided doses initially, increased to a maintenance dosage of 500 to 1,400 mg P.O. daily in divided doses	• Know that chlorpromazine is contraindicated in a pregnant or lactating client; a client with bone marrow depression or known hypersensitivity to the drug; a comatose client; a client receiving a high dosage of CNS depressants; or a child or adolescent with signs and symptoms of Reye's syndrome. • Administer with caution to an elderly or debilitated client or to one with cardiovascular or liver disease; a history of seizures; a chronic respiratory disorder, such as severe asthma or emphysema; acute respiratory infections; glaucoma; exposure to extreme heat or organophosphorus insecticides; or to a client receiving atropine or a related drug.

SELECTED PSYCHOTROPIC DRUGS   (continued)

Drug	Major indications	Usual adult dosages	Contraindications and precautions

Antipsychotic agents (continued)

Drug	Major indications	Usual adult dosages	Contraindications and precautions
fluphenazine (Prolixin)	Psychotic disorders	0.5 to 10 mg P.O. daily in divided doses every 6 to 8 hours, increasing cautiously to 20 mg	• Know that fluphenazine is contraindicated in clients with known hypersensitivity; blood dyscrasias or bone marrow depression; disorders accompanied by coma, brain damage, CNS depression, circulatory collapse, or cerebrovascular disease; and in those receiving adrenergic blocking agents or spinal or epidural anesthetics. • Administer with caution to clients with cardiac disease, encephalitis, Reye's syndrome, head injury, respiratory disease, seizure disorders, glaucoma, prostatic hypertrophy, urine retention, impaired renal or hepatic dysfunction, Parkinson's disease, pheochromocytoma, and hypocalcemia. • Be aware that some oral preparations contain tartrazine and may cause an allergic reaction in clients allergic to aspirin.
fluphenazine decanoate (Prolixin Decanoate)	Symptomatic relief of psychoses when compliance is a problem	12.5 to 25 mg I.M. or S.C. every 1 to 6 weeks initially, then 25 to 100 mg p.r.n. for maintenance	• Know that fluphenazine decanoate is contraindicated in a child under age 12, a comatose or severely depressed client, or one with known hypersensitivity to the drug, suspected or proven subcortical brain damage, blood dyscrasia, or liver damage. • Administer with caution to an elderly, debilitated, or pregnant client; a client undergoing surgery who takes large doses of fluphenazine; or one with cholestatic jaundice, dermatoses or other allergic reactions to phenothiazine derivatives, a seizure disorder, cardiovascular disease such as mitral insufficiency, pheochromocytoma, or exposure to extreme heat or organophosphorus insecticides.
perphenazine (Trilafon)	Psychosis	8 to 16 mg P.O. b.i.d., t.i.d., or q.i.d., increasing to 64 mg daily	• Know that perphenazine is contraindicated in clients with known hypersensitivity; blood dyscrasias or bone marrow depression; disorders accompanied by coma, brain damage, CNS depression, circulatory collapse, or cerebrovascular disease; and in those receiving adrenergic blocking agents or spinal or epidural anesthetics. • Administer with caution to clients with cardiac disease, encephalitis, Reye's syndrome, head injury, respiratory disease, seizure disorders, glaucoma, prostatic hypertrophy, urine retention, impaired renal or hepatic dysfunction, Parkinson's disease, pheochromocytoma, or hypocalcemia.

continued

SELECTED PSYCHOTROPIC DRUGS (continued)

Drug	Major indications	Usual adult dosages	Contraindications and precautions

Antipsychotic agents (continued)

Phenothiazines (continued)

Drug	Major indications	Usual adult dosages	Contraindications and precautions
thioridazine (Mellaril)	Psychoses, dysthymic disorder	50 to 100 mg P.O. t.i.d. up to 800 mg daily in divided doses	• Know that thioridazine is contraindicated in clients with known hypersensitivity; blood dyscrasias or bone marrow depression; disorders accompanied by coma, brain damage, CNS depression, circulatory collapse, or cerebrovascular disease; and in those receiving adrenergic blocking agents or spinal or epidural anesthetics. • Administer with caution to clients with cardiac disease, encephalitis, Reye's syndrome, head injury, respiratory disease, seizure disorders, glaucoma, prostatic hypertrophy, urine retention, Parkinson's disease, pheochromocytoma, or hypocalcemia.
trifluoperazine (Stelazine)	Anxiety states, schizophrenia and other psychotic disorders	1 to 2 mg P.O. b.i.d., increased as needed up to 40 mg daily; 1 to 2 mg I.M. every 4 to 6 hours as needed	• Know that trifluoperazine is contraindicated in clients with known hypersensitivity; blood dyscrasias or bone marrow depression; disorders accompanied by coma, brain damage, CNS depression, circulatory collapse, or cerebrovascular disease; and in those receiving adrenergic blocking agents or spinal or epidural anesthetics. • Administer with caution to clients with cardiac disease, encephalitis, Reye's syndrome, head injury, respiratory disease, seizure disorders, glaucoma, prostatic hypertrophy, urine retention, impaired renal or hepatic dysfunction, Parkinson's disease, pheochromocytoma, or hypocalcemia.

Thioxanthene

Drug	Major indications	Usual adult dosages	Contraindications and precautions
chlorprothixene (Taractan)	Psychotic disorders	10 mg P.O. t.i.d. or q.i.d. increasing gradually to a maximum of 600 mg daily	• Know that chlorprothixene is contraindicated in clients with known hypersensitivity; blood dyscrasias or bone marrow depression; disorders accompanied by coma, brain damage, CNS depression, circulatory collapse, or cerebrovascular disease. • Administer with caution to clients with cardiac disease, encephalitis, Reye's syndrome, head injury, respiratory disease, seizure disorders, glaucoma, prostatic hypertrophy, urine retention, impaired renal or hepatic dysfunction, Parkinson's disease, pheochromocytoma, or hypocalcemia.
	Agitation of severe neurosis, depression, schizophrenia	25 to 50 mg P.O. or I.M. t.i.d. or q.i.d. increasing as needed to a maximum of 600 mg daily	
thiothixene (Navane)	Acute agitation, psychosis	4 mg I.M. b.i.d. to q.i.d. to a maximum dosage of 30 mg; 2 mg P.O. t.i.d. increasing gradually to 15 mg daily to a maximum dosage of 60 mg	• Know that thiothixene is contraindicated in clients with known hypersensitivity; blood dyscrasias or bone marrow depression; or disorders accompanied by coma, brain damage, CNS depression, circulatory collapse, or cerebrovascular disease. • Administer with caution to clients with cardiac disease, encephalitis, Reye's syndrome, head injury, respiratory disease, seizure disorders, glaucoma, prostatic hypertrophy, urine retention, impaired renal or hepatic dysfunction, Parkinson's disease, pheochromocytoma, or hypocalcemia.

SELECTED PSYCHOTROPIC DRUGS *(continued)*

Drug	Major indications	Usual adult dosages	Contraindications and precautions
Sedative and hypnotic agents			
Barbiturates amobarbital (Amytal)	Sedative for anxiety and tension	30 to 50 mg P.O. or I.M. b.i.d. or t.i.d.	• Know that amobarbital is contraindicated in a pregnant client or one with porphyria or known hypersensitivity to the drug.
	Hypnotic for insomnia	65 to 200 mg P.O. or I.M. h.s.	
aprobarbital (Alurate)	Daytime sedative	40 mg P.O. t.i.d.	• Know that aprobarbital is contraindicated in a pregnant or lactating client or one with known hypersensitivity to the drug, porphyria, nephritis, renal insufficiency, or premonitory signs of hepatic coma.
	Hypnotic for insomnia	40 to 160 mg P.O. h.s.	• Administer with caution to a client with depression, suicidal tendencies, hepatic damage, or a history of drug abuse.
mephobarbital (Mebaral)	Daytime sedative	32 to 100 mg P.O. t.i.d. or q.i.d.	• Know that mephobarbital is contraindicated in a pregnant client or one with known hypersensitivity to the drug, porphyria, nephritis, renal insufficiency, or premonitory signs of hepatic coma. • Administer with caution to a lactating client or one with depression, suicidal tendencies, myasthenia gravis, myxedema, a history of drug abuse, or impaired hepatic, cardiac, or respiratory function.
pentobarbital (Nembutal)	Daytime sedative	20 to 40 mg P.O. b.i.d. to q.i.d.	• Know that pentobarbital is contraindicated in a pregnant client or one with porphyria or known hypersensitivity to the drug.
	Sedative before surgery	150 to 200 mg P.O. or I.M.	• Administer with caution to a lactating client or one with depression, suicidal tendencies, hepatic damage, or a history of drug abuse.
	Hypnotic for insomnia	100 mg P.O., 120 to 200 mg rectal, 100 to 200 mg I.M.	
phenobarbital (Barbita)	Daytime sedative	15 to 30 mg P.O. b.i.d. to q.i.d.	• Know that phenobarbital is contraindicated in a pregnant client or one with porphyria, nephritis, renal insufficiency, or known hypersensitivity to the drug.
	Sedative before surgery	100 to 200 mg I.M. 60 to 90 minutes before surgery	• Administer with caution to a lactating client or one with depression, suicidal tendencies, hepatic damage, or a history of drug abuse.
	Hypnotic for insomnia	100 to 320 mg P.O. or I.M. h.s.	
secobarbital (Seconal)	Daytime sedative	30 to 50 mg P.O. t.i.d. or q.i.d., 120 to 200 mg rectal	• Know that secobarbital is contraindicated in a pregnant client or one with porphyria or known hypersensitivity to the drug.
	Sedative before surgery	200 to 300 mg P.O. 1 to 2 hours before surgery	• Administer with caution to a lactating client or one with depression, suicidal tendencies, hepatic damage, or a history of drug abuse.
	Hypnotic for insomnia	100 to 200 mg P.O., 120 to 200 mg rectal, 100 to 200 mg I.M. h.s.	

continued

SELECTED PSYCHOTROPIC DRUGS *(continued)*

Drug	Major indications	Usual adult dosages	Contraindications and precautions

Sedative and hypnotic agents *(continued)*

Drug	Major indications	Usual adult dosages	Contraindications and precautions
Benzodiazepines estazolam (ProSom)	Hypnotic for insomnia	1 to 2 mg P.O. h.s.	• Know that estazolam is contraindicated in clients with history of hypersensitivity and during pregnancy. • Administer with caution to elderly or debilitated clients and those with hepatic impairment, compromised respiratory function, depression, impaired renal function, or sleep apnea.
flurazepam (Dalmane)	Hypnotic for insomnia	15 to 30 mg P.O. h.s.	• Know that flurazepam is contraindicated in a pregnant client or one with known hypersensitivity to the drug. • Administer with caution to a client with severe or latent depression, impaired renal or hepatic function, or chronic pulmonary insufficiency.
lorazepam (Ativan)	Sedative before surgery	0.05 mg/kg up to 4 mg I.M. 2 hours before operative procedure	• Know that lorazepam is contraindicated in a pregnant client or one with known hypersensitivity to the drug, acute narrow-angle glaucoma, a primary depressive disorder, or psychosis. • Administer with caution to a lactating or elderly client, one with impaired renal or hepatic function, or any client over a prolonged time.
	Hypnotic for insomnia from anxiety or transient situational stress, anxiety disorders	2 to 4 mg P.O. h.s.	
quazepam (Doral)	Hypnotic for insomnia	15 mg P.O. h.s. until the response is measured; then decreased to 7.5 mg, if possible	• Know that quazepam is contraindicated in a pregnant client or one with known hypersensitivity to the drug. • Administer with caution to a client with impaired renal or hepatic function.
temazepam (Restoril)	Hypnotic for insomnia	15 to 30 mg P.O. h.s.	• Know that temazepam is contraindicated in a pregnant client or one with known hypersensitivity to the drug. • Administer with caution to a lactating client or one with severe or latent depression, impaired renal or hepatic function, or chronic pulmonary insufficiency.
triazolam (Halcion)	Hypnotic for insomnia	0.125 to 0.25 mg P.O. h.s.	• Know that triazolam is contraindicated in a pregnant or lactating client or one with known hypersensitivity to the drug. • Administer with caution to a client with depression, impaired renal or hepatic function, or chronic pulmonary insufficiency.
Nonbenzodiazepines-nonbarbiturates chloral hydrate (Noctec)	Daytime sedative	250 mg P.O. or 325 mg rectal t.i.d. after meals	• Know that chloral hydrate is contraindicated in a client with known hypersensitivity to the drug, gastroenteritis, or ulcers. • Administer with caution to a pregnant or lactating client or one with depression, suicidal tendencies, or severe hepatic, renal, or cardiac disease.
	Hypnotic for insomnia	0.5 to 1 g P.O. or rectal 15 to 30 minutes before bedtime	

SELECTED PSYCHOTROPIC DRUGS *(continued)*

Drug	Major indications	Usual adult dosages	Contraindications and precautions
Sedative and hypnotic agents *(continued)*			
ethchlorvynol (Placidyl)	Daytime sedative	200 mg P.O. b.i.d. or t.i.d.	• Know that ethchlorvynol is contraindicated in a client with porphyria or known hypersensitivity to the drug.
	Hypnotic for insomnia	0.5 to 1 g P.O. h.s.	• Administer with caution to a pregnant or lactating client or one with suicidal tendencies, impaired renal or hepatic function, or a history of drug abuse.
glutethimide (Doriden)	Hypnotic for insomnia	250 to 500 mg P.O. h.s.	• Know that glutethimide is contraindicated in a client with porphyria, severe renal impairment, or known hypersensitivity to the drug.
			• Administer with caution to a pregnant or lactating client or one with depression, suicidal tendencies, or a history of drug abuse.
methyprylon (Noludar)	Hypnotic for insomnia	200 to 400 mg P.O. h.s.	• Know that methyprylon is contraindicated in a client with known hypersensitivity to the drug.
			• Administer with caution to a lactating client or one with porphyria or renal or hepatic impairment.
paraldehyde (Paral)	Sedative	5 to 10 ml P.O. or rectal	• Know that paraldehyde is contraindicated in a client with ulcerative gastroenteritis or known hypersensitivity to the drug.
	Hypnotic for insomnia	10 to 30 ml P.O. or rectal h.s.	• Administer with caution to a client with impaired hepatic function or a pulmonary disease, such as asthma.

Adapted from Baer, C.L., and Williams, B.R. (1992). *Clinical pharmacology in nursing, (2nd ed.).* Springhouse, PA: Springhouse Corp.

the agent used, effective antipsychotic therapy requires close observation of the client's behavior and drug effects.

Sedatives

Sedatives reduce activity or excitement, producing a calming effect, but they also induce drowsiness. When administered in large doses, sedatives are considered hypnotics, which induce a state resembling natural sleep. The three main classes of sedatives and hypnotics are benzodiazepines, barbiturates, and nonbenzodiazepine-nonbarbiturate agents. Benzodiazepines include five primary sedative and hypnotic agents: flurazepam (Dalmane), lorazepam (Ativan), quazepam (Doral), temazepam (Restoril), and triazolam (Halcion). These agents typically are preferred because of their effectiveness and safety; they cause few adverse reactions.

Barbiturates include amobarbital (Amytal), aprobarbital (Alurate), butabarbital (Butisal), pentobarbital (Nembutal), phenobarbital (Barbita), and secobarbital (Seconal). Like benzodiazepines, barbiturates are nonspecific central nervous system (CNS) depressants that produce various effects ranging from sedation to hypnosis, anesthesia, or coma. These agents have a high potential for physical and psychological dependence, abuse, and life-threatening toxicity with overdose. Adverse reactions are common and include CNS and respiratory depression.

Nonbenzodiazepine-nonbarbiturate agents include chloral hydrate (Noctec), ethchlorvynol (Placidyl), glutethimide (Doriden), methyprylon (Noludar), and paraldehyde (Paral). The most common adverse reactions are gastrointestinal distress and some hangover effects; respiratory depression also can occur.

Selected references

Baer, C.L., and Williams, B.R., (1992). *Clinical pharmacology and nursing* (2nd ed.). Springhouse, PA: Springhouse.

Burgess, A. (1990). *Psychiatric nursing in the hospital and the community.* Norwalk, CT: Appleton & Lange.

Janosik, E., and Davies, J.L. (1989). *Psychiatric-mental health nursing* (2nd ed.). Boston: Jones & Bartlett.

Johnson, B.S. (1989). *Psychiatric-mental health nursing* (2nd ed.). Philadelphia: Lippincott.

Stuart, G.W., and Sundeen, S.J. (1991). *Principles and practice of psychiatric nursing* (4th ed.). St. Louis: Mosby-Year Book.

Wilson, H.S. (1988). *Psychiatric nursing* (3rd ed.). Menlo Park, CA: Addison-Wesley.

INTRODUCTION
Stress and Mental Illness

Clinicians have long acknowledged that stress plays a major role in illness. Research has focused on gaining a clearer understanding of the mechanisms involved, attempting to define causal relationships between the brain and the body. Stress does not automatically lead to psychiatric or mental health problems. In fact, some stress is necessary to normal functioning. But when stress overwhelms a person's normal coping strategies, damaging physiologic and psychological changes can result.

Selye defines stress as a nonspecific response by the body to any demand made upon it. Stress varies in intensity depending on internal and external factors and the person's perception of the stress. Stressors include any physiologic, psychological, sociocultural, or environmental influence that requires an individual to change. Such change can be adaptive, restoring homeostasis, or maladaptive, leading to continued stress.

Stress can cause physiologic and psychological changes. Physiologic changes may include increased heart rate, headaches, fatigue, stomachaches, sleep disturbances, changes in appetite, and ulcers. Psychological changes include mood swings, irritability, depression, withdrawal, anger, forgetfulness, lack of interest, and an inability to concentrate or feel pleasure. Stress also can cause a person to question spiritual beliefs.

Because of the connection between the body and the mind, psychological stress can lead to physiologic stress and vice versa. Rage, for instance, stimulates the sympathetic branch of the autonomic nervous system, triggering the fight-or-flight response. A soothing emotion affects the parasympathetic branch, causing relaxation. Psychological stress also may suppress or stimulate the immune system by affecting neurotransmitter levels.

Several theorists attempt to explain the stress response, including Freud, Cannon, Selye, Lazarus, and Holmes and Rahe. Theories, including the cognitive and interpersonal theories, also examine stress. The interpersonal and cognitive theories are the basis for most of the psychosocial nursing theories.

Freud established some of the early links between physical and mental processes through his theory of psychosexual development, which explores developmental tasks related to specific physiologic functions. Freud described "conversion disorders" — physical disorders with no apparent organic cause — that responded to psychoanalysis. Such a physical disorder, he reasoned, symbolized an intrapsychic conflict produced by the client's inability to resolve conflicts at an earlier developmental phase.

The mind-body connection received further support when Cannon, an animal physiologist, described the fight-or-flight response. Cannon's work established the concept of homeostasis, thus laying the foundation for additional investigation into the physical responses to stress.

Selye's general adaptation syndrome theory describes an organized response involving three stages: alarm, resistance, and exhaustion. (See *Identifying stages of the general adaptation syndrome,* page 32.)

In the alarm stage, the person tries to adjust to a stressor that is perceived as life-threatening. The autonomic nervous system initiates the lifesaving fight-or-flight response. In the resistance stage, the person maintains a greater than normal resistance to stress. If adaptation to stress is successful, or if the stress diminishes or disappears, the person returns to normal. But if the stress continues, exhaustion results and the person can no longer resist the effects of stress. In this final stage, physical or emotional disorders may develop; in an extreme case, the person may die.

How much stress a person can handle before reaching the exhaustion stage varies. Factors affecting the ability to cope with stress include perception of the stressor, intelligence, health, personal hardiness and resiliency, family traits, family history of disease, genetic predisposition, environment, and social influences.

Lazarus also believes that the stress response occurs in three stages, but views each stage as a conscious evaluation of the stimulus — not as an automatic reaction. In the first stage, the person determines whether the stimulus is irrelevant or stressful; if it is stressful, the person decides whether it poses a threat or challenge. In the second stage, the person chooses coping strategies. In the third stage, the person reevaluates the situation and modifies coping strategies as needed.

Holmes and Rahe's theory suggests that all life events — whether positive, such as a marriage or vacation, or negative, such as a divorce — cause stress. As a result, their theory focuses not on a single stressor but on the cumulative effect of several stressors over a short period.

Holmes and Rahe created a social readjustment scale that ranks life events according to how much stress they cause, although the actual amount of stress will vary among individuals. The scale is a useful guide to identifying major stressors and determining the degree of stress in a person's life (see *Social readjustment rating scale,* page 33).

Cognitive theory examines thought rather than behavior. Whereas intrapsychic theory claims that unconscious drives guide a person's behavior and response to stress, cognitive theory holds that a person can consciously change behavior, including reac-

(Text continues on page 34.)

IDENTIFYING STAGES OF THE GENERAL ADAPTATION SYNDROME

A distinctive set of responses occurs during each of the three stages of the general adaptation syndrome. Use this checklist to help determine which stage your client is experiencing.

Alarm stage

In this stage, stress triggers both sympathetic and parasympathetic responses.

Sympathetic responses
- Anorexia, constipation, and flatulence
- Bronchodilation
- Decreased serum chloride
- Decreased urine output
- Hyperglycemia from glucose buildup
- Increased adrenal secretion
- Increased blood clotting
- Increased blood pressure
- Increased body temperature
- Increased cardiac contractility, heart rate, and cardiac output
- Increased gastric acid secretion
- Increased metabolic rate
- Increased respiratory rate
- Increased serum potassium, glucose, and lactate levels
- Inhibited micturition
- Mild dehydration
- Muscle tension
- Peripheral vasoconstriction
- Perspiration
- Protein catabolism from conversion of protein to glucose
- Pupil dilation
- Reduced intestinal motility
- Short-term increased resistance to inflammation and infection
- Sodium and water retention

Parasympathetic responses
- Bronchoconstriction
- Constricted, fixed pupils, leading to blurred vision
- Decreased cardiac contractility, heart rate, and cardiac output
- Decreased cognition
- Dyspnea
- Hyperventilation, leading to tremors and dizziness
- Hypoglycemia from depleted glycogen stores
- Increased gastrointestinal motility, possibly leading to diarrhea
- Involuntary or frequent urination
- Peripheral flushing
- Relaxed muscle tone
- Syncope

Resistance stage

In this stage, stress causes emotional, cognitive, and physiologic responses.

Emotional responses
- Aggressive behavior
- Alcohol and drug addiction
- Anger
- Criticism of others
- Crying
- Depression
- Emotional instability
- Feelings of helplessness
- Feelings of worthlessness
- Free-floating anxiety
- High-pitched voice
- Impatience
- Impulsive behavior
- Inability to love
- Inappropriate laughter
- Increased smoking

- Increased use of medications
- Irritability
- Low self-esteem
- Negative self-concept
- Neurotic behavior
- Overreaction to events
- Preoccupation with past events
- Psychosis
- Regressive behavior
- Strained relations with others
- Stuttering
- Suspicion
- Withdrawal

Cognitive responses
- Confusion
- Decreased awareness of external stimuli
- Decreased tolerance for ambiguity
- Disorientation
- Errors in judgment
- Forgetfulness
- Inability to concentrate, solve problems, or plan
- Inattention to detail or instructions
- Lack of initiative
- Misidentification of people
- Preoccupation
- Reduced fantasy, creativity, and perceptual field

Physiologic responses
- Adrenal cortex hypertrophy
- Agitation
- Diarrhea
- Dry mouth
- Elevated vital signs
- Emesis
- Fatigue
- Flatulence
- Headache and neck ache
- Increased natural killer-cell activity
- Increased susceptibility to disease
- Irregular elimination patterns
- Irregular sleep patterns
- Hyperchloremia
- Missed menstrual periods
- Muscle tightness, aches, tics, and tremors
- Nightmares
- Premenstrual tension
- Restlessness
- Sexual dysfunction
- Slumping posture
- Grinding of teeth
- Tight chest muscles, leading to dyspnea
- Tissue anabolism
- Urinary frequency
- Weakness

Exhaustion stage

In this final stage, a person may experience these responses.
- Intensified, then diminished, alarm response
- Severe anxiety, possibly leading to panic, neurosis, or psychosis
- Physical or emotional disorders
- Death

From: *Psychosocial crises*. Clinical Skillbuilders. Springhouse, PA: Springhouse Corp., 1992.

SOCIAL READJUSTMENT RATING SCALE

According to Holmes and Rahe, every event produces a certain amount of stress. Major life changes, such as the death of a family member, cause the most stress, but even seemingly minor events, such as a change in the number of family get-togethers, can cause some stress.

The rating scale below assigns a value to 43 life events. Any combination of events that pushes a client's total score above 150 can lead to a crisis. A score above 300 signals the possibility of a major life crisis.

(Note that the dollar amounts reflect the cost of living in 1967, when the rating scale was developed.)

Life event	Stress value	Life event	Stress value
Death of a spouse	100	Son or daughter leaving home	29
Divorce	73	Trouble with in-laws	29
Marital separation	65	Outstanding personal achievement	28
Jail term	63	Spouse begins or stops work	26
Death of a close family member	63	Beginning or end of school	26
Personal injury or illness	53	Change in living conditions	25
Marriage	50	Change in personal habits	24
Fired from job	47	Trouble with boss	23
Marital reconciliation	45	Change in work hours or conditions	20
Retirement	45	Change in residence	20
Change in health of a family member	44	Change in schools	20
Pregnancy	40	Change in recreation	19
Sexual difficulties	39	Change in church activities	19
New family member	39	Change in social activities	18
Business readjustment	39	Mortgage or loan less than $10,000	17
Change in financial status	38	Change in sleeping habits	16
Death of close friend	37	Change in number of family get-togethers	15
Change to different type of work	36	Change in eating habits	15
Change in number of arguments with spouse	35	Vacation	13
Mortgage over $10,000	31	Christmas	12
Foreclosure on mortgage or loan	30	Minor violations of the law	11
Change in responsibilities at work	29		

From Holmes, T.H., and Rahe, R.H. (1967). Social readjustment rating scale. *Journal of Psychosomatic Research.* 11(8), 216. Used with permission.

tions to stress—a change in thinking about a stressor results in more adaptive behavior.

Interpersonal theory focuses on a person's behavior with others. According to this theory, personality emerges in a person's interactions. A person relates to others in ways that bring about physical satisfaction (sufficient food, rest, physical contact, and sexual fulfillment) and social and emotional security. Stress results when a relationship no longer meets these needs and instead causes painful emotions.

Despite differences in perspective, all these theories agree on one basic point: a person experiencing stress tries to alleviate it. Protecting the self from serious discomfort involves unconscious defense mechanisms and conscious learned responses. Both help the individual cope with stressors by regulating emotional response and taking action to change the situation.

A person under stress may choose from four types of coping mechanisms: changing the environment by removing the stressor, developing ways to deal with the stressor, preventing neutral stimuli associated with a stressor from becoming stressors themselves, or looking for ways to divert attention from the stressor.

The effectiveness of a particular coping strategy depends on how and when a person uses it. Sometimes a strategy that has been successful in the past may no longer work. When this occurs, the person may need help to analyze the problem and adopt new coping strategies.

When coping strategies fail completely, the person may enter a crisis—a state of emotional disequilibrium that the person cannot correct. A crisis may be developmental or situational. Developmental crises stem from transitional changes that occur throughout life, such marriage, mid-life changes, and retirement. Situational crises occur in response to an unexpected event, such as illness or death. All crises are self-limiting, usually lasting no more than six weeks. They also have far-reaching effects. A person in crisis can adversely affect not only the family but the health care team.

A crisis that continues unabated can cause the person to become agitated, resistant, and combative, and can lead to long-term physical or mental disability, psychosis, and even suicide. But a crisis also can present possibilities for growth. A person in crisis may be more willing to accept help, especially with the realization that current coping mechanisms no longer work. Interventions focus on helping the person and family solve the immediate problem that triggered the crisis. These new coping skills then can be used to deal with stress that may arise in other situations.

Selected references

Cannon, W.B. (1929). *Bodily changes in pain, hunger, fear, and rage.* New York: Appleton-Century-Crofts.

Holmes, T.H., and Rahe, R.H. (1967). The social readjustment rating scale, *Journal of Psychosomatic Research* 11(8), 213-17.

Horney, K. (1972). *Our inner conflicts.* Norton: New York.

Lazarus, R. (1966). *Psychosocial stress and the coping process.* New York: McGraw-Hill.

Miller, T.W., (1988). Advances in understanding the impact of stressful life events on health. *Hospital and Community Psychiatry* 39, 615.

Pines, M. (1080). Psychological hardiness: The role of challenge in health, *Psychology Today* 14, 3-4.

Selye, H. (1956). *The stress of life.* New York: McGraw-Hill.

Tache, J., and Selye, H. (1985). On stress and coping mechanisms, *Issues in Mental Health Nursing* 7(1/4), 3-24.

INTRODUCTION
The Nursing Process in Psychiatric Nursing

The nurse's relationship with a client is documented through the nursing process—a system for making nursing decisions that includes assessment, nursing diagnosis, planning, implementation, and evaluation. The nursing process guides the nurse in providing quality care to the client and family in any setting. By following this process and supporting it with thorough documentation, the nurse can develop effective strategies for responding to the client's and family's current and potential needs while promoting mental health.

Assessment
The first step in the nursing process involves the orderly collection and careful interpretation of information about a client's health status. Information comes from interviews with the client or family members (subjective data) and from physical examination, medical records, diagnostic test results, and other medical or nursing sources (objective data). Together, subjective and objective data give the nurse information essential to developing an effective plan of care.

Psychiatric assessment is the scientific process of identifying a client's psychosocial problems, strengths, and concerns. Besides serving as a basis for psychiatric care, psychiatric assessment has broad nursing applications. Recognizing psychosocial problems and how they affect health is important in any clinical setting. Psychiatric assessment involves the psychiatric interview, mental status examination, physical examination, and diagnostic testing.

Psychiatric interview
A systematic psychiatric interview provides information about the client's behavioral disturbances, emotional and social history, and mental status. With this information, the nurse will be able to assess psychological functioning, understand coping methods and their effect on psychosocial growth, build a therapeutic relationship that encourages open communication, and develop a plan of care.

The client must feel comfortable enough in the interview to discuss problems. Before beginning the interview:
• explain the interview's purpose
• reassure the client that privacy will be maintained
• ask the client if a family member or friend should be present
• ask how the client wishes to be addressed
• find out which outcomes the client expects from the treatment.

The interview's success hinges on the nurse's ability to listen objectively and respond with empathy. Use these guidelines when interviewing psychiatric clients:

• Have clearly set goals—the interview is not a random discussion.
• Control personal values so that they do not compromise professional judgment.
• Pay attention to the client's reactions and any unspoken signals—look for signs of anxiety and distress and any topics the client avoids.
• Determine the client's cultural values and beliefs.
• Avoid making assumptions about how past events affected the client emotionally.
• Monitor personal reactions; watch for interference with interview goals.

Try to determine the chief complaint—what prompted the client to seek treatment. Some clients may not have a chief complaint—some identify several small problems, while others will insist nothing is wrong. A client with a medical problem typically fails to recognize depression or anxiety. When possible, discuss the client's complaint, including when the symptoms began, their severity, and if their onset was insidious or abrupt.

During the interview, obtain a psychosocial history, a psychiatric history, and a family history. The psychosocial history provides information about the client's mental and social status and function. Such a history includes information about the client's beliefs, relationships, life-style, coping skills, diet, sleeping patterns, and use of alcohol, drugs, and tobacco. The history should describe school, work, religious practices, community life, hobbies, and sexual activity. The psychosocial history also should explore how the client has coped with any significant changes, such as a recent divorce or death. Numerous assessment tools are available to help the nurse gather information about the client's psychosocial history (see Section III of this book for samples).

The psychiatric history explores previous psychological disorders; any episodes of violence, delusions, or attempts at suicide; and previous psychiatric treatment and its results. The family history explores family customs, child-rearing practices, and emotional support during childhood. It also includes information about family members' physical and emotional health, such as a history of substance abuse, alcoholism, suicide, violence, diabetes mellitus, or thyroid disorders.

Throughout the interview, gather information about the client's personality, including level of maturity; ego functioning, such as ability to control impulses, cope with stress, and maintain a sense of identity; strengths, such as talents and accomplishments; and ability to find emotional support.

Mental status examination

Usually part of the psychiatric interview, the mental status examination provides a means of assessing psychological dysfunction and identifying the causes of psychopathology. The nurse needs to understand the components of the examination to be able to interpret the physician's findings as well as plan appropriate nursing interventions. Various tools are available for mental status assessment; for an example, see *Folstein mini-mental state examination.*

The mental status examination assesses the client's level of consciousness, general appearance, behavior, speech, mood and affect, intellectual performance, judgment, insight, perception, and thought content.

Level of consciousness helps determine basic brain function — the client's response to stimulation, including the degree and quality of movement, content and coherence of speech, and level of eye opening and eye-to-eye contact. An impaired level of consciousness may indicate a tumor or abscess, an electrolyte or acid-base imbalance, or toxicity from liver or kidney failure or alcohol or drug use.

Appearance, including weight, coloring, skin condition, odor, body build, and obvious physical impairments, indicates the client's overall mental status. Note any discrepancies between objective observation and the client's feelings about his health. A disheveled appearance may indicate self-neglect or a preoccupation with other activities. Posture and gait also may reveal physical and emotional disorders — for example, a slumped posture may indicate depression, fatigue, or suspiciousness.

Behavior includes the client's demeanor and way of relating to others. When responding to questions, is the client cooperative, mistrustful, embarrassed, hostile, or too revealing? Body language, such as tenseness, rigidity, or restlessness, may be significant. An inability to sit still may indicate anxiety. Also watch for any extraordinary behavior, such as disconnected gestures that may indicate hallucinations.

Speech is observed for content and quality. Note any incoherencies, illogical or irrelevant replies, speech defects, excessively slow or fast speech, sudden interruptions, excessive volume, altered tone or modulation, slurring, excessive number of words, or minimal monosyllabic responses.

Mood and affect refer to an individual's pervading feeling and how it is expressed. Ask how the client feels and evaluate facial expression and posture.

Intellectual performance involves the ability to reason abstractly, make judgments, or solve problems. Various simple tests can be used to characterize the client's intellectual abilities. These tests evaluate orientation, immediate and delayed recall, recent and remote memory, attention level, comprehension, concept formation, and general knowledge.

Judgment is the ability to evaluate choices and draw a conclusion. *Insight* is the capacity for realistic self-assessment. *Perception* involves interpreting reality and using the senses.

Throughout the mental status examination, assess the client's thought patterns in terms of connection to reality, clarity, and progression in a logical sequence. Observe for indications of morbid thoughts and preoccupations; abnormal beliefs; suicidal, self-destructive, violent, or superstitious thoughts; recurring dreams; distorted perceptions of reality; and feelings of worthlessness or persecution.

Besides using information from the interview and the mental status examination, observe the client for significant behavior changes. Identify any departures from usual behavior patterns and compare them with the results of the interview and the client's history. Key signs and symptoms include changes in appetite, energy level, motivation, hygiene, self-image, self-esteem, sleep, sex drive, and competence.

Also assess for any signs of self-destructive behavior, including suicide attempts or threats. Keep in mind that not all self-destructive behavior is suicidal in intent. Some clients engage in self-destructive behavior because it helps them feel alive. A client who has lost touch with reality may commit self-harm, such as cutting or mutilating, to focus on physical pain, which may be less overwhelming than emotional distress. If the psychosocial interview or observation reveals any signs of hopelessness, assess the risk of suicide and protect the client from self-harm.

Physical examination

Because psychiatric problems may stem from organic causes or medical treatments, the nurse should conduct a physical assessment of all body systems (employing inspection, palpation, percussion, and auscultation). Although the extent of physical assessment depends on the client's needs, the health care setting, the nurse's level of training, and other factors, every client should be examined to obtain basic physiologic data. During any physical assessment, pay particular attention to areas associated with current complaints and past problems identified during the health history.

For the psychiatric client, assessment of the cranial nerves, cerebellar function, and sensory and motor systems is essential. A defect in perception may indicate cranial nerve dysfunction. A neurologic assessment will help determine whether a sensory defect results from a damaged nerve or a conversion disorder (a physical condition with no apparent organic cause).

The cerebellum controls equilibrium and muscle function, ensuring smooth, steady, and coordinated movement. An abnormality in cerebellar function may cause the client to depend on other people or mechanical devices for simple tasks, such as walking, bathing, or cooking. Loss of these abilities may create intense loneliness, sadness, or feelings of uselessness.

The sensory system carries impulses from the various areas of the body to the central nervous system, which registers and interprets them. Sensory functions

FOLSTEIN MINI-MENTAL STATE EXAMINATION

The Folstein Mini-Mental State Examination is the preferred tool for assessing the mental status of a client with suspected cognitive impairment. To perform the examination, ask the client to follow a series of simple commands that test the ability to understand and perform cognitive functions. Award a designated point value for successful completion of each instruction; then total the scores to determine the client's mental status. Scores of 26 to 30 indicate that the client is normal; 22 to 25, mildly impaired; and less than 22; significantly impaired.

Client instructions	Maximum score	Actual score
Orientation		
• Ask the client to name the year, season, date, day, and month. (Score one point for each correct response.)	5	_____
• Ask the client to name his state, city, street, and house address, and the room in which he is standing. (Score one point for each correct response.)	5	_____
Comprehension		
Name three objects, pausing 1 second between each name. Then ask the client to repeat all three names. (Score one point for each correct response.) Repeat this exercise until the client can correctly name all three objects (the client will be tested on his ability to recall this information later in the examination).	3	_____
Attention and calculation		
Ask the client to count backward by sevens, beginning at 100; have him stop after counting out five numbers. Alternatively, ask the client to spell "World" backward. (Score one point for each correct response.)	5	_____
Recall		
Ask the client to restate the name of the three objects previously identified in the examination. (Score one point for each correct response.)	3	_____
Language		
• Point to a pencil and a watch. Ask the client to identify each object. (Score one point for each correct response.)	2	_____
• Ask the client to repeat "No ifs, ands, or buts." (Score one point for a correct response.)	1	_____
• Ask the client to take a paper in the right hand, then fold the paper in half, then put the paper on the floor. (Score one point for each correct response to this three-part command.)	3	_____
• Ask the client to read and obey the written instruction "Close your eyes." (Score one point for a correct response.)	1	_____
• Ask the client to copy the following design. (Score one point for a correct response.)	1	_____

From: Folstein, M.F., et al. (1975). Mini-mental state: A practical method for grading the cognitive state of patients for the clinician, *Journal of Psychiatric Research* 12:196-97. Adapted with permission.

include simple touch, pain, temperature, stereognosis, and two-point discrimination. A sensory disorder occurring along the distribution pathway of a nerve is apt to have an organic cause; otherwise, suspect a somatoform disorder. The client with a sensory disturbance experiences severe psychological stress, becoming alternately demanding and withdrawn.

In the motor system, neurons carry impulses from the cerebrum to the skeletal muscles through the pyramidal and extrapyramidal motor tracts. Impulses traveling along the pyramidal tract stimulate individual muscles; those traveling along the extrapyramidal tract stimulate muscle groups. Motor system assessment includes observation of muscle tone, size, and strength. A client with a somatoform disorder may exhibit tics, tremors, or various paralyses with no apparent physiologic cause.

Diagnostic tests

Performing common diagnostic tests for the client with a suspected psychiatric disorder serves five purposes: it assists in accurate diagnosis, investigates any underlying physiologic disorders, establishes normal renal and hepatic function before the client takes prescribed psychotropic medications, monitors for therapeutic medication levels, and determines if the client is using a psychoactive substance. Diagnostic tests include invasive and noninvasive laboratory tests as well as psychological tests.

Laboratory tests may include a complete blood count, hemoglobin and hematocrit, and routine urinalysis. A complete blood count and hemoglobin and hematocrit help assess for an underlying condition, such as infection, anemia, and dehydration, that might cause or increase psychiatric symptoms. For example, an elevated hemoglobin value might indicate dehydration, which can cause delirium in an elderly or debilitated client. In addition, psychotropic medications may cause such conditions as aplastic anemia or leukopenia; consequently, regular blood counts are important. Urinalysis determines basic kidney function, an important consideration before the physician prescribes psychotropic medications because these drugs are excreted through the kidneys.

Toxicologic screening of the blood or urine commonly are ordered as part of the initial assessment. Such tests help determine the presence and level of drugs and can monitor blood levels of prescribed medications, such as lithium, to ensure therapeutic dosage.

Serum electrolytes may be checked because electrolyte disturbances can cause symptoms of mental confusion. Abnormal serum electrolyte levels may be a sign of certain psychiatric disorders. For example, an alcoholic client may have an elevated chloride level resulting from renal disease or metabolic acidosis, whereas an anorexic client may have a low chloride or potassium level from excessive vomiting. Some psychotropic medications can cause thirst; a client may have a low sodium level from excessive fluid intake.

Thyroid function tests may be ordered because signs of thyroid dysfunction are very similar to those of anxiety disorder, panic disorder, and depression. Thyroid studies are ordered before lithium is prescribed because the drug may induce hypothyroidism.

Liver function tests are ordered routinely for clients at high risk for liver disease (such as alcoholics and I.V. drug users) as well as to determine the liver's ability to filter medications from the blood.

Serology for sexually transmitted diseases and human immunodeficiency virus (HIV) testing may be ordered for clients who exhibit high-risk behaviors such as promiscuity, I.V. drug use, and unprotected sex. In addition, tertiary syphilis and acquired immunodeficiency syndrome can cause dementia. HIV-positive clients also may present with symptoms of depression.

Routine testing for most clients usually includes a chest X-ray and an electrocardiogram to rule out cardiopulmonary abnormalities or disease. An electroencephalogram may be performed to rule out brain abnormalities. The following diagnostic procedures also may be ordered to rule out physical causes (such as lesions, abscesses, atrophy, or arteriovenous abnormalities) for abnormal behavior:
• computed tomography, which provides a study of tissue density through radiologic and computer analysis
• magnetic resonance imaging, which provides detailed pictures of body structures on multiple planes
• positron emission tomography, which uses radioactive isotopes to maps the brain's metabolic activity, is useful in detecting such conditions as transient ischemia attacks, seizures, and head trauma, as well as the effects of drug therapy.

In addition to routine diagnostic tests, a client presenting with symptoms of depression may undergo a dexamethasone suppression test. Although not diagnostic for all depression, this test can reveal if low corticotropin levels may be the cause of the depression.

Additional assessment tools used specifically for the diagnosis of depression include rating scales, such as the Beck Depression Inventory (a 21-item self-rating scale, in which high scores indicate severe depression), the 20-item Zung Self-Rating Depression Scale, and the Geriatric Depression Scale (designed specifically for use with elderly individuals). Other psychological tests include the Stanford-Binet test, the Weschler Adult Intelligence Scale (revised), and the Minnesota Multiphasic Personality Inventory.

Noninvasive diagnostic tests specifically related to alcohol and drug abuse include:
• CAGE, a four-question tool in which two or three positive responses indicate alcoholism
• Michigan Alcoholism Screening Test, a 24-item timed test in which a score of five or better classifies the client as alcoholic
• Drug Use Questionnaire, used when drug use is suspected
• Cocaine Addiction Severity Test and Cocaine Assessment Profile, used when cocaine use is suspected.

Nursing diagnosis

After completing the assessment step, the nurse analyzes the subjective and objective data and formulates nursing diagnoses. In psychiatric nursing, the nurse uses diagnoses based on the North American Nursing Diagnosis Association (NANDA) taxonomy and the Psychiatric Nursing Diagnoses (PND) Taxonomy, and may consider medical diagnoses in the *Diagnostic and Statistical Manual of Mental Disorders, Third Edition, Revised* (DSM III-R).

A nursing diagnosis is a statement of an actual or potential health problem that a nurse is capable of treating and licensed to treat (Gordon, 1987). Determining one or more applicable nursing diagnoses for a client provides the basis for an individualized, effective nursing plan of care. Each diagnosis must be supported by clinical information obtained during assessment. (Complete care may involve collaborative treatment).

Nursing diagnoses provide a common language to convey the nursing management necessary for each client to any nurses involved in that client's care. To help ensure standardized nursing diagnosis terminology and usage, NANDA has formulated and classified a series of nursing diagnostic categories based on nine human response patterns (NANDA, 1990), including:

- exchanging (mutual giving and receiving)
- communicating (sending messages)
- relating (establishing bonds)
- valuing (assigning worth)
- choosing (selecting alternatives)
- moving (activity)
- perceiving (receiving information)
- knowing (meaning associated with information)
- feeling (subjective awareness of information).

Within each pattern are NANDA-approved nursing diagnostic categories. For example, the human response pattern devoted to relating includes such diagnostic categories as *sexual dysfunction* and *parental role conflict*. The complete list of NANDA diagnostic categories, arranged by human response pattern, is called the nursing diagnosis taxonomy. (For the complete list, see Appendix B, NANDA Diagnostic Categories Arranged by Gordon's Functional Health Patterns.) Assigning specific nursing diagnoses involves several steps, including grouping assessment data, choosing the appropriate category, and adding specific client information.

To help nurses classify psychiatric disorders, the American Nurses' Association (ANA) division of Psychiatric and Mental Health Nursing Practice supported a project to identify and develop a working list of the specific phenomena that concern psychiatric and mental health nurses. A panel of specialists in specific age and diagnostic client groups convened to develop a conceptual classification system. The classification system is called the *ANA Classification of Phenomena of Concern to Psychiatric and Mental Health Nursing,* also referred to as *Psychiatric Nursing Diagnoses, First Edi-*

tion. (For more information, see Appendix C, Psychiatric Nursing Taxonomy.)

The standard interdisciplinary psychiatric diagnosis serves the mental health team in labeling a client's disorder. (The nursing diagnosis assists the nurse in conceptualizing the client's human response that nursing can address.) The official guide to psychiatric classification is the American Psychiatric Association's DSM III-R. This classification system reflects the medical model, but also includes descriptive, behavioral, and social understandings of mental disorders. Because interdisciplinary health care teams use the DSM III-R, the nurse should have a general understanding of the system.

Planning

After formulating appropriate nursing diagnoses, the nurse develops a plan of care appropriate for the client and family. Effective planning focuses on the client's specific needs, considers strengths and weaknesses, encourages the client's participation in setting achievable goals and in the care itself, includes feasible interventions, and is within the scope of applicable nursing practice acts.

Planning involves three basic steps: setting and prioritizing goals, formulating nursing interventions, and developing a plan of care.

The nurse sets one or more goals for each applicable diagnosis. A goal—the desired client outcome after nursing care—states what the nurse and client will do to minimize or eliminate a problem. Appropriate goals help the nurse select nursing interventions and also serve as criteria for evaluating the interventions. Goals should relate directly to the nursing diagnoses and reflect the desires of the client, family, and nurse, who work together to formulate them. Setting goals with the client and family helps ensure appropriate and realistic care planning, encourages client involvement, and gives the client a sense of control.

An effective goal statement, or outcome criterion, is measurable, realistic, and stated so that the client and family understand it. It should include the desired client behavior and predicted outcome, measurement criteria, a specified time for attainment or reevaluation, and any other conditions under which the behavior will occur.

After goals are formulated, the nurse works with the client and family to prioritize them. This involves ranking the nursing diagnoses and goals in an accepted order (such as Maslow's hierarchy of needs).

Goals may be short- or long-term. Short-term goals may take priority over long-term ones. When prioritizing goals, the nurse and client should account for possible effects of the client's ethnic and cultural background, socioeconomic status, and other factors that might influence goal achievement.

Next, the nurse formulates interventions to achieve each short- and long-term goal. These interventions will include strategies, actions, or activities that help the client reach established goals by diminishing or resolving problems identified in the nursing diagnoses. The nurse and client should work together to formulate interventions, analyzing possible strategies and choosing those best suited to the client's circumstances. Interventions may be collaborative, including nursing and medical care, physical therapy, nutritional counseling, and social services.

Effective nursing interventions must be based on both sound nursing practice and research. Such a knowledge base provides the proper rationales to support nursing interventions.

The nurse develops a nursing plan of care by integrating each step of the nursing process: collecting and analyzing health history and physical assessment data, selecting nursing diagnoses, setting and prioritizing goals, formulating interventions, and evaluating outcomes. The plan of care, which can be revised and updated as needed, acts as a written guide for and documentation of the client's care. Also, it helps ensure continuity of care when the client interacts with other members of the health care team.

The format of nursing plans of care varies among health care facilities and sometimes among units in the same facility. All plans of care, however, include written nursing diagnoses, goals, interventions, and evaluation criteria. Standardized care plans have evolved as a time-saving and efficient method of ensuring documentation. A standardized care plan incorporates the major aspects of nursing care required by clients with a similar problem, while allowing alterations to reflect individual differences.

Implementation

Implementation involves working with the client and family to accomplish the designated interventions and move toward the desired outcomes. Effective implementation requires a sound understanding of the plan of care and collaborative interactions among the client, family, and other members of the health care team, as needed. The implementation phase begins as soon as the plan of care is completed and ends when the established goals are achieved. Before and during implementation of any intervention, the nurse reassesses the client to ensure that planned interventions continue to be appropriate. Periodic reassessment helps ensure a flexible, individualized, and effective plan of care.

To implement nursing interventions effectively, the nurse will use four types of skills:
- cognitive skills, based on knowledge of current clinical practice and basic sciences
- affective skills, including verbal and nonverbal communication and empathy
- psychomotor skills, involving both mental and physical activity and encompassing traditional nursing actions (such as taking vital signs and administering medications) and more complex procedures
- organizational skills, such as counseling, managing, and delegating.

Evaluation

Through evaluation, the nurse obtains additional subjective and objective assessment data relating to the goals identified in the planning stage. The nurse uses these data to determine whether goals have been met totally, met partially, or remain unmet. Although evaluation is the final step in the nursing process, it actually occurs throughout, particularly during implementation, where the nurse continually reassesses the effect of interventions. Evaluation is directly linked to and must be based on the goals developed from each nursing diagnosis.

When all goals for a particular nursing diagnosis have been met, the nurse and client may decide that the diagnosis is no longer valid. The nurse then documents when and how the goals were met and may delete the diagnosis from the nursing plan of care. Alternatively, the nurse and client may judge a goal met but still feel that the nursing diagnosis requires other goals; they then would retain it in the plan of care.

If goals have been only partially met or remain unmet by the target date, the nurse must reevaluate the plan of care. Reevaluation involves deciding whether the initial plan was appropriate, whether the assigned timeframe was realistic, whether the goals were realistic and measurable, and whether other factors interfered. Based on this information, the nurse can clarify or amend the assessment data, reexamine and correct the nursing diagnoses as necessary, establish new goals reflecting the revised diagnoses, and devise new interventions for achieving these goals. The nurse then adds the revised plan of care to the original document and records the rationale for these revisions in the nursing notes.

Selected references

Alfaro, R. (1990). *Applying nursing diagnosis and nursing process: A step-by-step guide* (2nd ed.). Philadelphia: Lippincott.

Barry, P.D. (1989). *Psychosocial nursing assessment and intervention* (2nd ed.). Philadelphia: Lippincott.

Carpenito, L. (1989). *Nursing diagnosis: Application to clinical practice* (3rd ed.). Philadelphia: Lippincott.

Folstein, M.F., et al. (1975). Mini-mental state: A practical method for grading the cognitive state of patients for the clinician, *Journal of Psychiatric Research* 12(3), 189-98.

Gordon, M. (1987). *Nursing diagnosis: Process and application* (2nd ed.). New York: McGraw-Hill.

Talbott, J.A., et al. (1988). *Textbook of psychiatry.* Washington, DC: American Psychiatric Association.

Townsend, M.C. (1988). *Nursing diagnoses in psychiatric nursing.* Philadelphia: F.A. Davis.

Section II: Plans of Care

General Anxiety Disorders

DSM III-R classifications
300.00 Anxiety disorder not otherwise specified
300.02 Generalized anxiety disorder

Psychiatric nursing diagnostic class
Anxiety

Introduction
Generalized anxiety disorder is characterized by unrealistic or excessive worry about life circumstances. This disorder lasts at least 6 months. The residual classification *anxiety disorders not otherwise specified* covers those disorders that do not conform to the classification criteria for any other specific anxiety disorder (generalized anxiety disorder, phobic and panic disorders, obsessive-compulsive disorder, and post-traumatic stress disorder). Management for the two anxiety disorder classifications covered in this plan of care is the same.

ETIOLOGY AND PRECIPITATING FACTORS
Currently, no one etiology thoroughly explains all of the psychophysiologic manifestations of anxiety as it relates to generalized anxiety disorder and anxiety disorders not otherwise specified. Therefore, brief descriptions follow of four major categories of causation theories: behavioral, biological, familial, and psychodynamic.

Behavioral theorists believe anxiety is a learned, conditioned response to specific stimuli. For example, children who are beaten whenever the father becomes drunk may develop anxiety whenever the father begins to drink. Behaviorists also believe that because anxiety is a learned response, it can be unlearned. According to behavioral theory, taking steps that remove or reduce anxiety-triggering factors and produce positive action can alleviate anxiety at an early point.

Although no definitive conclusions about biological causes of anxiety yet exist, biological theorists are producing increasingly significant support for hypotheses that relate manifestations of anxiety to physiologic abnormalities. General health affects the individual's predisposition to anxiety. Typically, anxiety accompanies certain physical disorders and is associated with others, including hyperthyroidism, hypoglycemia, and severe pulmonary disease. Anxiety also may exacerbate some disorders, such as hypertension, heart disease, and peptic ulcer. Much current research focuses on the functions of the peripheral autonomic nervous system and the hypothalamus. Other research is directed at neurotransmitter system disruption and at increases in autonomic nervous system discharges.

Theorists who explore the structure and function of the family suggest that individuals with dysfunctional behavior may represent familial dysfunction. For example, the individual who becomes anxious responds to stresses within the family, as when an adolescent develops severe anxiety from discord between the parents. Reasons for familial dysfunction and the resultant stress vary and may include addiction, chronic illness, financial difficulty, and communication problems.

Sigmund Freud proposed that anxiety signals potentially overwhelming threats to the ego (the conscious personality in contact with reality) in its role as mediator between the demands of the id (unconscious, instinctive drives and impulses) and those of the superego (conscious, culturally acquired restrictions). Although Harry Stack Sullivan based his work on Freudian psychology, he proposed that anxiety resulted from interpersonal conflicts involving approval versus disapproval from the mothering figure. Hildegard Peplau suggested that anxiety itself was a threat to an individual's security and that this threat could exist in the psychic as well as the biological realm. She also indicated that anxiety could be communicated interpersonally—that is, an individual can sense anxiety in another person and become anxious in turn—and that it could develop whenever situations or factors interfered with an individual's meeting of basic human needs.

Assessment guidelines
NURSING HISTORY (Functional health pattern findings)
The client may report or exhibit one or more of the findings grouped here according to functional health patterns.

Health perception—health management pattern
• extreme concern over general health
• exaggerated worry over daily life circumstances
• worry over medication compliance, follow-up visits, and inability to follow through
• fear of "going crazy"
• inability to control feelings
• numerous somatic complaints, with or without diagnostic validation
• overuse or underuse of health care system to ease anxiety symptoms

Nutritional-metabolic pattern
• worry over eating behaviors, such as using food to calm or soothe self
• weight gain or loss
• changes in appetite, including anorexia and binges

Elimination pattern
• concern over GI system disturbances, such as pain, flatulence, diarrhea, nausea, constipation, vomiting, and intestinal bleeding
• frequent urination
• concern over increased sweating, cold and clammy skin, or both

Activity-exercise pattern
• restlessness or trembling
• concern about being easily fatigued
• difficulty in accomplishing normal daily activities
• concern about inability to participate in and enjoy leisure activities
• concern about any limitations and restrictions of activity caused by disease or condition
• withdrawn or apathetic behavior

Sleep-rest pattern
• concern about falling or staying asleep and nightmares
• feeling fatigued after sleep
• concern about use or abuse of sleep aids, such as alcohol, benzodiazepines, and hypnotics

Cognitive-perceptual pattern
• difficulty concentrating
• difficulty with understanding and reacting to external stimuli
• worry over inability to think clearly
• distorted perceptions

Self-perception–self-concept pattern
• concern over being indecisive and dependent
• perception of self as being highly anxious
• perception of self as being incompetent and powerless
• concerns about body image, self-esteem, and self-worth

Role-relationship pattern
• intense concern over relationships with family and friends
• rumination over engaging in social situations with friends, fellow employees, or family
• concern over the lack of response to or support of life-style changes from family and friends
• concern about a distressful work situation
• concern about how community members and neighbors may respond to the disease or condition

Sexual-reproductive pattern
• dissatisfaction with sexual relations
• difficulty with intimacy
• concern about involvement in high-risk sexual behavior, such as unprotected sex or promiscuity
• concern about involvement with high-risk partners, including I.V. drug users, homosexual or bisexual partners, and strangers

Coping–stress tolerance pattern
• pervasive muscle tension
• constant irritability, feeling on edge or keyed up
• contant shakiness, trembling, or twitching
• concern over experiencing an exaggerated startle response (hypervigilance)
• denial of clearly manifest anxiety
• inability to identify those persons or measures that alleviate rather than exacerbate the condition
• belief that significant life-style changes are contributing to feeling out of control

Value-belief pattern
• feeling powerless to achieve life goals
• desire to increase or decrease involvement in spirituality or religion
• concern over impaired ability to believe in anything or anyone
• disbelief about present situation

PHYSICAL FINDINGS
The client may report or exhibit one or more of the following physical findings.

Cardiovascular
• cold, clammy skin
• elevated blood pressure
• hot and cold flashes
• increased heart rate
• palpitations
• sweating
• tingling sensation

Respiratory
• increased respiratory rate
• shortness of breath
• smothering sensation
• choking sensation

Gastrointestinal
• dry mouth
• abdominal distress
• nausea
• vomiting
• diarrhea
• difficulty swallowing

Genitourinary
• frequent urination

PHYSICAL DISORDERS ASSOCIATED WITH ANXIETY

Anxiety may result from certain physical disorders and may exacerbate others. Here are some common examples:

Cardiovascular disorders
- Arrhythmias
- Cardiomyopathies
- Congestive heart failure
- Coronary insufficiency
- Mitral valve prolapse
- Myocardial infarction

Endocrine disorders
- Adrenal insufficiency
- Carcinoid syndrome
- Cushing's syndrome
- Hyperparathyroidism
- Hyperthyroidism
- Hypoglycemia
- Hypothyroidism

Gastrointestinal disorders
- Colitis
- Irritable bowel syndrome
- Peptic ulcer disease

Metabolic disorders
- Hypocalcemia
- Hypokalemia
- Hyponatremia

Neurologic disorders
- Essential tremor
- Huntington's chorea
- Multiple sclerosis
- Parkinson's disease
- Seizure disorders
- Vestibular dysfunction

Respiratory disorders
- Asthma
- Chronic obstructive pulmonary disease
- Hyperventilation syndrome
- Pneumothorax
- Pulmonary edema
- Pulmonary embolism

From *Psychosocial crises.* Clinical Skillbuilders. Springhouse, PA: Springhouse Corp. 1992.

Musculoskeletal
- increased fatigue
- muscle aches, pains, or soreness
- muscle tension
- restlessness
- shakiness
- trembling
- twitching

Neurologic
- dilated pupils
- dizziness or faintness
- light-headedness
- paresthesia
- restlessness
- insomnia

Psychological
- feeling keyed up or on edge
- inability to concentrate
- irritability
- blank mind

Potential complications

Undiagnosed medical reasons for anxiety could lead to physical deterioration and a delay in obtaining appropriate treatment (see *Physical disorders associated with anxiety*).

Nursing diagnosis: *Anxiety related to real or perceived threat to physical integrity or self-concept*

NURSING PRIORITY: To help the client recognize the anxiety and use effective coping strategies

Interventions

1. Establish and maintain trust with the client while using active listening and showing empathy and respect.

Rationales

1. These strategies may alleviate any perceived threats that the client feels, thereby decreasing the client's anxiety level.

2. Recognize and manage your own anxiety or negative feelings that may occur in response to the client's resistance to recommended changes (see *Sympathetic and parasympathetic responses to anxiety*).

3. Identify client behaviors that produce anxiety in others. Explore these behaviors with the client as the therapy progresses.

4. Encourage the client to keep a daily journal and to make entries recording feelings, behaviors, stressors, coping strategies, and degrees of anxiety relief achieved. Help the client to describe any anxiety associated with specific activities or events, such as work, relationships, and holidays.

5. Identify the types and significance of stressors in the client's life.

2. Anxiety and negative feelings in response to the client's resistance to recommended changes can inhibit the nurse's problem-solving abilities, thereby blocking effective interventions.

3. Identifying and exploring such behaviors can facilitate client growth and change and may help the client to recognize how such negative behavior affects others.

4. Developing effective coping strategies requires that the client recognize anxiety and its attendant feelings and overcome resistance to change. Recording feelings, stressors, and coping strategies in a journal may facilitate self-awareness and help to clarify the client's resistance patterns. Describing anxiety in specific situations can help the client to identify its causes and prevent free-floating anxiety (anxiety without identifiable cause), which if untreated can cause progressive dysfunction.

5. Identifying stressors and determining their significance helps the client understand which stressors play a positive role and which play a negative role (for example, job-related stress can help motivate performance and raise self-esteem, whereas family tension resulting from continual parental arguing can lead to feelings of personal failure in a child).

SYMPATHETIC AND PARASYMPATHETIC RESPONSES TO ANXIETY

Because clients with anxiety can provoke anxiety in others, nurses should learn to recognize physical signs and symptoms of anxiety in themselves and take necessary measures to prevent their exacerbation. This chart identifies common sympathetic and parasympathetic responses to anxiety that may occur.

Body system	Sympathetic response	Parasympathetic response
Cardiovascular	• palpitations • increased heart rate • increased blood pressure	• faintness or fainting • decreased blood pressure • decreased pulse rate
Respiratory	• rapid, shallow breathing • shortness of breath • feeling of pressure in the chest • lump in the throat • gasping • choking sensation	• none
Gastrointestinal	• loss of appetite • revulsion toward food • abdominal discomfort	• abdominal pain • nausea • heartburn • diarrhea
Genitourinary	• none	• pressure in lower abdomen • urinary frequency
Integumentary	• facial flushing • localized or general sweating • itching • hot and cold spells • pallor	• none

From *Psychosocial crises*. Clinical Skillbuilders. Springhouse, PA: Springhouse Corp., 1992.

SHORT-TERM MEDICATION THERAPY

Short-term drug therapy forms an important part of the treatment plan for some clients who suffer from anxiety. This chart includes the most commonly prescribed antianxiety agents along with their recommended dosages. Nursing considerations for all drugs are provided.

Drug and dosages

alprazolam (Xanax)	0.5 mg P.O. t.i.d.
buspirone (BuSpar)	5 to 10 mg P.O. t.i.d.
chlordiazepoxide (Libritabs)	5 to 25 mg P.O. t.i.d. or q.i.d.
clorazepate (Tranxene)	15 to 60 mg P.O. daily.
diazepam (Valium)	2 to 10 mg P.O. b.i.d. to q.i.d.
halazepam (Paxipam)	20 to 40 mg P.O. t.i.d. or q.i.d.
hydroxyzine (Vistaril)	25 to 100 mg P.O. t.i.d. or q.i.d.
lorazepam (Ativan)	2 to 6 mg P.O. daily in divided doses
oxazepam (Serax)	10 to 30 mg P.O. t.i.d. or q.i.d.
prazepam (Centrax)	20 to 40 mg P.O. daily in divided doses

Nursing considerations

• If your client is pregnant, make sure her physician knows of her condition.

• Instruct your client to take the medication as prescribed and not to stop taking it abruptly.

• Monitor the client's vital signs during the initial treatment.

• If your client is also receiving another central nervous system (CNS) depressant or an anticholinergic, monitor for additive effects, including drowsiness, dry mouth, and constipation.

• Periodically monitor the client's complete blood count and liver function.

• When reviewing laboratory studies, watch for increased levels of serum bilirubin; aspartate aminotransferase (AST), formerly SGOT; and alanine aminotransferase (ALT), formerly SGPT.

• If treatment with the antianxiety drug will continue after discharge, teach your client to avoid alcohol and other CNS depressants, and to call the physician before taking any over-the-counter medications.

From *Psychosocial crises.* Clinical Skillbuilders. Springhouse, PA: Springhouse Corp., 1992.

---

6. Help the client to develop new, adaptive coping strategies by first exploring past methods used to reduce anxiety. Identify both effective and ineffective strategies, as well as destructive or overused ones. Explore the negative consequences of the ineffective strategies, and work with the client to suggest new, productive ones.

6. Learning new, adaptive coping strategies enables the client to use available resources and to accept personal responsibility for making and maintaining positive changes.

7. Encourage the client to participate in an exercise or physical activity program.

7. Exercise is a healthful and effective means of decreasing the physical manifestations of anxiety.

8. Encourage proper nutrition, and direct the client to record dietary intake in daily journal entries.

8. Food, stimulants (such as nicotine and caffeine), and depressants (such as alcohol) may initially help to suppress the client's anxiety. However, if overused, they can cause additional problems—compulsive overeating, nicotine or caffeine addiction, and alcoholism—which may require treatment. Journal records can provide evidence of how the client uses food and drink to cope with anxiety.

9. If appropriate, use role playing in a supervised, safe environment.

9. Role playing allows the client to rehearse new coping strategies. Many coping skills require practice, feedback, and fine-tuning before the client feels comfortable using them.

10. Teach the client relaxation techniques, such as guided imagery (recalling a pleasant, serene scene to induce relaxation), meditation, muscle relaxation (conscious tensing and relaxing of each muscle group), biofeedback (monitoring the reduction of tension that occurs during relaxation techniques), and hypnosis.

10. These techniques can help alleviate the emotional distress that accompanies anxiety and may decrease anxiety-related symptoms.

11. Administer medication, as ordered (see *Short-term medication therapy*). Monitor drug levels and report any signs of adverse reactions.

11. Antianxiety (anxiolytic) medications can relieve the physical symptoms of anxiety; however, they can cause significant adverse reactions, such as dizziness, drowsiness, insomnia, and dependency.

CLIENT-FAMILY GUIDELINES FOR USING BENZODIAZEPINES

Benzodiazepines are commonly prescribed for clients with anxiety disorders. Here are some general guidelines to follow.

Prescibed medication: _____

Precautions
• Do not drink alcohol while taking this medication or during the next few days after stopping the medication.
• Take only the amount of medication prescibed—no more and no less.
• Do not abruptly stop taking the medication without your physician's approval.
• Expect some drowsiness while taking this medication. Do not drive a car, operate machinery, or perform tasks that require alertness until you have completely adjusted to taking the medication.
• Notify your physician if you are pregnant or intend to become pregnant while using this medication.

Drug interactions
This medication may interact with other prescribed or over-the-counter drugs.
• Notify your physician before taking any pain relievers, sleeping aids, cough or cold medication, tranquilizers, or depression medication.
• Do not drink alcohol while taking this medication.
• Avoid excessive caffeine, which can counteract the effects of the medication.

Adverse reactions
This medication may cause drowsiness. If this becomes a problem, contact your physician.

If you forget a dose
Contact your physician or pharmacist immediately if you miss a prescribed dose.

Additional instructions

_____

_____

_____

Adapted from guidelines established by Thomas Jefferson University Hospital, Philadelphia, 1992. Used with permission.

12. As necessary, provide instruction about the medication regimen. Monitor the client's self-administration, and, when appropriate, provide written instructions for managing any adverse reactions, indicating when to call the physician (see *Client-family guidelines for using benzodiazepines*).

12. Adequate information about the prescribed anxiolytic enables the client and family to take appropriate action should adverse reactions occur.

Nursing diagnosis: *Ineffective individual coping related to inadequate coping strategies, inadequate support systems, high anxiety level, personal vulnerability or fragility, or multiple stressors*

NURSING PRIORITY: To help the client identify ineffective coping behavior and negative consequences of this behavior

Interventions

1. Assess the client's stressors and any factors that may cause stress, including negative self-concept, disapproval by others, inadequate problem-solving skills, loss or grief, inadequate support system, sudden life-style changes, a recent change in health status, and moral or ethical conflict.

2. Assess the client's developmental level and functional capacity to determine ability to cope with anxiety.

3. Identify any chemical substances (such as alcohol or drugs) and potentially compulsive behaviors (involving eating, gambling, sexual behaviors, smoking, spending, or working) that the client might be using to suppress anxiety.

4. Observe and monitor the client's behavior. Describe and clarify your observations for the client in clear, objective terms. Monitor complaints of physical disturbances. Clarify discrepancies among behavioral, cognitive, and physical manifestations of anxiety.

5. Provide the client with information and instructions for problem-solving techniques that can decrease negative and automatic responses to anxiety-provoking situations. For example, instruct the client to record events that precede anxiety attacks and then avoid those events.

6. Help the client to evaluate daily routines and stressors in family, work, and social relationships and situations.

7. Collaborate with treatment team members on providing the client with referrals for group, family, or marital therapy, as well as information about support groups, spiritual resources, and financial assistance.

Rationales

1. Identifying the degree and impact of stressors and contributing factors can guide the nurse in developing appropriate treatment, especially for a client with multiple stressors or a high stress level. Such a client may become physically or emotionally ill, and coping abilities may regress.

2. Developmental and functional levels determine how a client can cope with stress. For example, a young boy might cry and run to his mother when anxious, whereas an adolescent might turn to peers or drugs. In addition, how well a person copes is affected by current events in the person's life. A client working full-time while going to school may not have time to continue activities or sports that in the past helped to decrease anxiety.

3. Drugs and compulsive behaviors are commonly used to suppress anxiety; however, overuse can interfere with the client's ability to manage anxiety. Chemical substances or compulsive behaviors then become stressors rather than effective methods of reducing stress.

4. This procedure can help the nurse avoid making judgmental evaluations while increasing the client's awareness. Anxiety-ridden clients typically have more somatic complaints that need assessment, such as headaches, stomachaches, and nonspecific complaints of pain.

5. This method gives the client an opportunity to learn and practice new coping skills.

6. Examining relationships and situations that may be contributing to the client's anxiety allows the client to make informed, conscious changes rather than impulsive ones.

7. The client and family may need various types of support to continue improvement.

Nursing diagnosis: *Self-esteem disturbance related to altered body image, inability to cope, loss or grief, or unmet expectations*

NURSING PRIORITY: To help the client develop and maintain an enhanced self-esteem

Interventions

1. Establish a trusting, supportive relationship with the client.

2. Set up opportunities for the client to interact socially with others. Though you will want to avoid overprotecting the client, take care not to make too many demands initially.

3. Help the client to describe self-image and to identify any factors that threaten that self-image.

4. Through a discussion of past incidents, help the client to recognize personal strengths and capabilities in coping with previous anxiety-provoking situations.

5. Use role playing to help the client discover and rehearse coping strategies that can be used in threatening or anxiety-provoking situations.

Rationales

1. A trusting relationship between the nurse and client can put the client at ease. This in turn may help the client establish a positive sense of self.

2. Structured interactions can develop the client's ability to socialize. They also can help the client to realize that others have similar social needs.

3. This self-examination may give the client a better sense of reality, which may have been distorted by increased anxiety.

4. These discussions should acknowledge the client's previous successes and abilities to cope with anxiety.

5. Allowing the patient to act out situations and practice well-defined coping strategies can diminish anticipatory anxiety and improve self-esteem.

Nursing diagnosis: *Impaired social interaction and social isolation related to altered mental status, altered sensory and perceptual status, inadequate personal resources, lack of social support, self-esteem disturbance, or unsuccessful social interactions*

NURSING PRIORITY: To help the client recognize anxiety and identify factors that lead to impaired social interaction and social isolation

Interventions

1. Encourage the client to discuss and analyze reasons for and feelings about social isolation.

2. Encourage the client to identify what causes the anxiety that inhibits social interaction.

3. Express a positive regard for the client.

4. Assess the client's use of coping skills and defense mechanisms.

Rationales

1. Discussing reasons for and feelings about being alone can help the client differentiate between choosing to be alone for enjoyment and purposefully isolating oneself from society.

2. Identifying specific causes can guide the client in adapting strategies to deal with anxiety in social situations.

3. Doing so communicates a belief in the client and establishes a safe, secure environment in which the client can feel comfortable about disclosing thoughts, fears, and feelings.

4. Knowing when and to what degree defense mechanisms are used allows the client to make informed choices when changing behavior. It also helps the client develop adaptive social interaction skills.

5. Recommend that the client participate in educational programs directed at conflict areas or skill deficiencies. Such programs may address assertiveness skills, body awareness, managing multiple commitments, and stress-management strategies.

5. Participating in educational programs can instill in the client a sense that an anxiety-related disorder is a manageable condition and not something that need be suffered in isolation or forever.

Nursing diagnosis: *Sleep pattern disturbance related to physiologic disturbance, psychological stress, or thought intrusion*

NURSING PRIORITY: To help the client recognize the relationship between anxiety and the sleep disturbance, and identify appropriate interventions that promote normal sleep patterns

Interventions

1. Identify the sleep pattern disturbance and assess the client's usual sleep rituals.

2. Encourage the client to restrict stimulant and depressant intake before bedtime.

3. Teach the client relaxation techniques to use at bedtime.

4. Teach the client methods to decrease the amount of waking time spent in bed.

5. Encourage the client to increase daytime activities, participate in an exercise program, and avoid exercise 2 hours before bedtime.

6. Teach the client about the prescribed sedative or hypnotic. Encourage the client to use the drug only as directed and to keep a journal describing responses to the behavioral interventions and the drug and how both affect sleep.

Rationales

1. Identifying usual sleep rituals in clients with sleep pattern disturbances can help determine specific sleep-inducing strategies. For example, the client may learn that drinking a glass of warm milk before retiring promotes relaxation.

2. Stimulants (such as caffeine and nicotine) and depressants (such as alcohol) interfere with the normal sleep cycle and can contribute to a sleep pattern disturbance.

3. Relaxation techniques reduce anxious feelings and muscle tension, thereby improving the ability to sleep.

4. Having a concrete plan to manage sleep disturbance can alleviate any immediate anxiety the client has about falling asleep.

5. Regular, moderate exercise increases body fatigue and the desire to rest and sleep without stimulating the client too much before going to bed.

6. Sedatives and hypnotics interfere with non-rapid eye movement (NREM) and rapid eye movement (REM) sleep and alter the quality of rest. A significant problem of rebound insomnia, characterized by intense dreaming, nightmares, and increased sleep disruption, can develop.

Nursing diagnosis: *Ineffective family coping related to extended disability that produces significant family strain, misinformation or lack of knowledge about the client's condition, transient family disorganization, and role disruptions*

NURSING PRIORITY: To help the client's family recognize their own needs for support and identify and use resources effectively

Interventions

1. Assess the learning needs of the client's family members.

Rationales

1. Lack of knowledge or misunderstanding of the client's behavior can disrupt the way the family normally interacts. This disruption may escalate anxiety in family members.

2. Identify the client's role in the family, and determine how the condition has altered the family function and organization.

3. Explain to the family the client's needs and behaviors.

4. Clarify with the family which members are experiencing problems and which need to be involved in solving the problems.

5. Encourage the family to develop problem-solving and decision-making skills.

6. Refer family members to appropriate resources, including support groups, financial counseling and support, family therapy, and spiritual counseling.

2. Family organization and function may be influenced significantly by a member who is unable to contribute positively or fulfill usual roles.

3. Understanding the client's needs and behaviors as well as the nature of the condition or disease can help other family members cope with the situation.

4. Understanding who needs help and why enables family members to understand their responsibilities better. It also encourages family members to ask for and offer help in a mutually beneficial manner.

5. Doing so allows the family to learn and use new strategies for coping with conflicts and for preventing anxiety-provoking situations.

6. The family may require additional assistance and support to maintain family integrity and functioning.

Outcome criteria

As treatment progresses, the client, family, or both should be able to:
• verbalize awareness of anxiety
• identify effective coping mechanisms to manage anxiety-provoking situations
• identify ineffective coping behaviors and consequences
• demonstrate problem-solving and decision-making skills to manage increased anxiety levels
• participate in activities that enhance interactions and decrease social isolation
• identify and use appropriate interventions to facilitate sleep
• report improvement in sleep patterns
• recognize support needs, seek assistance, and use resources appropriately.

Discharge criteria

Nursing documentation indicates that the client:
• has demonstrated an increased ability to recognize anxiety symptoms
• can use newly learned skills to manage anxiety-provoking situations
• understands the diagnosis, treatment, and expected outcomes
• is aware of available group, family, or marital support resources and their referrals
• can use alternative coping skills
• has scheduled follow-up appointments.

Nursing documentation also indicates that the family:
• understands the client's diagnosis, treatment, and expected outcome

• has been referred to appropriate group, family, and other support services
• can use alternative coping skills
• has scheduled necessary follow-up appointments.

Selected references

Adams, A., and Dixey, D. (1988). Running an anxiety management group. *Health Visitor*, 61(12), 375-376.

American Psychiatric Association (APA). (1987). *Diagnostic and statistical manual of mental disorders* (3rd ed., rev.) Washington, DC: APA Press.

Barlow, D.H. (1988). *Anxiety and its disorders: The nature and treatment of anxiety and panic*. New York: Guilford Press.

Barlow, D.H., Blanchard, E.B., Vermilyea, J.A., Vermilyea, B., and DiNardo, P.A. (1986). Generalized anxiety and generalized anxiety disorder: Description and reconceptualization. *American Journal of Psychiatry*, 143(1), 40-44.

Barry, P. (1989). *Psychosocial nursing assessment and intervention: The care of the physically ill patient*. Philadelphia: Lippincott.

Beeber, L.S. (1989). Update on medications for the treatment of anxiety. *Journal of Psychosocial Nursing and Mental Health Services*, 27(10), 42-43.

Borysenko, J. (1987). *Minding the body, mending the mind*. Redding, MA: Addison-Wesley.

Carpenito, L.J. (1991). *Nursing diagnosis: Application to clinical practice* (4th ed.). Philadelphia: Lippincott.

Derogatis, L.R., and Wise, T.N. (1989). *Anxiety and depressive disorders in the medical patient*. Washington, DC: APA Press.

Grainger-Knowles, R.D. (1990). The patient with anxiety. In S. Lewis, et al, (Eds.), *Manual of psychoso-*

cial nursing interventions: Promoting mental health in medical-surgical settings. Philadelphia: Saunders.

King, J.V. (1988). A holistic technique to lower anxiety: Relaxation with guided imagery. *Journal of Holistic Nursing,* 6(1), 16-20.

Kusher, M.G., Sher, K.J., and Beitman, B.D. (1990). The relation between alcohol problems and the anxiety disorders. *American Journal of Psychiatry,* 147(6), 685-95.

Noyes, R., Clarkson, C., Crowe, R.R., Yates, W.R., and McChesney, C.M. (1987). A family study of generalized anxiety disorder. *American Journal of Psychiatry,* 144(8), 1019-1024.

Scandrett, S.L., Bean, J.L., Breeden, S., and Powell, S. (1986). A comparative study of biofeedback and progressive relaxation in anxious patients. *Issues in mental health nursing,* 8(3), 255-271.

Sheehan, D.V., Raj, A.B., Harnett-Sheehan, K., and Soto, S. (1990). Adinazolam sustained release formulation in the treatment of generalized anxiety disorder. *Journal of Anxiety Disorders,* 4(3), 239-246.

Taylor-Loughran, A.E., O'Brien, M.E., LaChapelle, R., and Rangel, S. (1989). Defining characteristics of the nursing diagnoses fear and anxiety: A validation study. *Applied Nursing Research,* 2(4), 178-186.

Todd, B. (1989). Disabling anxiety. *Geriatric Nursing,* 10(3), 152-156.

Townsend, M.C. (1990). *Drug guide for psychiatric nursing.* Philadelphia: Davis.

Whitley, G.G. (1989). Anxiety: Defining the diagnosis. *Journal of Psychosocial Nursing and Mental Health Services,* 27(10), 6-8, 10-12, 37-38.

Williams, R.L., Karacan, I., and Moore, C.A. (1988). *Sleep disorders: Diagnosis and treatment* (2nd ed.). New York: John Wiley & Sons.

Phobic and Panic Disorders

DSM III-R classifications
Phobic disorders
300.22 Agoraphobia without history of panic disorder
300.23 Social phobia
300.29 Simple phobia
Panic disorders
300.01 Panic disorder without agoraphobia
300.21 Panic disorder with agoraphobia

Psychiatric nursing diagnostic class
Anxiety

Introduction
Phobic disorders
Phobic disorders are characterized by a persistent, irrational fear of a specific activity, object, or situation. These disorders, which affect about 5% of the population, are classified as *agoraphobia without history of panic disorder, social phobia,* and *simple phobia.*

Agoraphobia without history of panic disorder is relatively rare because agoraphobia usually is accompanied by panic. The prognoses for this disorder vary. Less severely disturbed individuals may experience remissions and exacerbations of symptoms, whereas those more severely affected may suffer lifetime disability. Generally, agoraphobic individuals, who often have a history of generalized anxiety as well, limit travel and social activity.

Social phobia is characterized by a persistent fear of being scrutinized by others. Individuals with social phobias may avoid eating, drinking, or speaking in public.

Simple phobia is an isolated fear of one object or activity. This common phobia includes the fear of heights, thunder, lightning, closed spaces, and certain animals. Though a simple phobia usually causes minimal impairment, it can become incapacitating with prolonged or frequent exposure to the feared object or activity.

Panic disorders
Panic disorders are characterized by recurrent, unpredictable attacks of intense apprehension or terror. Such panic attacks can render an individual unable to control a situation or to perform even simple tasks. Behavior can be further complicated by an anticipatory fear of helplessness or of losing control. In its most severe state, a panic attack can produce such symptoms as chest pain, numbness, and shortness of breath, which are typically associated with a heart attack (see *Recognizing a panic attack,* page 54).

Panic disorders occur with or without agoraphobia. Panic disorders with agoraphobia are especially debilitating because they typically lead to severe social, work, and travel restrictions.

ETIOLOGY AND PRECIPITATING FACTORS
Explanations of etiology and precipitating factors for phobic and panic disorders remain controversial. Most research continues to focus on the biological and psychological causes of panic.

Biological explanations for panic include the sodium lactate infusion hypothesis, hypocalcemia theory, focal brain abnormality theory, and defective biochemical trigger theory. These theories claim that panic is the product of physical vulnerability or an actual defect.

The sodium lactate infusion hypothesis first challenged the belief that panic attacks were induced solely by exogenous stimuli. During laboratory experiments, subjects without diagnosed anxiety developed minor discomfort evidenced by tremors and paresthesias when injected with sodium lactate. However, when sodium lactate was injected into subjects with diagnosed anxiety, panic ensued.

The hypocalcemia theory is an outgrowth of the sodium lactate infusion experiments. During those experiments, researchers administered calcium in addition to sodium lactate and observed a significantly diminished incidence and severity of panic symptoms among subjects with diagnosed anxiety.

The focal brain abnormality theory claims that lactate-sensitive individuals have abnormally high oxygen metabolism, blood flow, and blood volume in the right side of the parahippocampal region of the brain. These individuals have demonstrated additional brain changes in the focal area even when they were not suffering an active panic attack.

The defective biochemical trigger theory claims that individuals with panic disorders have a basic metabolic defect that produces an oversensitivity to particular chemical messengers in the blood. As these messengers penetrate the locus ceruleus—the principal noradrenergic nucleus in the central nervous system— large amounts of norepinephrine are released, thereby triggering emotional and physical responses.

Psychological theorists regard anxiety as an outward sign of internal conflict and identify certain basic predisposing factors in the etiology of panic disorders. These factors include a history of childhood separation anxiety; sudden loss of a family member or loved one; and a series of stressful life events, such as a job change, marriage, divorce, and birth of a child. Commonly, those with panic disorder have a history of one or more of these factors. Furthermore, research in-

---

RECOGNIZING A PANIC ATTACK

A panic attack is a brief period of intense apprehension or fear; it may last from minutes to hours. A history of four attacks within 4 weeks that are unrelated to extreme physical exertion, life-threatening situations, or phobias confirm panic disorder.

During a panic attack, the client will display four or more of these signs and symptoms:

- chest pains
- palpitations
- dyspnea
- choking or smothering feeling
- vertigo, dizziness, or unsteadiness
- feelings of faintness
- depersonalization or feeling of unreality
- tingling in the hands and feet
- shaking or trembling
- hot and cold flashes
- diaphoresis
- fear of going crazy, dying, or being out of control during a panic attack
- nausea or abdominal distress.

From *Professional guide to diseases* (4th ed.). Springhouse, PA: Springhouse Corp., 1992.

---

dicates that over 80% of clients with panic disorder experienced an intensely stressful life event shortly before their initial panic attack.

Other psychological theorists postulate that panic disorders are related to the stress experienced during late adolescence or early adulthood. During this period, the individual addresses numerous psychological issues, such as independence, separation from parents, and career and relationship choices, any of which may contribute to the development of panic disorders.

Assessment guidelines
NURSING HISTORY (Functional health pattern findings)
The client may report or exhibit one or more of the findings grouped here according to functional health patterns.

Health perception–health management pattern
- extreme concern over general health
- persistent fear of some object or situation that poses no actual danger
- fear of "going crazy"
- numerous somatic complaints, with or without diagnostic validation
- inability to move, speak, or identify ways of decreasing anxiety
- worry over medication compliance, follow-up visits, and inability to control feelings

- inability to control feelings
- overuse or underuse of health care system to ease panic symptoms

Nutritional-metabolic pattern
- concern over eating behaviors, such as using food to suppress feelings
- significant weight fluctuations

Elimination pattern
- concern over GI system disturbances, such as nausea, pain, diarrhea, and vomiting
- frequent urination
- concern over increased sweating, cold and clammy skin, or both

Activity-exercise pattern
- restlessness or trembling
- fear of situations that consistently lead to panic attacks, helplessness, and humiliation
- concern about inability to participate in and enjoy leisure activities
- manipulation of environment and dependence on others to avoid confrontation with certain situations or objects
- concern about limitations and self-imposed activity restrictions caused by inability to predict panic attacks
- difficulty accomplishing normal daily activities

Sleep-rest pattern
- concern about falling or staying asleep and nightmares
- concern about use or abuse of sleep aids, such as alcohol, benzodiazepines, and hypnotics
- feeling fatigued after sleep
- fatigue and inability to function during the day

Cognitive-perceptual pattern
- difficulty concentrating
- worry over inability to think clearly
- distorted thinking and inability to test reality
- difficulty with understanding and reacting to external stimuli

Self-perception–self-concept pattern
- perception of self as being highly anxious
- dread and certainty that death is near
- perception of self as being incompetent and powerless

Role-relationship pattern
- concern over relationships with family or loved ones
- concern over the lack of response to or support of life-style changes from family or loved ones

Sexual-reproductive pattern
- dissatisfaction with sexual relations
- difficulty with intimacy

Coping–stress tolerance pattern
• pervasive muscle tension
• constant irritability, feeling on edge or keyed up
• shakiness, trembling, or twitching
• feeling unreal or depersonalized
• belief that significant life-style changes are contributing to feeling out of control

Value-belief pattern
• feeling powerless to achieve life goals
• disbelief about present situation
• concern over inability to believe in anything or anyone

PHYSICAL FINDINGS
The client may report or exhibit one or more of the following physical findings.

Cardiovascular
• chest pain or discomfort
• elevated blood pressure
• hot and cold flashes or chills
• increased heart rate
• palpitations
• sweating
• syncope
• tachycardia

Respiratory
• choking sensation
• dyspnea
• hyperventilation
• increased respiratory rate
• shortness of breath
• smothering sensation

Gastrointestinal
• abdominal distress
• diarrhea
• difficulty swallowing
• dry mouth
• lump in throat
• nausea
• vomiting

Musculoskeletal
• muscle aches
• muscle tension
• restlessness
• shakiness
• trembling

Neurologic
• dilated pupils
• dizziness or faintness
• light-headedness
• paresthesia
• inability to fall asleep or difficulty staying asleep
• vertigo or unsteadiness

Psychological
• fear of losing control or dying
• feeling keyed up or on edge
• feeling unreal or depersonalized
• inability to concentrate or focus
• irritability
• blank mind
• perceptual field deficits

Potential complications
Undiagnosed medical reasons for phobic or panic symptoms can lead to physical deterioration. If left untreated, these disorders can lead to increasing social withdrawal and isolation, which may severely impair the client's social and work life.

Nursing diagnosis: *Anxiety related to confrontation with feared object or situation*

NURSING PRIORITY: To help the client become desensitized to the phobic object or situation

Interventions
1. Help the client to identify the feared object or situation.

Rationales
1. Identifying the phobic object or situation can enable the client to avoid or at least limit contact with it. This limited contact can be especially helpful initially when the nurse is developing a definitive treatment program.

2. Help the client to identify the original anxiety-provoking conflict.

2. Identifying the original conflict can focus the client's attention and diminish or eliminate displacement of anxiety onto other objects or situations.

3. Teach assertiveness skills (for example, making "I" statements, such as "I feel," "I want," or "I need") that reduce submissive and fearful responses.

3. Such strategies enable the client to experiment with new ways of coping and discard old ways, which may be perpetuating the phobic response.

4. Explore the client's anticipatory thinking about the feared object or situation.

4. Anticipating a future or imminent phobic reaction can escalate the physiological manifestations of fear. Identifying anticipatory thinking enables the client to make the necessary changes to stop it.

5. Teach the client relaxation and thought-stopping techniques, such as progressive muscle relaxation and guided imagery. Provide time for practice sessions using role-playing scenarios.

5. Relaxation techniques enable the client to alleviate anxiety's negative consequences. Thought-stopping techniques provide the client with a means of recognizing a negative feeling and its accompanying thought and then stopping that thought and replacing it with a positive one. By role playing, the client can rehearse ways to relax while confronting a feared object or situation.

6. Encourage the client to imagine encountering the feared situation or object and then taking steps to alleviate that fear. Encourage the client to describe the coping process step-by-step.

6. Examining specific behaviors and coping strategies can increase the client's sense of control and strengthen skill mastery.

7. Collaborate with the client and multidisciplinary team to develop and implement a systematic desensitization program.

7. A well-developed desensitization program, one in which the client is systematically exposed to the feared object or situation in a controlled and supportive environment, may diminish the client's fear.

8. Collaborate with the client and multidisciplinary team to assess the need for pharmacologic intervention.

8. The appropriate use of antiphobic or antipanic agents can relieve the physical symptoms associated with phobic and panic disorders.

9. Administer antiphobic or antipanic agents, such as antianxiety agents (benzodiazepines), tricyclic antidepressants (amitriptyline [Elavil], doxepin [Sinequan]), or monoamine oxidase inhibitors (isocarboxazid [Marplan], phenelzine [Nardil]) as indicated. Monitor the client's response, and observe for adverse reactions.

9. These agents have a significant calming effect and may facilitate the client's ability to change behavior by reducing anxiety during desensitization sessions. Educating the client about both the positive effects and adverse reactions (including nausea, dry mouth, dizziness, and potential dependency) facilitates compliance.

Nursing diagnosis: *Ineffective breathing pattern related to choking or smothering sensation, shortness of breath, or hyperventilation associated with panic*

NURSING PRIORITY: To help the client restore a normal breathing pattern

Interventions

1. Remain with the client while maintaining a calm, supportive but direct approach.

2. Assess the client's respiratory status by determining respiratory rate and ability to breathe and by noting the color of lips and nail beds.

3. Loosen all of the client's tight clothing, including ties, collars, and belts.

4. During an acute attack, demonstrate slow- and deep-breathing techniques and breathe along with the client.

Rationales

1. The client needs simple directions and reassurance that suffocation or death are not imminent.

2. Any sign of hyperventilation, difficulty breathing, or cyanosis indicates hypoxia, which requires immediate medical attention.

3. Decreasing bodily restrictions helps to decrease choking and suffocating sensations.

4. Active participation and role modeling can be effective when instructing a client with an impaired or restricted perceptual field.

5. If necessary, instruct the client to breathe into a paper bag to counteract hyperventilation during an acute attack.

5. This procedure maintains normal acid-base balance by normalizing carbon dioxide levels and preventing respiratory acidosis, which can cause depressed respirations.

Nursing diagnosis: *Powerlessness related to a perceived inability to maintain control over a situation*

NURSING PRIORITY: To help the client verbalize about the situation and exhibit more control in life

Interventions

1. Encourage the client to assume responsibility for establishing and maintaining self-care practices.

2. Help the client to establish realistic, achievable goals.

3. Explore ways in which cultural values and religious beliefs might support helpless and dependent behavior.

4. Continue to clarify the client's unmet goals (for example, the client's inability to assume responsibility for an increase in dependence).

5. Help the client to identify areas in life that are beyond personal control.

6. Encourage the client to investigate and use self-help and support groups.

Rationales

1. The client who can assume responsibility for self-care practices will probably feel more in control.

2. Realistic goals should make the client more comfortable with the treatment. Achieving goals builds self-confidence.

3. A person's interpretation of cultural values and religious beliefs sometimes reinforces a sense of rigidity, shame, guilt, self-protection, and self-deprecation, as well as a distorted sense of reality. By becoming aware of how these value systems can work negatively, the client may gain a better sense of self-control.

4. The client should become more adept at modifying behavior as personal insight deepens.

5. Recognizing such limitations promotes acceptance of what cannot be changed and allows the client to focus on resolvable issues.

6. Incorporating additional outside support can reinforce the client's self-management and control.

Nursing diagnosis: *Sensory-perceptual alteration related to diminished perceptual field during panic-level anxiety*

NURSING PRIORITY: To ensure the client's safety during panic attacks

Interventions

1. Remain with and reassure the client that you are both safe, that you will remain, and that the attack will end.

2. Speak to the client in simple, one-step sentences.

3. Decrease environmental stimuli (for example, by dimming lights or closing doors). If necessary, move the client to a quieter, smaller area.

Rationales

1. During a panic attack, a client typically fears being abandoned. Remaining with the client and offering reassurance that the attack will end provides the first measure of security needed to decrease anxiety.

2. The client's severely restricted perceptual field limits the ability to comprehend complicated thoughts and sentences.

3. Exposure to environmental stimuli can escalate anxious behavior, especially in someone with an impaired ability to deal with such stimuli. A smaller, quieter area can make the client feel more secure.

Nursing diagnosis: *Altered family processes related to the inability of family members to express feelings*

NURSING PRIORITY: To help family members verbalize and demonstrate feelings of intimacy

Interventions

1. Help individual family members to define and clarify their roles and relationships within the family.

2. Teach family members assertiveness techniques to express thoughts, feelings, and needs. Include the use of "I" statements, such as "I feel" and "I need."

3. Teach family members how to express what they need from each other to feel loved, cared for, and emotionally supported. For example, teach them to tell each other when they are frightened or when they need a hug. Demonstrate these behaviors and have family members practice them.

Rationales

1. Increasing the family's knowledge about family system dynamics can facilitate self-appraisal and ongoing redefinition of family functioning.

2. Encouraging such open expression helps family members to identify their feelings and needs and to work through some of their built-up resentment. Open discussions also provide insight into how deeply the client's illness has disrupted their normal family structure.

3. Although the family is traditionally viewed as the primary group in which feelings of intimacy and caring are nurtured and fostered, many families have difficulty recognizing the lack of support and do not know how to ask for help from one another.

Outcome criteria

As treatment progresses, the client, family, or both should be able to:
• verbalize signs and symptoms of increasing anxiety
• identify effective coping strategies to maintain anxiety at a manageable level
• control disabling fear when exposed to the phobic object, activity, or situation
• use breathing techniques to decrease anxiety
• recognize support needs, seek assistance, and use resources appropriately.

Discharge criteria

Nursing documentation indicates that the client:
• has expressed an ability to recognize symptoms of phobia or panic
• can use newly learned skills to manage phobia- or panic-provoking situations
• understands the diagnosis, treatment, and expected outcomes
• is aware of available group, family, or marital support resources
• has arranged for scheduled follow-up appointments.

Nursing documentation also indicates that the family:
• understands the client's diagnosis, treatment, and expected outcomes
• has been referred to appropriate group, family, or marital support resources
• can use alternative coping skills
• has scheduled necessary follow-up appointments.

Selected references

Adler, C.M., Craske, M.G., and Barlow, D.H. (1987). Relaxation induced panic (RIP): When resting isn't peaceful. *Integrative Psychiatry*, 5, 94-112.

American Psychiatric Association (APA). (1987). *Diagnostic and statistical manual of mental disorders* (3rd ed., rev.). Washington, DC: APA Press.

Babior, S., and Goldman, C. (1990). *Overcoming panic attacks: Strategies to free yourself from the anxiety trap*. Minneapolis: Compcare Publishers.

Baker, J.M. (1991). Clients with anxiety disorders. In G.K. McFarland and M.D. Thomas (Eds.), *Psychiatric mental health nursing: Application of the nursing process*. Philadelphia: Lippincott.

Balon, R., Jordan, M., Pohl, R., and Yeragani, V.K. (1989). Family history of anxiety disorders in control subjects with lactate-induced panic attacks. *American Journal of Psychiatry*, 146(10), 1304-1306.

Barlow, D.H. (1988). *Anxiety and its disorders: The nature and treatment of anxiety and panic*. New York: Guilford Press.

Barlow, D.H., and Cerry, J.A. (1988). *Psychological treatment of panic*. New York: Guilford Press.

Charney, D.S., Woods, S., Goodman, W., and Heninger, G. (1987). Neurobiological mechanisms of panic anxiety. *American Journal of Psychiatry*, 144(8), 1030-1036.

Charney, D.S., and Woods, S.W. (1989). Benzodiazepine treatment of panic disorder: A comparison of alprazolam and/or lorazepam. *Journal of Clinical Psychiatry*, 50(11), 418-423.

Edlund, M.J., Swann, A.C., and Clothier, J. (1987). Patients with panic attacks and abnormal EEG results. *American Journal of Psychiatry,* 144(4), 508-509.

Fava, M., Anderson, K., and Rosenbaum, J.F. (1990). "Anger attacks": Possible variants of panic and major depressive disorders. *American Journal of Psychiatry,* 147(7), 867-870.

Fontaine, K.L. (1991). Psychologic responses to anxiety. In J.S. Cook and K.L. Fontaine (Eds.), *Essentials in mental health nursing* (2nd ed.) New York: Addison-Wesley.

Goldberg, R., Morris, P., Christian, F., and Badger, J. (1990). Panic disorder in cardiac outpatients. *Psychosomatics,* 31(2), 168-173.

Heimberg, R.G., and Barlow, D.H. (1988). Psychosocial treatments for social phobia. *Psychosomatics,* 29(1), 27-37.

King, J.V. (1988). A holistic technique to lower anxiety: Relaxation with guided imagery. *Journal of Holistic Nursing,* 6(1), 16-20.

Laraia, M.I., Stuart, G.W., and Best, C.L. (1989). Behavioral treatment of panic-related disorders: A review. *Archives of Psychiatric Nursing,* 3(3), 125-133.

Marks, I.M. (1987). Behavioral aspects of panic disorder. *American Journal of Psychiatry,* 144(9), 1160-65.

Marks, I.M. (1987). *Fears, phobias & rituals: Panic, anxiety & their disorders.* New York: Oxford University Press.

Matuzas, W., Al Sadir, J., Uhlenhuth, E., and Glass, R. (1987). Mitral valve prolapse and thyroid abnormalities in patients with panic attacks. *American Journal of Psychiatry,* 144 (4), 493-496.

Pollard, C.A., Detrick, P., Flynn, T., and Frank, M. (1990). Panic attacks and related disorders in alcohol-dependent, depressed and non-clinical samples. *Journal of Nervous and Mental Disease,* 178(3), 180-185.

Townsend, M.C. (1990). *Drug guide for psychiatric nursing.* Philadelphia: Davis.

Walker, J.R., Norton, G.R., and Ross, C.A. (1991). *Panic disorder and agoraphobia: A comprehensive guide for the practitioner.* Pacific Grove, CA: Brooks/Cole Publishing.

Zal, H.M. (1990). *Panic disorder: The great pretender.* New York: Plenum Press.

Obsessive-Compulsive Disorder

DSM III-R classification
300.30 Obsessive-compulsive disorder

Psychiatric nursing diagnostic class
Anxiety

Introduction

Obsessive-compulsive disorder is characterized by a compulsive response to an obsessive thought or impulse (obsession). The individual usually considers the obsession to be unacceptable or irrational but also feels powerless to control its persistent intrusion into consciousness. Fear that the obsession may actually be enacted generates considerable anxiety, and compulsive acts are attempts to allay this anxiety.

Compulsive behaviors are as diverse as the people who display them. The individual may perform repetitive acts or engage in seemingly purposeless behavior to divert the conscious mind from its obsession. Such behaviors include frequent hand or body washing, constant counting, an overemphasis on cleanliness, checking and rechecking lights or gas stoves before leaving the house, and masturbation. The prevalence of obsessive-compulsive disorder is not known; however, it occurs most frequently in individuals in their mid-twenties.

ETIOLOGY AND PRECIPITATING FACTORS

Obsessive-compulsive disorder commonly is initiated by a situation or event that produces or reactivates an internal conflict. The individual usually regards the situation or event with distinct ambivalence, especially if it has elicited an aggressive response.

In many cases, the activating situation or event occurs early in life. In fact, almost 50% of diagnosed obsessive-compulsive clients claim that they first experienced symptoms during childhood. Unlike children with most other psychological disorders, those with obsessive-compulsive disorder continue to display the same symptoms as adults. Additionally, 20% of diagnosed clients have a family member with the disorder.

While continuing to examine psychological triggers, researchers studying obsessive-compulsive disorder are beginning to focus on biological causes. Serum testing results have shown a serotonin deficiency, which may cause repetitive behavior.

Assessment guidelines

NURSING HISTORY (Functional health pattern findings)

The client may report or exhibit one or more of the findings grouped here according to functional health patterns.

Health perception–health management pattern
• extreme concern about diet, germs, and disease
• concern about or evidence of inadequate attention to health care needs
• extreme concern over general health
• exaggerated worry over daily life circumstances
• worry over medication compliance, follow-up visits, and inability to follow through
• fear of "going crazy"
• inability to control feelings
• numerous somatic complaints, with or without diagnostic validation
• overuse or underuse of health care system to ease anxiety symptoms

Nutritional-metabolic pattern
• weight loss resulting from fear of contaminated food or ritualistic behaviors that interfere with meal time and eating ability
• weight gain resulting from compulsive eating
• worry over eating behaviors, such as using food to calm or soothe self
• changes in appetite, including anorexia and binges

Elimination pattern
• constipation resulting from fear of contacting excrement
• concern over GI system disturbances, such as pain, flatulence, diarrhea, nausea, constipation, vomiting, and intestinal bleeding
• frequent urination
• concern over increased sweating, cold and clammy skin, or both

Activity-exercise pattern
• concern about compulsive behavior interfering with personal, occupational, scholastic, and social functioning
• restlessness or trembling
• concern about being easily fatigued
• difficulty in accomplishing normal daily activities
• concern about inability to participate in and enjoy leisure activities
• concern about any limitations and restrictions of activity caused by disease or condition
• withdrawn or apathetic behavior

Sleep-rest pattern
• decreased sleep resulting from obsessive thoughts or impulses
• inability to relax because of constant activity resulting from an inability to prevent intrusive obsessive thoughts or impulses
• concern about falling or staying asleep and nightmares
• feeling fatigued after sleep
• concern about use or abuse of sleep aids, such as alcohol, benzodiazepines, and hypnotics

Cognitive-perceptual pattern
• concern about the disturbing nature of obsessions
• awareness of illogical thoughts and behavior and of the inability to control them
• self-destructive or aggressive ideas or impulses
• difficulty concentrating
• difficulty understanding and reacting to external stimuli
• worry over inability to think clearly
• distorted perceptions

Self-perception–self-concept pattern
• low self-esteem and feelings of powerlessness resulting from the inability to control thoughts and behavior
• feelings of worthlessness secondary to feeling unclean
• concern over inability to meet expectations
• concern over being indecisive and dependent
• perception of self as being highly anxious
• perception of self as being incompetent
• concerns about body image

Role-relationship pattern
• disturbance in interpersonal relationships
• diminished ability to meet occupational, functional, interpersonal, or parental expectations
• intense concern over relationships with family and friends
• rumination over engaging in social situations with friends, fellow employees, or family
• concern over the lack of response to or support of life-style changes from family and friends
• concern about a distressful work situation
• concern about how community members and neighbors may respond to the disease or condition

Sexual-reproductive pattern
• fear of intimate contact with others resulting from fear of contamination and disease
• sexual dysfunction
• compulsive or ritualistic sexual activity, such as compulsive masturbation, excessive fascination with pornography, or use of others as sex objects
• dissatisfaction with sexual relations
• difficulty with intimacy
• concern about involvement in high-risk sexual behavior, such as unprotected sex or promiscuity

• concern about involvement with high-risk partners, including I.V. drug users, homosexual or bisexual partners, and strangers

Coping–stress tolerance pattern
• feeling overwhelmed
• avoiding social situations
• concern over increasing frequency and duration of compulsive behaviors
• pervasive muscle tension
• constant irritability, feeling on edge or keyed up
• constant shakiness, trembling, or twitching
• concern over experiencing an exaggerated startle response (hypervigilance)
• denial of clearly manifest anxiety
• inability to identify those persons or measures that alleviate rather than exacerbate the condition
• belief that significant life-style changes are contributing to feeling out of control

Value-belief pattern
• fear of condemnation
• feelings of powerlessness, hopelessness, or unworthiness
• concern that the condition is punishment for sin or previous acts
• over-reliance on or identification with religious themes associated with ritualistic behavior
• desire to increase or decrease involvement in spirituality or religion
• concern over impaired ability to believe in anything or anyone
• disbelief about present situation

PHYSICAL FINDINGS
The client may report or exhibit one or more of the following physical findings.

Cardiovascular
• cold, clammy skin
• elevated blood pressure
• hot and cold flashes
• increased heart rate
• palpitations
• sweating
• tingling

Respiratory
• increased respiratory rate
• shortness of breath
• smothering sensation
• choking sensation

Gastrointestinal
• dry mouth
• abdominal distress
• nausea
• vomiting

- diarrhea
- difficulty swallowing

Genitourinary
- frequent urination

Integumentary
- skin irritation from constant washing

Musculoskeletal
- increased fatigue
- muscle aches, pains, or soreness
- muscle tension
- restlessness
- shakiness
- trembling
- twitching

Neurologic
- dilated pupils
- dizziness or faintness
- light-headedness
- paresthesia
- restlessness
- inability to sleep or to stay asleep

Psychological
- feeling keyed up or on edge
- inability to concentrate
- irritability
- blank mind

Potential complications
Untreated, obsessive-compulsive disorder can lead to aggressive behavior toward self or others as well as depression, skin breakdown from obsessive washing, and infection caused by skin breakdown.

Nursing diagnosis: *Ineffective individual coping related to checking and rechecking actions or other ritualistic behaviors*

NURSING PRIORITY: To help the client gradually decrease ritualistic behavior and learn alternative strategies for coping with stress and anxiety

Interventions

1. Assess the degree of interference with daily functions by determining how much time the client spends on compulsive behaviors. Involvement of 1 hour or less a day on such behavior is considered mild interference; 1 to 3 hours per day, moderate; 3 to 5 hours per day, severe; and almost constant involvement, extreme.

2. As part of the structured care, provide the client with time for rituals and compulsive behaviors without focusing attention on them. As the client's anxiety abates, gradually decrease the time allowed for these behaviors.

3. Encourage the client to verbalize feelings and to discuss the maladaptive or disruptive nature of the behavior.

4. Have the client help to develop the plan of care and set realistic goals and expectations.

5. Establish behavioral contracts in which the client agrees to refrain from certain behaviors in exchange for certain rewards. (For example, if the client decreases the number of hand washings after meals from 50 to 40 times, the client can walk outside with a staff member.)

Rationales

1. As the involvement level increases, the client typically has less time to devote to normal daily functions. A client exhibiting severe or extreme involvement will be unable to use adaptive problem-solving skills.

2. Allowing time for the client's compulsive behaviors can decrease anxiety, thereby decreasing the need for rituals and compulsions. Furthermore, acknowledging the client's feelings and fears helps establish a trusting nurse-client relationship.

3. A frank discussion about the condition and feelings can help the client develop a more realistic perspective about the behavior. Such discussion also fosters trust between the nurse and client.

4. Such participation can increase the client's self-esteem and sense of control while decreasing anxiety and frustration.

5. Positive reinforcements for nonritualistic behaviors enhance the client's self-esteem and encourage the continuation of those behaviors.

6. Provide realistic, alternative coping methods, such as social interaction, occupational therapy, diversionary activities, relaxation, and self-help support groups.

6. Success with new behaviors and coping methods can increase self-esteem, decrease feelings of powerlessness, provide structure, and reinforce behavioral change. Self-help support groups provide both support and the opportunity for the client to talk about fears.

7. Respond positively when the client makes productive behavioral adaptations to cope with anxiety.

7. Reinforcing the successful use of new behaviors increases the client's self-esteem and feelings of control.

8. Gradually begin to set limits on the frequency and duration of compulsive behaviors.

8. Reducing the time allowed for compulsive behaviors can give the client a sense that treatment is progressing. Furthermore, limiting such behaviors decreases the potential for client injury.

9. Encourage the client to talk about the cause of and need for the compulsive behavior. Also encourage the client to describe feelings just before and during such behavior.

9. As the client's understanding of the behavior, its causes, and personal feelings about it become clearer, the client will be better able to choose more appropriate adaptive behaviors.

Nursing diagnosis: *Potential for impaired skin integrity related to ritualistic behaviors involving cleaning, such as hand washing, scrubbing, teeth brushing, and showering*

NURSING PRIORITY: To help the client maintain intact skin to prevent infection

Interventions

1. Assess the client's skin integrity.

2. Encourage the client to use only a mild soap and skin cream during ritualistic behaviors involving cleaning.

Rationales

1. Assessment is necessary to ensure that the client's behaviors are not compromising the integumentary system.

2. Using a mild soap and skin cream can prevent or minimize trauma to the integumentary system until the client can alter the compulsive behavior.

Nursing diagnosis: *Altered family processes related to inability to express feelings and develop intimate relationships*

NURSING PRIORITY: To facilitate the family's participation in a therapy program

Interventions

1. Help family members to define and clarify their relationships with one another.

2. Help family members to identify their feelings and to understand the importance of sharing those feelings with each other.

3. Teach family members assertiveness techniques, and rehearse these techniques with them.

Rationales

1. Making the client and family more aware of how families function can enable them to continually evaluate and, if necessary, redefine their relationships.

2. Families that are aware of and able to deal with emotions function more positively. Clearly expressing and communicating feelings also enhances family functioning.

3. Family members need to assume responsibility for their own thoughts and feelings rather than blame others.

4. Teach the family about obsessive-compulsive behavior and ways they can assist the client, such as through use of relaxation and behavioral modification.

4. Adequate information about obsessive-compulsive disorder enables the family to better understand the client's condition and behavior. By reinforcing client relaxation, using behavioral contracts, helping the client recognize anxious behavior, and praising appropriate coping strategies, family members can enhance the client's self-esteem and feelings of control.

Outcome criteria

As treatment progresses, the client, family, or both should be able to:
• identify signs and symptoms of increasing anxiety
• demonstrate alternative methods of coping
• verbalize feelings of improved self-esteem
• demonstrate improved social skills
• report an absence of physical symptoms, such as constipation, skin irritations, and sleep disturbances
• recognize support needs, seek assistance, and use resources appropriately.

Discharge criteria

Nursing documentation indicates that the client:
• has demonstrated an increased ability to recognize obsessive-compulsive symptoms
• uses alternative coping methods
• reports a reduction or an absence of intrusive thoughts
• displays an increased ability to use social skills
• reports a positive mood change
• is aware of aftercare options and plans
• has improved sleep and elimination patterns
• can maintain skin integrity.

Nursing documentation also indicates that the family:
• understands the client's condition and needs
• has planned for the client's aftercare
• reports improvements in family relationships
• reports improved sleep patterns
• reports a decrease in or absence of suicidal or homicidal impulses.

Selected references

DeSilva, P. (1986). Obsessional-compulsive imagery. *Behaviour Research and Therapy*, 24(3), 333-350.

DeVeaugh-Geiss, J., Landace, P., and Katz, P. (1989). The treatment of obsessive-compulsive disorder with clomipramine. *Psychiatric Annals*, 19(2), 97-101.

Farid, B.T. (1986). Obsessional symptomatology and adverse mood states. *British Journal of Psychiatry*, 149, 108-112.

Goodwin, G., and Guze, S. (1989). *Psychiatric Diagnosis* (4th ed.). New York: Oxford University Press.

Hand, I. (1988). Obsessive-compulsive patients and their families. In I.R.H. Falloon (Ed.), *Handbook of behavioral family therapy*. New York: Guilford Press.

Insel, T.R., and Akiskal, H.S. (1986). Obsessive-compulsive disorder with psychotic features: A phenomenologic analysis. *American Journal of Psychiatry*, 143(12), 1527-1533.

Levenkron, S. (1991). *Obsessive-compulsive disorders: Treating and understanding crippling habits*. New York: Warner Books.

Nicholi, A.M., Jr. (1988). *The New Harvard Guide to Psychiatry*. Cambridge, MA: The Belknap Press of Harvard University Press.

Paquette, M., Neal, M., and Roderick, C. (1991). *Psychiatric Nursing Diagnosis and Care Plans for the DSM-III-R*. Boston: Jones & Bartlett.

Price, L., Goodman, W., Charney, D., and Rasmussen, S. (1987). Treatment of severe obsessive-compulsive disorder with fluvoxamine. *American Journal of Psychiatry*, 144(8), 1059-61.

Rapaport, J.L. (1989). *The boy who couldn't stop washing: The experience & treatment of obsessive-compulsive disorder*. New York: Dutton.

Turner, S.M., and Beidel, D.C. (1988). *Treating obsessive-compulsive disorder*. New York: Pergamon Books.

ANXIETY DISORDERS
Post-traumatic Stress Disorder

DSM III-R classification
309.89 Post-traumatic stress disorder

Psychiatric nursing diagnostic class
Anxiety

Introduction
Post-traumatic stress disorder (PTSD) affects individuals who have experienced traumatic events that generally fall outside the spectrum of normal human experience. Such events include military combat, hostage situations, natural disasters, rape, criminal assaults, and domestic abuse or violence. Rescue workers and health care providers also may develop PTSD.

After the traumatic event, the individual typically experiences anxiety characterized by elevated autonomic responses (such as a rapid pulse and an increased respiratory rate) and a cognitive impairment that makes concentrating difficult and alters memory. In addition, the individual persistently reexperiences the traumatic event and suppresses emotional responsiveness. These latter behaviors are hallmark PTSD symptoms.

The traumatic event usually is reexperienced in one or more of the following ways: recurrent and intrusive distressing recollections, recurrent and distressing dreams, a sudden acting or feeling as if the event were recurring, or intense psychological distress when exposed to such events as anniversaries that resemble or symbolize the original event.

ETIOLOGY AND PRECIPITATING FACTORS
An individual suffering from PTSD considers the traumatic experience to be a threat to physical integrity, self-concept, or both. Consequently, the person develops severe anxiety that cannot be managed by normal coping strategies and becomes psychologically vulnerable. This vulnerability may be demonstrated by either excessive or inadequate self-control. The person who exhibits excessive self-control uses punitive strategies, such as assuming guilt for the traumatic event. The person who exhibits inadequate self-control continually behaves impulsively, such as suddenly quitting a job and moving to another state.

Assessment guidelines
NURSING HISTORY (Functional health pattern findings)
The client may report or exhibit one or more of the findings grouped here according to functional health patterns.

Health perception–health management pattern
- extreme concern about "going crazy"
- fear of being confined in a hospital
- extreme concern over general health
- exaggerated worry over daily life circumstances
- worry over medication compliance, follow-up visits, and inability to follow through
- inability to control feelings
- numerous somatic complaints, with or without diagnostic validation
- overuse or underuse of health care system to ease anxiety symptoms

Nutritional-metabolic pattern
- concern over eating behaviors, such as using food to suppress feelings
- concern over weight fluctuations
- inattentiveness to dental problems
- changes in appetite, including anorexia and binges

Elimination pattern
- concern over GI system disturbances, such as pain, flatulence, diarrhea, nausea, constipation, vomiting, and intestinal bleeding
- frequent urination
- concern over increased sweating, cold and clammy skin, or both

Activity-exercise pattern
- agitation and restlessness
- concern about fluctuations in energy and activity level
- decreasing interest and participation in leisure or social activities
- trembling
- concern about being easily fatigued
- difficulty accomplishing normal daily activities
- concern about any limitations and restrictions of activity caused by disease or condition
- withdrawn or apathetic behavior

Sleep-rest pattern
- feeling fatigued after sleep
- dreams or nightmares of traumatic event
- sleep disturbances, such as falling asleep but not staying asleep or awakening early in the morning
- use or dependence on sleep aids, such as alcohol, benzodiazepines, or hypnotics
- concern about use or abuse of sleep aids

Cognitive-perceptual pattern
- memory impairment
- difficulty concentrating
- acute or chronic pain

- difficulty learning
- difficulty understanding and reacting to external stimuli
- worry over inability to think clearly
- distorted perceptions

Self-perception–self-concept pattern
- anxiety or feelings of inadequacy
- feeling detached or estranged from others
- feelings of having no control over life
- concern over being indecisive and dependent
- perception of self as being highly anxious
- perception of self as being incompetent and powerless
- concerns about body image, self-esteem, and self-worth

Role-relationship pattern
- concern over inability to maintain relationships with loved ones
- inability to maintain consistent or rewarding employment
- concern about feeling alone and not being involved in the community
- intense concern over relationships with family and friends
- rumination over engaging in social situations with friends, fellow employees, or family
- concern over the lack of response to or support of life-style changes from family and friends
- concern about a distressful work situation
- concern about how community members and neighbors may respond to the disease or condition

Sexual-reproductive pattern
- decrease in sexual desire
- difficulties with sexual performance or satisfaction
- dissatisfaction with sexual relations
- difficulty with intimacy
- concern about involvement in high-risk sexual behavior, such as unprotected sex or promiscuity
- concern about involvement with high-risk partners, including I.V. drug users, homosexual or bisexual partners, and strangers

Coping–stress tolerance pattern
- feeling tense most of the time
- flashbacks or recurrences of traumatic event
- significant number of stressful events during the last year
- inability to cope
- feelings of "going crazy"
- pervasive muscle tension
- constant irritability, feeling on edge or keyed up
- constant shakiness, trembling, or twitching
- concern over experiencing an exaggerated startle response (hypervigilance)
- denial of clearly manifest anxiety
- inability to identify those persons or measures that alleviate rather than exacerbate the condition

- belief that significant life-style changes are contributing to feeling out of control

Value-belief pattern
- inability to achieve goals in life
- desire to increase or decrease involvement in spirituality or religion
- concern over impaired ability to believe in anything or anyone
- disbelief about present situation

PHYSICAL FINDINGS
The client may report or exhibit one or more of the following physical findings.

Cardiovascular
- excessive perspiration
- increased heart rate
- cold, clammy skin
- elevated blood pressure
- hot and cold flashes
- palpitations
- tingling sensation

Respiratory
- hyperventilation
- increased respiratory rate
- shortness of breath
- smothering sensation
- choking sensation

Gastrointestinal
- abdominal distress
- diarrhea
- nausea
- gastric ulcers
- dry mouth
- vomiting
- difficulty swallowing

Genitourinary
- frequent urination

Musculoskeletal
- muscle aches, pains, or soreness
- muscle tension
- restlessness
- trembling
- fatigue
- shakiness
- twitching

Neurologic
- headaches
- hyperalertness
- hypervigilance
- memory impairment
- inability to sleep or to remain asleep
- startle reactions

- tremors or tics
- dilated pupils
- dizziness or faintness
- light-headedness
- paresthesia
- restlessness

Psychological
- anger
- anxiety at or around the time of year that the traumatic event occurred
- feeling constricted
- diminished interest in life activities or work
- feeling detached or estranged
- sleep-induced hypnagogic hallucinations (such as might occur when a veteran falls asleep and reexperiences a bombing incident)
- hypnopompic hallucinations, or dreams that continue after waking (such as those that make an ex-hostage continue to feel as if he is being held hostage after awaking from a dream about the experience)

- nightmares
- recurrent dreams about the traumatic event
- illusions of being back in the traumatic situation (such as might occur when a veteran hears a car backfire and thinks he is back in combat)
- intrusive thoughts of the traumatic event
- general numbing of emotional responsiveness
- self-hatred
- significant irritability
- social withdrawal
- substance abuse or dependence
- sudden acting or feeling as if the traumatic event were recurring
- survivor guilt
- feeling keyed up or on edge
- inability to concentrate
- blank mind

Potential complications
Undiagnosed or untreated PTSD can lead to substance abuse or dependence, violent behavior, and suicide.

Nursing diagnosis: *Post-trauma response related to the subjective experience of an overwhelming traumatic event, such as disaster, war, rape, torture, catastrophic illness, injury, assault, being held hostage, or of vicarious traumatization*

NURSING PRIORITY: To assess the traumatic event and degree of client anxiety to determine the seriousness of the perceived threat

Interventions

1. Observe for and identify any physical injury to the client.

2. Identify the client's symptoms (such as numbness, headache, nausea, palpitations, or chest tightness), and ensure that they are anxiety related and not the products of a physiologic condition.

3. Identify any physical effects of the traumatic event on the client. Such effects might include disfigurement, chronic physical conditions, and disabilities.

4. Identify and document the client's psychological responses (such as shock, anger, panic, bewilderment, and confusion) and emotional changes. Observe for emotional instability evidenced by crying, alternating calm and agitation, hysteria, and statements of self-blame or disbelief concerning the incident.

5. Identify the client's cultural beliefs and ethnic background.

Rationales

1. Physical injuries can occur during a traumatic event as well as during a recurrence of that event.

2. Anxiety-related symptoms must be differentiated from medical symptoms so that appropriate treatment can be instituted.

3. Sequelae from the traumatic event may significantly interfere with normal daily functioning. They also may serve as constant reminders of the event.

4. The behavioral range following a traumatic event is naturally broad; however, such responses must be managed or they will become repetitive and chronic.

5. Knowing the client's cultural beliefs and ethnic background can help the nurse better understand responses to both the event and treatment. For example, a male client whose culture emphasizes macho behavior may have particular difficulty coping with a frightening experience that caused him to run away.

6. Determine the degree of disorganization in the client's thinking and coping.

6. Evaluating the client's thinking and coping abilities helps the nurse determine the degree of intervention necessary during hospitalization, crises, follow-up care, and support group therapy.

7. Observe for verbal and nonverbal expressions of survivor guilt (self-blame or guilt over having survived the traumatic event) and for signs of increasing anxiety.

7. Self-blame, guilt, and increasing anxiety indicate a decreased coping ability. Should these symptoms occur and escalate during the initial interview, the nurse should assess the client's suicide potential and institute suicide precautions if necessary.

Nursing diagnosis: *Powerlessness related to a life-style of helplessness, inadequate problem-solving and coping skills, and overwhelming anxiety*

NURSING PRIORITY: To help the client regain control over feelings and behaviors

Interventions

1. Assess the client's previous coping abilities.

2. Explore cultural and religious beliefs that support helpless behavior as well as those that might be used to support the client.

3. Collaborate with the client to establish realistic, achievable goals for an effective plan of care.

4. Help the client to identify feelings of powerlessness as well as factors that contribute to these feelings.

5. Teach the client strategies to diffuse intense stress and escalating anxiety. Such strategies include deep breathing, using thought-stopping techniques to interrupt irrational thinking, counting to refocus energy, and reviewing the situation with a staff or family member or friend. Rehearse the strategies with the client.

6. Encourage the client to participate in group psychotherapy and self-help support groups.

Rationales

1. Acknowledging any past success that the client has had in dealing with the condition fosters self-confidence and self-control. It also reminds the client that other behavior exists.

2. Cultural and religious beliefs need to be examined in terms of the rigidity, shame, guilt, and sense of powerlessness they can instill. Understanding the influence of such beliefs can enable the client to see that feelings have certain rationales and that they are not beyond control. Positive cultural and religious beliefs, such as those that promote self-control and self-determination, can help the client regain a sense of control.

3. Involvement in the plan of care can enhance the client's sense of control.

4. Identifying stressors that contribute to or trigger feelings of powerlessness can enhance client self-confidence and self-control.

5. These strategies provide alternative coping methods for feelings of powerlessness and can increase the client's sense of self-management.

6. Participating in such groups enables the client to learn and share new coping strategies with peers who have experienced similar traumatic events and reactions.

Nursing diagnosis: *Sleep pattern disturbance related to recurrent nightmares, dreams of personal death, or fear of reexperiencing the traumatic event*

NURSING PRIORITY: To help the client establish a restful environment to increase hours of refreshing sleep

Interventions

1. Gather information from the client, loved ones, or family members to assess the client's usual sleep pattern and any changes in that pattern that have occurred since the traumatic event.

2. Assess the client's usual sleep-related behaviors, such as time of retiring and rising, bedtime rituals, alcohol and sleep aid use, and caffeine intake before bedtime.

3. Teach the client effective sleep measures, such as retiring and rising at regular times, avoiding naps, and avoiding caffeine and alcohol in the evening. Encourage the client to remain fairly active during the early evening and not to spend most of the night on the couch resting or watching television.

4. Arrange a quiet, restful environment that is not too warm and that has no direct light.

5. Encourage the client to install a dim night-light in the bedroom.

6. Help the client to develop an individualized relaxation program. Demonstrate and rehearse such techniques as self-hypnosis, imagery, and muscle relaxation.

7. Refer the client to a support group concerned with similar traumatic events.

8. In collaboration with the client and physician, select, administer, and monitor a hypnotic-sedative for short-term intervention.

Rationales

1. Both subjective and objective information can help the nurse assess the client's specific sleep disturbance and focus interventions.

2. Knowing when the client goes to bed and arises and usual bedtime rituals can help the nurse evaluate potential difficulties. For example, alcohol and sleep aids interfere with the rapid-eye-movement (REM) sleep cycle, thereby preventing refreshing sleep. Coffee, exercise, or animated conversations before bed can cause restlessness and interfere with sleep.

3. Taking measures to modify behaviors and promote sleep can help decrease the client's anxiety about sleeplessness.

4. These measures can facilitate a sleep-inducing environment.

5. Should the client awake quickly from a nightmare, a night-light promotes orientation, thereby reducing overwhelming fear.

6. These strategies can produce both physical and mental relaxation, which may decrease the client's anxiety and induce sleep. Relaxation can reduce the incidence of nightmares.

7. Exploring trauma-related nightmares and fears in a supportive and understanding environment can help diminish the client's feelings of isolation and loneliness.

8. The client may require short-term psychopharmacotherapy to decrease exhaustion, fatigue, or fear and to induce sleep. However, frequent assessments are necessary to prevent the client from overusing or relying on the medication.

Nursing diagnosis: *Self-esteem disturbance related to the traumatic experience*

NURSING PRIORITY: To help enhance the client's self-esteem

Interventions

1. Discuss with the client any experiences related to community response to the traumatic event. (For example, a Vietnam veteran might recall his reception upon returning home or complain of a perceived lack of recognition on Veterans Day.)

Rationales

1. Relating these experiences can give the client an opportunity to explore specific events of prejudicial behavior.

2. Explore cultural and social values that might contribute to the client's lowered self-esteem.

2. Cultural and social values can instill a sense of shame related to certain traumatic events, such as rape. Helping the client to dissociate these views from personal feelings may enhance self-esteem.

Nursing diagnosis: *Potential for violence, self-directed or directed toward others, related to the inability to verbalize feelings*

NURSING PRIORITY: To ensure the safety of the client and others

Interventions

1. Teach the client to recognize early warning signs of impending violence. Verbal signs include the content of remarks and tone of voice. Nonverbal signs include trembling, sweating, pacing, hypervigilance, rapid startle reaction, pounding of clenched fists, and angry facial expressions.

2. Explore with the client the relation between high anxiety and hostile behaviors.

3. Help the client to identify and remove the causes of escalating anxiety.

4. Help the client to understand and verbalize the reasons for angry, vengeful, retaliatory feelings.

5. Help the client to discover and rehearse different methods for expressing feelings.

6. Remain calm and nonthreatening during a client crisis.

7. Provide for and monitor the client's use of immediate, safe outlets for the physical expression of tension. Such outlets might include a punching bag and gloves, walking, or exercising.

8. Determine the probability of impending violence while removing potential weapons or dangerous objects.

9. Ensure clear access to the client and a safe exit route for the staff when managing a potentially violent episode.

Rationales

1. Early identification can help de-escalate the violence cycle and prevent loss of control.

2. High anxiety can increase underlying hostility and lead to a loss of control.

3. Preventing anxiety escalation can help halt the violence cycle.

4. Verbal expression of anger can diminish the need for physical outbursts. This in turn can decrease the incidence of rejection or disapproval by others.

5. The client needs to find rational, acceptable ways to manage feelings rather than resort to destructive, violent behavior.

6. During any interaction with an angry, hostile, or threatening client, the nurse must remember to control personal anxieties. Should the nurse become fearful or avoid the client, the situation will escalate. Loss of objectivity can result in a nurse-client power struggle, which increases anxiety and worsens the crisis.

7. The client needs to discharge the physical energy that high-level anxiety produces; however, the nurse must be present to prevent self-injury, property damage, or injury to others.

8. The nurse must limit the possibility of harm or injury to both the client and others in the area.

9. The nurse and health care team must collaborate to ensure a safe, injury-free intervention during a violent episode. An effective strategy is for one member to talk to the client while other team members prepare for specific tasks should restraints be necessary. This approach reinforces that the client is in a safe, controlled environment.

Nursing diagnosis: *Spiritual distress related to the client's perception of the world as threatening after the traumatic event*

NURSING PRIORITY: To help the client manage personal fears

Interventions	Rationales
1. Encourage the client, loved ones, and family to express feelings about the traumatic event.	1. Doing so prevents suppression or denial of feelings.
2. Collaborate with the client, family members, and a religious counselor to discover the reasons for the traumatic event.	2. Understanding that such events occur for specific reasons can help the client accept that he was not a random victim; this in turn can give the client a more positive outlook on life.
3. Discuss support systems available to both the client and family members.	3. Knowing that support is available can make the client and family feel more connected to others and diminish feelings of isolation.
4. Determine whether the client's spiritual practices are adversely affecting treatment.	4. Understanding the client's spiritual or religious beliefs can help the nurse determine any conflict between such beliefs and treatment.

Outcome criteria

As treatment progresses, the client, family, or both should be able to:
• state that intrusive memories produce less anxiety
• demonstrate an ability to manage emotional reactions
• demonstrate appropriate life-style changes and actively pursue support from other family members
• express a sense of control over the present situation
• help make decisions about present and future care
• verbalize an understanding of any sleep disorder and identify relevant interventions to facilitate sleep
• identify effective coping methods for alleviating negative self-perception
• identify factors that lead to violence
• demonstrate increased self-control
• verbalize an increased sense of self-esteem and hope for the future.

Discharge criteria

Nursing documentation indicates that the client:
• has demonstrated an increased ability to recognize the impact of intrusive thoughts or memories and to use strategies that diminish that impact
• can effectively use strategies that diminish feelings of powerlessness
• has demonstrated a willingness to participate in the plan of care and decision making
• can effectively use methods that facilitate sleep
• can use alternative coping skills
• is aware of available group, family, or marital support resources
• understands the importance of and participates in an ongoing therapy program

• understands the prescribed drug regimen
• understands how to obtain emergency help.

Nursing documentation also indicates that the family:
• can cope with the client's illness
• is aware of community organizations that can help them meet legal or financial needs
• has been referred to appropriate family, group, or marital support resources
• can administer the client's prescribed drug regimen if necessary
• can identify client behaviors that indicate the client's need for immediate assistance.

Selected references

American Psychiatric Association (APA). (1987). *Diagnostic and statistical manual of mental disorders* (3rd ed. rev.). Washington, DC: APA Press.

Burge, S.K. (1988). Post-traumatic stress disorder in victims of rape. *Journal of Traumatic Stress,* 1(9), 193-210.

Carroll, E.M., Foy, D.W., Cannon, B.J., and Zwier, G. (1991). Assessment issues involving the families of trauma victims. *Journal of Traumatic Stress,* 4(1), 25-40.

Doenges, M.E., and Moorhouse, M.F. (1991). *Nurse's pocket guide: Nursing diagnoses with interventions* (3rd ed.). Philadelphia: Davis.

Figley, C.R. (1988). A five-phase treatment of post-traumatic stress disorder in families. *Journal of Traumatic Stress,* 1(1), 127-141.

Figley, C.R. (1989). *Helping traumatized families.* San Francisco: Josey-Bass.

Flach, F. (1989). *Stress and its management.* New York: Norton.

Friedman, M.J. (1991). Biological approaches to the diagnosis and treatment of post-traumatic disorder. *Journal of Traumatic Stress,* 4(1), 67-91.

Glaubman, H., Mikulincer, M., Porat, A., Wasserman, O., and Birger, M. (1990). Sleep of chronic post-traumatic patients. *Journal of Traumatic Stress,* 3(2), 255-263.

Horowitz, M. (1986). *Stress response syndromes* (2nd ed.). Northvale, NJ: Jason Aronson.

Inman, D.J., Silver, S.M., and Doghramji, K. (1990). Sleep disturbance in post-traumatic stress disorder: A comparison with non-PTSD insomnia. *Journal of Traumatic Stress,* 3(3), 429-437.

Kolb, L.C. (1987). A Neuropsychological hypothesis explaining post-traumatic stress disorders. *American Journal of Psychiatry,* 144(8), 989-995.

Lyons, J.A. (1991). Issues to consider in assessing the effects of trauma: Introduction. *Journal of Traumatic Stress,* 4(1), 3-6.

Lyons, J.A. (1991). Strategies for assessing the potential for positive adjustment following trauma. *Journal of Traumatic Stress,* 4(1), 93-111.

Marmar, C.R., and Freeman, M. (1988). Brief dynamic psychotherapy of post-traumatic stress disorders: Management of narcissistic regression. *Journal of Traumatic Stress,* 1(3), 323-337.

McCormack, A., Burgess, A.W., and Hartman, C. (1988). Familial abuse and post-traumatic stress disorder. *Journal of Traumatic Stress,* 1(2), 231-242.

Murphy, S. (1988). Mediating effects of intrapersonal and social support on mental health 1 and 3 years after a natural disaster. *Journal of Traumatic Stress,* 1(2), 155-172.

Ochberg, F.M. (1988). *Post-traumatic therapy and victims of violence.* New York: Brunner/Mazel Publishers.

Rinear, E.E. (1988). Psychosocial aspects of parental response patterns to the death of a child by homicide. *Journal of Traumatic Stress,* 1(3), 305-322.

Tanaka, K. (1988). Development of a tool for assessing post-trauma response. *Archives of Psychiatric Nursing,* 2(6), 350-356.

Van der Kolk, B.A. (1988). The trauma spectrum: The interaction of biological and social events in the genesis of the trauma response. *Journal of Traumatic Stress,* 1(3), 273-290.

Williams, R.L., Karacan, I., and Moore, C.A. (1988). *Sleep disorders: Diagnosis and treatment* (2nd ed.). New York: John Wiley & Sons.

Bipolar Disorders

DSM III-R classifications
296.4x Bipolar disorder, manic
296.5x Bipolar disorder, depressed
296.6x Bipolar disorder, mixed
296.70 Bipolar disorder not otherwise specified
301.13 Cyclothymia

Psychiatric nursing diagnostic class
Mood disturbance

Introduction

A recurrent illness that typically begins with depression, *bipolar disorder* affects about 1% of the United States population. Most individuals subsequently experience both depression and mania, although 10% to 20% experience only mania. It occurs almost equally in men and women, with the onset usually in the late teens to early twenties. Episodes occur more frequently in the early stages of the illness than in later stages, when they seem to stabilize. Bipolar disorder is further classified as manic, depressed, mixed, and not otherwise specified. *Cyclothymia,* a chronic mood disturbance, is considered by some to be a mild bipolar disorder and therefore is included here.

Bipolar disorder, manic
The manic form is characterized by manic states ranging from hypomania to frank mania to delirious mania (Goodwin and Jamison, 1990). Hypomania is characterized by emotional instability, euphoria and irritability, overconfidence, grandiosity, and increased motor activity. Hypomanic individuals may exhibit increased goal-directed thinking and may become more productive and creative. They rarely lose the ability to carry out social roles and almost never require hospitalization.

In individuals with frank mania, irritability turns into hostility and anger, thoughts become loose and disorganized, and hallucinations and delusions commonly occur. Individuals with frank mania frequently require hospitalization to protect themselves and those around them from harm.

Delirious mania is characterized by frenzied activity, delirium, confusion, and incoherent thought processes. Delirious mania symptoms closely resemble those of schizophrenia or organic psychosis. The family's ability to provide information about the incidence, course, and severity of illness is crucial to making an accurate diagnosis.

Bipolar disorder, depressed
The depressed form of this disorder is distinguished by the occurrence of one or more manic episodes at some time during the illness. Individuals commonly experience symptoms at a young age and are physically inactive, sleep excessively, and are prone to suicide. They also are likely to experience hallucinations and delusions. Other symptoms include decreased energy, decreased sexual interest, decreased thought and speech rate, pessimism, hopelessness, suicidal ideation, and lack of interest or pleasure.

Bipolar disorder, mixed
The mixed form of bipolar disorder can be thought of as either a transitional state between the depressed and manic forms or as a separate state having a mixture of symptoms. Individuals with this mood disorder typically exhibit the full spectrum of both manic and depressive symptoms; however, the symptoms may occur intermixed or alternate every few days.

Bipolar disorder not otherwise specified
This category (sometimes referred to as Bipolar II) includes bipolar disorders that do not meet criteria for other specific bipolar disorders but that involve manic or hypomanic behaviors. Disorders that involve at least one hypomanic or one major depressive episode fall into this category.

Cyclothymia
Cyclothymia refers to a chronic adult mood disorder of at least 2 years' duration that resembles bipolar disorder but does not meet the criteria for the major depressive or manic form in terms of severity and duration. Some investigators believe cyclothymia is really a mild bipolar disorder. Little or no impairment of occupational functioning occurs during cyclothymia, and self-medication with psychoactive substances is common.

ETIOLOGY AND PRECIPITATING FACTORS
Classical psychoanalytic theory suggests that a trauma or loss in the oral phase of childhood development leads to bipolar disorders. According to Sigmund Freud, this trauma disrupts ego development, and the unhindered, stricter superego forces the weaker, underdeveloped ego into an unconscious conflict, leaving little time or energy for the individual to enjoy life, resulting in depression. Consequently, manic behavior is seen as a defense against depression.

The object relations theory builds on the classical psychoanalytic concepts developed by Freud. According to this theory, the traumatic separation of the infant from the maternal figure during the first 6 months of life causes the infant to experience grief and mourning, which in turn disturbs the ego's development. Upon reaching adulthood, the individual develops an intense love-hate ambivalence toward loved ones. The negative side of the love-hate ambivalence is expressed as depression; the positive side, as mania.

Family theories suggest that parents who suffer from chronic low self-esteem may project this onto their children, commonly in the form of unrealistically high expectations for success. The anger accompanying this scenario manifests as depression or mania in the child.

Evidence exists to support a genetic developmental theory of bipolar disorder. Studies comparing twins, adopted individuals, and whole families have shown that genetic factors—more so than postnatal environmental factors—are significantly related to the disorder's occurrence. Researchers, however, have been unable to identify a consistent genetic link that would explain bipolar disorder development to the exclusion of other theories.

Another widely accepted biological explanation for bipolar disorder involves biogenic amines. Biogenic amines, such as norepinephrine and serotonin, are the principal neurotransmitters of the limbic system in the midbrain. The limbic system regulates sleep, arousal, sexual function, emotional states, and appetite. Researchers have discovered that antidepressants enhance amine transmission in the brain and subsequently have claimed that depression may be caused by dysregulation of biogenic amine transmission in the limbic system.

The kindling-sensitization hypothesis represents an important link between biological and psychosocial causation theories of bipolar disorder. Kindling is a process by which the limbic system shows an increasing electrical response, or seizure, to a repetitive stimulus. Eventually, this process becomes self-driven. Psychosocial stress may be the stimulus that initiates this process in individuals predisposed to bipolar disorder, thereby causing illness. The efficacy of antiseizure medications for some individuals seems to support this hypothesis. The implication is that early medication along with psychosocial support may protect the brain from emotionally disruptive influences and reduce the occurrence of bipolar episodes.

Assessment guidelines
NURSING HISTORY (Functional health pattern findings)
The client may report or exhibit one or more of the findings grouped here according to functional health patterns.

Health perception–health management pattern
- euphoria over being in the best health ever
- overconfidence in managing health-related issues
- denial of need for health care attention
- noncompliance with medication regimen
- excessive drug or alcohol use
- exaggerated lack of concern over health-related issues

Nutritional-metabolic pattern
- inadequate or irregular food and fluid intake
- significant weight loss
- appetite loss
- short attention span during meals

Elimination pattern
- abdominal distress, including pain, flatulence, indigestion, and nausea
- excessive, frequent urination
- increased perspiration

Activity-exercise pattern
- restlessness and boundless energy
- excessive time spent exercising
- denial of fatigue
- sexual promiscuity, excessive spending, irresponsible enterprises, or other activities that have a high potential for painful or unpleasant consequences
- psychomotor agitation
- poor personal hygiene

Sleep-rest pattern
- decreased need for sleep
- feeling rested after only 2 or 3 hours of sleep
- drug or alcohol use to aid sleep
- disrupted sleep with initial, middle, or late insomnia
- nightmares, illusions, or hallucinations during the night

Cognitive-perceptual pattern
- confusion
- racing thoughts
- being easily distracted
- decreased short-term memory
- difficulty concentrating
- illusions or hallucinations
- disorganized, incoherent, and accelerated speech
- poor impulse control
- poor judgment
- grandiose, unrealistic ambitions
- denial of feeling painful stimuli
- slowed reactions

Self-perception–self-concept pattern
- perception of self as being magically omnipotent
- intolerance of criticism
- lack of shame or guilt
- history of angry or aggressive outbursts

Role-relationship pattern
- grandiose delusions about special relationships with political, religious, or entertainment figures or with God
- inappropriate enthusiasm during social interactions and an increased involvement in social groups

• concern over the lack of support shown by family and loved ones concerning life-style or behavioral changes
• intrusive, demanding, or domineering behaviors
• isolated, stressful living circumstances
• frequent, angry outbursts directed at loved ones
• manipulative and limit-testing behaviors

Sexual-reproductive pattern
• involvement in multiple sexual encounters
• concern about involvement in high-risk sexual behavior, such as promiscuity
• concern about involvement with high-risk partners, including bisexual or homosexual partners, and I.V. drug users
• irregular menstrual periods or other menstrual cycle changes
• disrupted relations with spouse or loved one
• difficulty with issues of dependence and independence
• difficulty with intimacy
• difficulty doing things for others
• fear of social isolation

Coping–stress tolerance pattern
• increased irritability and tension
• drug or alcohol use
• loss of control
• exaggerated startle response (hypervigilance)
• engagement in significant, stressful situations before symptom exacerbation
• inability to identify what may be helpful

Value-belief pattern
• grandiose delusions involving religious themes
• exaggerated feelings of power
• denial of illness and nonparticipation in care
• inability to trust anyone
• inability to control situation
• feelings of hopelessness about the condition
• concern about real or perceived personal failures

PHYSICAL FINDINGS
The client may report or exhibit one or more of the following physical findings.

Cardiovascular
• hypotension or hypertension
• palpitations
• sweating
• rapid heart rate
• irregular rhythm

Respiratory
• increased respiratory rate
• shortness of breath

Gastrointestinal
• abdominal pain
• diarrhea
• dry mouth
• flatulence
• heartburn
• indigestion
• nausea
• vomiting

Genitourinary
• menstrual irregularities
• increased sex drive
• sexually transmitted diseases
• frequent urination

Integumentary
• changes in hair amount, texture, and distribution
• changes in nail growth and texture
• rashes or scales
• pigmentation and skin temperature changes

Musculoskeletal
• aches or pains
• cramping
• fractures
• muscle weakness
• numbness
• tingling
• tremors
• twitching

Neurologic
• agitation
• dizziness

Psychological
• alternating euphoria and irritability
• delusions
• decreased ability to concentrate
• extreme self-confidence
• impaired judgment
• lack of insight

Potential complications
If left untreated, bipolar disorder can lead to exhaustion and poor judgment, which in turn can lead to financial problems, unrealistic decisions, and alcohol or drug abuse.

Nursing diagnosis: *Potential for violence, self-directed or directed at others, related to poor impulse control or cognitive and perceptual changes*

NURSING PRIORITY: To maintain the client's safety

Interventions

1. Provide a safe environment for the client by removing potentially dangerous items, such as sharp objects and belts, and rearranging furniture as needed.

2. Intervene at the beginning stages of agitation, and frequently assess the client's agitation level.

3. Communicate in simple, direct sentences.

4. Allow the client to resume interactions with other clients gradually as behavior improves.

5. When feasible, encourage the client to participate in decision making. Avoid arguing with the client.

6. When feasible, develop with the client written behavioral plans that clearly state limits on undesirable or destructive behavior as well as rewards for appropriate, positive behavior.

7. Address client needs promptly.

8. Administer antimanic medications as ordered (see *Reviewing antimanic drugs*). Monitor the client's response, and assess for any adverse reactions. For the client taking lithium, see *Client-family guidelines for using lithium,* page 78.

9. Encourage the client to identify and discuss conditions that cause anger and agitation.

10. Monitor rapid mood shifts and behavioral changes, paying special attention to depressive thoughts and feelings.

Rationales

1. The client whose thinking is impaired and who is behaving in a psychotic manner can be a physical threat to self and others. Removing potentially destructive implements can help prevent violent incidents.

2. Intervening when agitation begins can help prevent the situation from escalating and can allow the nurse to treat the client in a less restrictive manner. Such intervention may include speaking in a calm, reassuring voice; decreasing stimulation by having the client limit interactions with others; and restricting the client to one room if necessary.

3. The impulsive, agitated, and easily distracted client cannot process complex messages. Simple, clear directions can help ease client agitation.

4. Gradually resuming interactions with others promotes, reinforces, and enhances the client's self-esteem and sense of self-control.

5. Participating in treatment can increase the client's sense of control. Arguing can escalate an agitated client's behavior and may increase the sense of powerlessness.

6. Plans that clearly spell out behavioral limits discourage nurse-client power struggles, limit manipulative client behaviors, and enhance continuity of care. A plan that provides positive reinforcement for desirable behavior increases the client's desire to repeat that behavior.

7. The agitated and impulsive client cannot tolerate waiting. Unnecessary delays and delayed gratification can provoke client violence.

8. Neuroleptics, benzodiazepines, and lithium—all indicated for mania—have different actions and potential adverse effects. Careful monitoring of the client's response and of blood levels decreases the risk of adverse effects or toxic reactions and allows for more accurate titration.

9. Knowing the conditions and factors that cause agitation can enable the client to recognize when such episodes might occur, which in turn allows the client to implement alternative coping methods.

10. Emotional instability and impulsive behavior may lead to suicidal gestures or aggressive outbursts. Monitoring mood swings and related behavioral changes can protect the client and others in the area from danger.

REVIEWING ANTIMANIC DRUGS

Drug and dosage	Adverse reactions	Nursing considerations
lithium carbonate (Eskalith), lithium citrate (Cibalith-S) 600 to 1,800 mg	**Blood:** Leukocytosis **CNS:** Tremors, drowsiness, headache, confusion, restlessness, dizziness, psychomotor retardation, stupor, lethargy, syncope, coma, seizures, electroencephalogram changes, impaired speech, ataxia, weakness, incoordination, hyperexcitability **CV:** Electrocardiogram changes, arrhythmias, hypotension, peripheral circulatory collapse, allergic vasculitis, peripheral edema **EENT:** Tinnitus, visual disturbances **GI:** Nausea, vomiting, anorexia, diarrhea, dry mouth, thirst, metallic taste **GU:** Polyuria, glycosuria, renal toxicity, nephrogenic diabetes insipidus **Metabolic:** Transient hyperglycemia, goiter, hypothyroidism, hyponatremia **Skin:** Pruritus, rash, diminished or lost sensation, dryness and thinning of hair	• Observe the client for signs of lithium toxicity: diarrhea, vomiting, slurred speech, dizziness, muscle twitching, tremors, urine retention, and hypotension. • Instruct the client to take lithium with meals or just after meals to decrease gastric irritation. • Warn against reducing dietary salt intake. • Advise the client to avoid excessive exercise and perspiration. • Instruct the client to follow the physician's instructions regarding regular lithium blood level determinations. • Tell the client to report any symptoms of recurring illness. • Warn against taking any over-the-counter medications without first consulting a physician. • Advise female clients to report pregnancy promptly so that dosage can be carefully regulated and to avoid breast-feeding after delivery.

From: *Psychiatric problems.* NurseReview. Springhouse, PA: Springhouse Corp., 1990.

Nursing diagnosis: *Sleep pattern disturbance related to hyperactivity and perceived lack of need for sleep*

NURSING PRIORITY: To help the client reestablish a regular and restful sleep pattern

Interventions	Rationales
1. Establish a distraction-free environment at bedtime.	1. A quiet, comfortable environment induces relaxation and decreases the client's attention to stimuli.
2. Restrict the client's caffeine and nicotine intake.	2. Stimulants can interfere with normal sleep and exacerbate the client's manic symptoms.
3. Establish a daily morning and afternoon exercise routine. Discourage strenuous evening activity 2 hours before bedtime.	3. Daily exercise induces fatigue and promotes sleep. Strenuous evening activity may energize the client and interfere with sleep.
4. Administer prescribed medications as ordered, and monitor the client's response.	4. Medications may assist in reestablishing a normal sleep pattern and reduce the client's restlessness.
5. Establish with the client a bedtime routine to manage any sleep disturbance.	5. Establishing a planned bedtime routine helps to alleviate client anxiety, frustration, and irritability associated with a sleep disturbance.
6. Offer warm milk and a snack at bedtime.	6. A bedtime snack can help the client to relax. Warm milk contains tryptophan, a substance useful in insomnia treatment.

CLIENT-FAMILY GUIDELINES FOR USING LITHIUM

Lithium is commonly prescribed for clients with bipolar disorder. Here are some general guidelines to follow.

Prescribed medication: _____

Precautions
- Always take this medication with food or milk.
- Maintain adequate fluid and salt intake while taking this medication, especially during hot weather or during activities that cause you to sweat.
- Notify your physician if you are pregnant or intend to become pregnant while using this medication.
- Alert your physician if you have any vomiting, diarrhea, or flulike symptoms while taking this medication.
- If you are taking Lithobid tablets, do not crush or cut the tablet.

Drug interactions
This medication may interact with other prescribed or over-the-counter drugs. Be sure to alert all of the health care providers you see that you are taking lithium.
- Do not drink large quantities of caffeine-containing beverages (such as coffee, tea, and colas) while taking lithium. These substances may reduce the effect of the medication.
- Do not use baking soda (sodium bicarbonate) as an antacid while taking lithium.
- Use a normal amount of table salt in your food unless otherwise directed by your physician.

Adverse reactions
This medication may cause the following adverse reactions. Alert your physician if any of these becomes a problem:

- nausea
- shakiness and tremor
- increased thirst
- dry mouth
- increased urination
- metallic taste
- weight gain
- swelling of hands and feet
- drowsiness
- skin rash.

When to call your physician
Withhold your next dose and contact your physician immediately if you experience any of the following problems:

- vomiting
- diarrhea
- jerking muscles
- slurred speech
- dizziness
- unsteadiness
- blurred vision
- headache.

If you forget a dose
Follow these guidelines if you forget to take a dose of medication:
- If your next dose is more than 2 hours away, take the lithium immediately.
- If your next dose is less than 2 hours away, do not take the missed dose.

NOTE: Never double a dose. Instead, go back to your regular dosing schedule. If you have any questions about this, check with your physician.

Blood testing
Your physician may order a blood test from time to time to check the level of lithium in your body. If a blood test is ordered, keep in mind that the test will be done in the morning, about 10 to 14 hours after your last dose. Do not take your usual morning dose of lithium until after the blood test. You may have breakfast before this blood test.

Adapted from guidelines established by Thomas Jefferson University Hospital, Philadelphia, 1992. Used with permission.

Nursing diagnosis: *Altered nutrition, less than body requirements, related to increased metabolic rate, distractibility, and poor attention span*

NURSING PRIORITY: To help the client establish better eating habits and maintain proper nutrition

Interventions	Rationales
1. Monitor the client's serum electrolyte and albumin levels, weight, and fluid intake and output status daily.	1. This enables the nurse to determine the client's fluid and electrolyte status, ongoing nutritional needs, and hydration status.
2. Offer small, frequent meals of high-calorie foods. Include foods that the client likes as well as those that can be eaten while moving about.	2. The manic client has a generally high metabolic rate and may be too distracted to eat complete meals. Foods that can be eaten while moving around may be indicated for the client who is too agitated to sit long enough to eat a meal.
3. Serve the client meals in an area with few distractions.	3. Reducing mealtime distractions encourages the client to focus attention on eating.

Nursing diagnosis: *Impaired social interaction related to impulsive behavior, distractibility, impaired judgment, cognitive or perceptual changes, and paranoid ideation*

NURSING PRIORITY: To protect the client from harmful consequences of poor and diffuse personal and social boundaries and to enhance the establishment and maintenance of interpersonal relationships

Interventions	Rationales
1. Intervene as needed to protect the client from harmful social interactions.	1. The manic client typically does not recognize the intrusive, demanding nature of personal interactions. The nurse can diffuse potentially violent outbursts by intervening during such interactions.
2. Approach the client in a nondefensive, casual manner, and explain any refusals of irrational or inappropriate requests.	2. The manic client is highly sensitive to communication styles, which inadvertently may trigger impulsive, angry responses. By providing rationales for refusing irrational requests, the nurse can discourage such responses.
3. Discuss the impact the client's behaviors and verbal messages have on others, and encourage the use of more appropriate interacting styles.	3. The nurse may be able to encourage the manic client to use a heightened sensitivity to nonverbal behavior and verbal messages to explore the impact of behavior on others. As concentration and attention span improve, the client should be better able to accept feedback regarding interacting style.

Nursing diagnosis: *Sensory-perceptual alterations related to decreased ability to concentrate, racing thoughts, distractibility, flight of ideas, hallucinations, delusions, sleep deprivation, or anxiety*

NURSING PRIORITY: To orient the client to reality, maintain a safe environment for the client and others, and encourage realistic, goal-directed thinking

Interventions

1. Frequently orient the client to reality, speaking in a clear, simple manner.

2. Provide the client with a relaxing area with decreased environmental stimulation.

3. Gradually integrate the client into a social environment while observing for changes in tolerance of such activity.

4. Design a daily schedule appropriate to the client's mental status. Reevaluate the schedule and add activities as the client's ability to process and tolerate stimuli improves.

5. Be sensitive to the client's physical and psychological boundaries during interaction. (For example, use physical contact cautiously and clearly distinguish your own experiences from the client's in conversation.)

Rationales

1. Frequently orientating the client to reality helps reduce potential agitation resulting from confused perceptions and thoughts.

2. An environment free from distractions decreases anxiety and reduces the potential for agitation or hyperactivity.

3. Interacting with others can decrease the client's feelings of isolation and allow for nonpressured participation in a social environment.

4. An established daily schedule defines both client and staff expectations of behavior and guides daily planning. It also keeps client choices to a minimum, which in turn avoids agitation.

5. Clearly separating the client from others, including the nurse, decreases client confusion, reduces paranoia and anxiety, and shows respect for the client's territorial space.

Nursing diagnosis: *Self-esteem disturbance related to delusions and grandiosity*

NURSING PRIORITY: To help the client plan for recovery and develop a realistic sense of abilities and self-esteem

Interventions

1. Establish minimum standards of self-care and provide guidance, assistance, and support as needed. Reevaluate and revise standards as the client's functioning level increases.

2. Address the client in a respectful, dignified manner while helping to maintain personal privacy.

3. Offer the client choices related to treatment, and encourage participation in the treatment plan.

4. Reinforce the client's successes and gains made toward achieving personal goals.

Rationales

1. Establishing standards encourages the client to assume personal responsibility, promotes independent functioning, and enhances self-worth.

2. By behaving respectfully, the nurse can enhance the client's sense of self-worth.

3. The client who participates in treatment should develop an increased sense of control and value.

4. Acknowledging accomplishments and efforts toward achieving goals reinforces the client's sense of self-worth.

Nursing diagnosis: *Powerlessness related to feelings of hopelessness and perceived lack of control over life situations, self, and illness*

NURSING PRIORITY: To help the client regain a sense of self-control as well as control over life situation and illness

Interventions

1. Collaborate with the client to develop and implement the treatment plan.

2. Discuss with the client early signs and symptoms, such as increased activity, little appetite, or decreased need for sleep, that may indicate a recurrence of the illness. With the client, develop early intervention strategies.

3. Provide the hospitalized client with opportunities to demonstrate self-control. For example, instruct the client to ask for quiet time when becoming overstimulated.

4. Explore the client's feelings of hopelessness and identify misperceptions, distortions, and irrational beliefs.

5. Help the client set realistic, attainable goals for the present and future.

Rationales

1. Helping to make treatment-related decisions can enhance the client's sense of control over self and the illness.

2. Making the client aware of early symptoms of the illness and developing steps to minimize its recurrence can help to avoid future hospitalization resulting from an acute episode.

3. Such opportunities to rehearse self-control can foster confidence in personal abilities.

4. Doing so helps the client differentiate between irrational and real concerns. It also enables the client to examine the accuracy of perceptions and helps to increase positive thinking.

5. Setting realistic goals can increase the client's sense of self-control while eliminating distorted, unattainable objectives.

Nursing diagnosis: *Altered family processes related to role changes, economic crisis, or lack of knowledge about the client's illness*

NURSING PRIORITY: To teach family members about bipolar disorder while encouraging discussion of thoughts and feelings about how the client's and the family's behaviors affect one another

Interventions

1. Assess the family's external support network and encourage participation in family therapy and support groups.

2. Assess communication patterns and boundaries within the family.

3. Observe interaction patterns within the family, and discuss their influence on the client and family functioning.

4. Provide the family with information regarding bipolar disorder and the client's treatment and prognosis.

Rationales

1. External support networks can provide a safe, nurturing environment for the expression of fears and concerns. Such groups encourage the formation of friendships based on common interests.

2. Knowing basic information about the family's functioning, the ability of family members to resolve problems, and the family's impact on the client can help the nurse develop a more effective treatment plan.

3. Both the client and family need to be aware of how the client's behaviors affect family relationships in order to adapt to necessary changes.

4. Such knowledge may relieve guilt, encourage discussion of issues, and increase the family's ability to detect early signs of the disorder's degeneration.

Outcome criteria

As treatment progresses, the client, family, or both should be able to:
• report feeling rested and having reestablished a regular sleep pattern
• report and demonstrate increasing mood stability
• identify early signs and symptoms of decompensation and verbalize an appropriate plan of action
• remain free from harm
• reestablish an adequate fluid and electrolyte balance, demonstrate a stable weight, and verbalize the need to eat
• recognize and control intrusive, demanding behavior in social situations and interact effectively and appropriately
• recognize how interaction styles affect the family and identify more constructive ways to interact
• verbalize realistic, goal-directed thinking related to abilities, recovery, and control of condition
• verbalize and demonstrate a sense of personal control
• discuss the disorder as a biological condition triggered by stressors
• recognize the need for and benefit of outside support systems and use them appropriately.

Discharge criteria

Nursing documentation indicates that the client:
• has demonstrated stable mood, thoughts, perceptions, and behavior
• can interact appropriately with others and care for self
• can recognize early signs of illness recurrence and implement an appropriate plan of action
• can use effective coping methods
• understands the need for follow-up care and is willing to comply with recommended treatment
• knows when and how to use emergency services
• is aware of appropriate community resources.

Nursing documentation also indicates that the family:
• is maintaining a stable sleep cycle and nutritional status
• has scheduled necessary follow-up appointments
• has been referred to the appropriate community resources
• understands the potential problems that can develop during the transition from inpatient to outpatient care.

Selected references

American Psychiatric Association (APA) (1987). *Diagnostic and statistical manual of mental disorders* (3rd ed., rev.). Washington, DC: APA Press.

Bauer, M., and Frazer, A. (1991). Mood disorders and their treatment. In A. Frazer, A. Winokur, and P. Molinoff (Eds.), *Biology of normal and abnormal brain function*. New York: Raven Press.

Doenges, M., Townsend, M., and Moorhouse, M. (1989). *Psychiatric care plans: Guidelines for patient care*. Philadelphia: Davis.

Georgotas, A., and Cancro, R. (Eds.) (1988). *Depression and mania*. New York: Elsevier.

Goodwin, F., and Jamison, K. (1990). *Manic depressive illness*. New York: Oxford University Press.

Hirschfeld, R., and Goodwin, F. (1988). Mood disorders. In J. Talbott, R. Hales, and S. Yudofsky (Eds.), *Textbook of psychiatry*. Washington, DC: APA Press.

Kaplan, H., and Sadock, B. (1991). *Synopsis of psychiatry* (6th ed.). Baltimore: Williams & Wilkins.

Klerman, G. (1987). The classification of bipolar disorders. *Psychiatric Annals, 17*(1), 13-17.

McEnany, G. (1990). Psychobiological indices of bipolar mood disorder: Future trends in nursing care. *Archives of Psychiatric Nursing, 4*(1), 29-38.

McFarland, G., and Thomas, M. (1991). *Psychiatric mental health nursing*. Philadelphia: Lippincott.

Post, R., Rubinow, D., and Ballenger, J. (1986). Conditioning and sensitisation in the longitudinal course of affective illness. *British Journal of Psychiatry, 149*, 191-201.

Simmons-Alling, S. (1987). New approaches to managing affective disorders. *Archives of Psychiatric Nursing, 1*(4), 219-224.

Stuart, G., and Sundeen, S. (1991). *Principles and practice of psychiatric nursing*, (4th ed.). St. Louis: Mosby.

Thomas, M.D., Sanger, E., Wolf-Wilets, V., and Davis Whitney, J. (1988). Nursing diagnosis of patients with manic and thought disorders. *Archives of Psychiatric Nursing, 2*(6), 339-344.

Tirrell, C., and DeForest, D. (1987). Neuroendocrine factors in affective disorders. *Archives of Psychiatric Nursing, 1*(4), 225-229.

Townsend, M.C. (1990). *Drug guide for psychiatric nursing*. Philadelphia: Davis.

Wehr, T.A., Sack, D.A., Rosenthal, N.E., et al. (1988). Rapid cycling affective disorder. *American Journal of Psychiatry, 145*(2), 179, 184.

MOOD DISORDERS

Depressive Disorders

DSM III-R classifications
296.2x Major depression, single episode
296.3x Major depression, recurrent
300.40 Dysthymia

Psychiatric nursing diagnostic class
Mood disturbance

Introduction

Major depression is a mood disturbance in which the major symptoms—depressed mood and loss of interest or pleasure in all or almost all activities—occur daily for at least 2 weeks. Related symptoms include appetite disturbance, sleep disturbance, weight changes, psychomotor agitation or retardation, low energy, decreased libido, feelings of worthlessness, difficulty concentrating, recurrent thoughts of death, and suicidal ideation or suicide attempts. Major depression can occur during infancy, represented by failure-to-thrive syndrome, and throughout adulthood.

Major depression may be classified as a single episode (one occurrence) or as recurrent (two or more depressive episodes separated by at least 2 months). *Dysthymia* is a chronic mood disorder characterized by a depressed mood during most of the day and lasting at least 2 years.

Before diagnosing a depressive disorder, the physician must first rule out organic factors (see *Diseases that cause depression* and *Drugs that cause depression*, page 84) and establish that the depressive response is not just a normal reaction to loss, referred to as uncomplicated bereavement.

ETIOLOGY AND PRECIPITATING FACTORS
Freudian theory maintains that a rigid superego strictly controls the joyful, free-spirited id, resulting in anger and resentment that is not permitted outward expression. The unacceptable anger is internalized, leading to depression.

Interpersonal and family system theories emphasize the individual's role within the family system. According to these theories, interpersonal difficulties, dysfunctional family communication, and abusive lifestyle patterns cause depression.

The cognitive theory of depression maintains that the depressed individual has learned to function from a negative, self-defeating point of view. This negative distortion of reality results from irrational beliefs, dysfunctional assumptions, overgeneralizations, magnification, personalization, and "all-or-nothing" thinking.

The most widely accepted biological theory of depressive disorders maintains that depression results from an inadequate amount or transmission of specific

---

DISEASES THAT CAUSE DEPRESSION

The following list includes some diseases and disorders that can cause or aggravate depression.

Endocrine disorders
• Hypothyroiditis
• Hyperthyroidism
• Hyperparathyroidism
• Cushing's disease
• Menopause
• Diabetes
• Adrenal insufficiency

Gastrointestinal disorders
• Chronic abdominal pain
• Colitis
• Islet cell adenoma
• Hepatitis

Metabolic disorders
• Electrolyte imbalance
• Uremia
• Hypercalcemia
• Gout
• Pernicious anemia
• Porphyria

Neurologic disorders
• Seizure disorders
• Alzheimer's type dementia
• Parkinson's disease
• Multiple sclerosis
• Head injury
• Brain tumors
• Chronic pain
• Migraine headache

Nutritional disorders
• Vitamin B_{12} deficiency
• Iron deficiency
• Obesity
• Inanition
• Dehydration

Miscellaneous disorders
• Systemic lupus erythematosus
• Urinary tract infection
• Bilateral cataracts
• Hypertension
• Rheumatoid arthritis
• Sinus arrhythmias
• Influenza
• Alcoholism

---

neurohormones, including norepinephrine, serotonin, dopamine, and acetylcholine. Other studies strongly indicate that genetic factors influence depression; however, the exact mechanism of genetic transfer is still under investigation.

DRUGS THAT CAUSE DEPRESSION

Antihypertensives
- clonidine (Catapres)
- guanethidine (Ismelin)
- hydralazine (Apresoline)
- methyldopa (Aldomet)
- propranolol (Inderal)
- reserpine (Serpasil)

Stimulants
- amphetamines
- cocaine
- methylphenidate (Ritalin)

Steroids
- cortisone (Cortone)
- dexamethasone (Decadron)

Antiparkinsonian drugs
- levodopa (Larodopa)
- carbidopa-levodopa (Sinemet)

Hormones
- estrogen (Premarin)
- progesterone (Gesterol)

Miscellaneous drugs
- barbiturates
- benzodiazepines
- cimetidine (Tagamet)
- digitalis
- narcotics
- neuroleptics

Assessment guidelines

NURSING HISTORY (Functional health pattern findings)

The client may report or exhibit one or more of the findings grouped here according to functional health patterns.

Health perception–health maintenance pattern
- concern over somatic complaints
- increased irritability

Nutritional-metabolic pattern
- decreased or increased appetite
- weight loss or gain

Elimination pattern
- decreased motility or constipation

Activity-exercise pattern
- increased fatigue
- decreased libido
- psychomotor retardation
- withdrawal from daily life activities
- decreased ability to enjoy life or to function at work

Sleep-rest pattern
- early morning awakening and depression
- difficulty falling asleep
- hypersomnia as a method of withdrawal
- alcohol or drug use to induce sleep

Cognitive-perceptual pattern
- difficulty concentrating
- difficulty making decisions
- ruminating thoughts (continually dwelling on the same topic)
- impoverished thinking
- distorted perceptions (such as "everyone hates me" or "nobody loves me")

Self-perception–self-concept pattern
- preoccupation with self
- low self-esteem
- feelings of inadequacy or guilt
- increased irritability
- perception of self as being worthless or incompetent

Role-relationship pattern
- dependence upon spouse or loved one
- perception of self as a burden to spouse or loved one
- feelings of worthlessness at work

Sexual-reproductive pattern
- decreased libido
- difficulty with intimacy
- fertility, reproductive, or menstrual disturbances

Coping–stress tolerance pattern
- considering suicide as coping mechanism
- suicidal ideation or gestures
- difficulty coping
- inability to reach reasonable solutions to problems

Value-belief pattern
- feelings of powerlessness or hopelessness in achieving life goals

PHYSICAL FINDINGS

The client may report or exhibit one or more of the following physical findings.

Cardiovascular
- elevated blood pressure

Respiratory
- increased respiratory rate
- increased sighing
- shortness of breath

Gastrointestinal
- abdominal distress
- anorexia
- constipation
- diarrhea
- increased appetite
- weight gain or loss

Musculoskeletal
- fatigue
- lethargy
- muscle tension, aches, pains

Neurologic
- agitation
- memory difficulties
- restlessness
- sleep disturbance (such as difficulty sleeping, early morning awakening, or excessive sleeping)
- slowed thinking

Psychological
- anhedonia
- crying or tearfulness
- delusions
- difficulty concentrating
- restlessness
- excessive concern with physical health
- feelings of inadequacy
- feelings of worthlessness, shame, or guilt
- indecisiveness
- loss of interest in environment
- preoccupation with certain thoughts
- social withdrawal
- suicidal thoughts

Potential complications

An undiagnosed medical reason for depressive symptoms could lead to physical deterioration and delay in obtaining appropriate treatment. Such reasons may include an undiagnosed disease or disorder that produces depressive symptoms or depression induced by prescription or over-the-counter medications. Note that drug-induced depression is especially important when counseling alcoholics or clients taking benzodiazepines or antiparkinsonian agents.

Nursing diagnosis: *Ineffective individual coping related to depression in response to identifiable stressors*

NURSING PRIORITY: To help the client develop positive coping mechanisms and understand how stress affects the condition

Interventions

1. Encourage the client to identify events that cause unpleasant emotional responses. Help the client to distinguish between extraneous issues and relevant stressors.

2. Assess real, significant losses that the client has experienced. Also identify cultural and social factors that may have determined how the client coped with these losses.

3. Assess the client's support network.

Rationales

1. Gaining insight about how certain events can affect feelings is an important step in developing self-control. Organizing and ranking stressors can enhance the client's sense of control.

2. Cultural and social values can negatively affect how people cope with grief and loss. (For example, a person may feel that crying over or mourning the death of a loved one is socially unacceptable. Such suppression and denial of feelings can lead to depression.)

3. A support network including family and friends can help the client recover from depression.

4. Assess the client's alcohol and drug use as well as the suicide potential.

4. Alcohol or drug use is an ineffective coping method. In fact, alcohol, a depressant, can increase depression. Other drugs may mask the client's feelings but do not remove the depression's cause. A depressed client is at higher risk for suicide, especially one who sees no way out of the situation. Alcohol or drug use increases the risk for suicide in such clients.

5. Help improve the client's self-esteem by suggesting simple, success-oriented tasks.

5. Low self-esteem commonly accompanies depression. Giving the client simple, success-oriented tasks can increase feelings of self-worth.

6. Collaborate with the multidisciplinary team to determine and monitor appropriate pharmacologic and other somatic therapies, such as electroconvulsive therapy or phototherapy. (For a list of antidepressant medications, see *Selected psychotropic drugs,* pages 18 to 29. Also see *MAO inhibitors: Food and drug interactions,* for a list of substances to avoid while taking monoamine oxidase [MAO] inhibitors.) Make sure the client and family receive clear guidelines for using tricyclic antidepressants or MAO inhibitors before the client is discharged from the unit (see *Client-family guidelines for using tricyclic antidepressants,* page 88, and *Client-family guidelines for using monoamine oxidase inhibitors,* page 89).

6. The client may require a combination of therapies to relieve depression. Some forms of depression respond well to medication, whereas others may need electroconvulsive therapy or other treatments.

Nursing diagnosis: *Potential for self-directed violence*

NURSING PRIORITY: To ensure the client's safety, paying specific attention to suicide prevention

Interventions

1. Periodically evaluate the client's risk for suicide. Suicide clues include making vague references to others as being "better off without me," giving away objects, feelings of hopelessness, withdrawn behavior, and impulsive gestures.

Rationales

1. Suicide methods vary with the seriousness of the intent. (For example, taking an overdose of medication in the presence of others is a much less lethal attempt than driving a car into a highway barrier.)

2. Assess the suicide potential if the client suddenly appears in a better mood.

2. A depressed client may be at greater risk for suicide when the depression begins to lift because there is more energy to carry out the attempt.

3. Implement suicide precautions, such as a written contract with the client, to ensure safety.

3. A written contract with the client can represent concrete commitments to self-preservation.

4. If in a psychiatric setting, check the client's condition every 15 minutes. Be alert to potentially lethal items, administer medications in liquid or injectable form, and check packages brought to the client; if in a nonpsychiatric unit, consult with a psychiatric clinical nurse specialist and employ all of the safety precautions listed above.

4. Suicidal clients typically are hospitalized when they are no longer competent to maintain their own safety. During the hospital stay, the nurse is legally responsible to ensure the client's safety.

MAO INHIBITORS: FOOD AND DRUG INTERACTIONS

MAO inhibitors interact with numerous foods, beverages, and other drugs. Some interactions can cause severe and even life-threatening complications. Use the following list as a guide for avoiding dangerous interactions. Follow manufacturer's guidelines when administering these drugs to clients.

Foods and beverages	Drugs
Alcohol (especially beer and Chianti)	Amphetamines
Avocados	Anesthesia, general and local
Bananas	Anorexiants
Caviar	Antiallergy drugs
Cheese (particularly, aged)	Antiasthmatic drugs
Coffee	Antihistamines
Cola	Antihypertensive drugs
Chicken liver	Antiparkinson drugs
Chocolate	Barbiturates
Fava beans	Cocaine
Figs, canned	Cold remedies
Fish, dried	Meperidine (Demerol)
Meat, especially if unrefrigerated or fermented	Metrizamide (Amipaque)
Meat tenderizers	Narcotics
Pickled herring	
Raisins	
Sausages, fermented	
Sour cream	
Soy sauce	
Tea	
Yeast supplements	
Yogurt	

From *Psychosocial problems*. NurseReview. Springhouse, PA: Springhouse Corp., 1990.

Nursing diagnosis: *Decisional conflict related to an inability to concentrate and a need for perfection*

NURSING PRIORITY: To help the client recognize and use the ability to make logical decisions

Interventions

1. Assess the client's impairment level.

2. Help the client to identify one decision that has to be made.

3. Help the client develop and rehearse problem-solving skills.

4. Implement safe, structured activities involving limited demands on the client, such as occupational therapy.

5. Encourage the client to delay making major life decisions until the depressive disorder has improved. Help the client to set reasonable time tables for such decisions.

Rationales

1. The nurse must determine the degree of impairment before planning appropriate interventions.

2. Focusing on one decision at a time can decrease the client's feelings of being overwhelmed and helpless.

3. Developing new skills presents the client with alternative behavior and can help point out the inadequacies of old behaviors.

4. Directed activities can facilitate initial decision-making as the client develops these skills. Such activities increase self-confidence and self-esteem.

5. Making rational major life decisions requires optimal psychophysiologic functioning.

(Text continues on page 90.)

CLIENT-FAMILY GUIDELINES FOR USING TRICYCLIC ANTIDEPRESSANTS

Antidepressants are commonly prescribed for clients with depressive disorders. Here are some general guidelines.

Prescribed medication: _____

Precautions
- Do not drink alcohol while taking this medication or during the first week after stopping the medication.
- Expect some drowsiness while taking this medication. Do not drive a car, operate machinery, or perform tasks that require alertness until you have completely adjusted to taking the medication.
- Do not abruptly stop taking this medicine without your physician's approval. If your physician tells you to stop taking the medication, be sure to follow the above precautions for 1 week because some of the drug will still be in your body.
- Notify your physician if you are pregnant or intend to become pregnant while using this medication.

Drug interactions
This medication may interact with other prescribed or over-the-counter drugs.
- Notify your physician before taking any pain relievers, sleeping aids, cough or cold medication, tranquilizers, or other depression medication.
- Do not drink alcohol while taking this medication.

Adverse reactions
This medication may cause the following:
- dry mouth
- constipation
- dizziness
- increased appetite for sweets.
- tremors
- sedation.

When to call your physician
Most people experience few or no adverse reactions from this medication. However, any medicine can sometimes cause problems. Call your physician if you develop any of the following:
- blurred vision
- sore throat
- fainting
- confusion
- fever
- mouth sores
- eye pain
- skin rash
- problems urinating.

If you forget a dose
Contact your physician or pharmacist immediately if you miss a prescribed dose.

Additional instructions

_____

_____

_____

_____

Adapted from guidelines established by Thomas Jefferson University Hospital, Philadelphia, 1992. Used with permission.

CLIENT-FAMILY GUIDELINES FOR USING MONOAMINE OXIDASE INHIBITORS

Monoamine oxidase (MAO) inhibitors are commonly prescribed for clients with depressive disorders. Here are some general guidelines.

Prescribed medication: _____

Precautions
- Follow a restricted diet carefully while taking this medication and during the first 3 weeks after stopping the medication. Failure to follow the diet may result in a dangerous increase in your blood pressure.
- Do not take any prescription or nonprescription medications without your physician's knowledge. Such medications also may cause a dangerous change in blood pressure.
- Expect some drowsiness or blurred vision while taking this medication. Use caution when driving or performing other tasks that require alertness.
- Expect some dizziness, weakness, or faintness when arising from a lying or sitting position. Rise slowly until you completely adjust to taking the medication.
- Notify your physician if you are pregnant or intend to become pregnant while using this medication.

Drug interactions
This medication may cause a dangerous interaction with other prescription or over-the-counter drugs. Refer to the precautions above, and check with your physician before taking any other medications.

Adverse reactions
- This medication may cause sleeping problems. Do not take doses late in the day.
- Other effects may include restlessness, constipation, vomiting, headache, and dry mouth. Alert your physician if these become a problem.

When to call the physician
Contact your physician immediately if you develop any of the following symptoms of increasing blood pressure:
- severe headache
- stiff neck
- chest pain
- rapid heartbeat
- nausea and vomiting
- sweating.

Notify your physician if you experience:
- problems urinating
- darkening of the urine
- rash
- itching
- swelling of the hands or feet
- any other unusual problems.

If you forget a dose
Contact your physician or pharmacist if you miss a prescribed dose.

Additional instructions

_____

_____

_____

Adapted from guidelines established by Thomas Jefferson University Hospital, Philadelphia, 1992. Used with permission.

Nursing diagnosis: *Diversional activity deficit related to inability to be gratified because of overwhelming depressive feelings*

NURSING PRIORITY: To promote the client's engagement in satisfying diversional activities within the scope of psychophysiologic limitations

Interventions

1. Determine the client's ability and interest to participate in available activities, such as helping to plan a unit party.

2. Motivate the client to participate in activities by jointly selecting personally meaningful activities that provide immediate gratification and ensure success.

3. Encourage the client to assist in scheduling required as well as optional activities. Encourage the client to gradually assume more responsibility for the daily schedule.

4. Do not make changes in the daily schedule without first conferring and negotiating with the client.

Rationales

1. A severely depressed or physically impaired client may not have the psychic or physical energy to initiate and participate in activities.

2. Helping the client to select and participate in such activities can decrease feelings of inadequacy and incompetence.

3. Client involvement reestablishes feelings of control and self-reliance.

4. The nurse and other staff members must adhere to their commitments and thereby serve as role models for responsible behavior.

Outcome criteria

As treatment progresses, the client, family, or both should be able to:
• identify ineffective coping behaviors and consequences
• express feelings and thoughts directly
• demonstrate mastery in problem solving
• comply voluntarily with signing and adhering to a safety contract
• control impulses for self-harm
• acknowledge feelings of anxiety and distress related to making decisions
• make decisions and state satisfaction with decisions
• engage in satisfying activities within personal limitations.

Discharge criteria

Nursing documentation indicates that the client:
• no longer indulges in suicidal ideation or self-harm behaviors
• has demonstrated improved coping mechanisms, relaxation techniques, and direct communication skills
• has demonstrated a willingness to enlist family involvement in ongoing treatment
• is aware of available support resources
• understands the potential adverse effects associated with drug therapy, electroconvulsive therapy, phototherapy, and sleep deprivation therapy.

Nursing documentation also indicates that the family:
• has demonstrated a willingness to involve themselves in the client's treatment
• has been referred to the appropriate group or family support resources in the community
• understands when, how, and why to contact the health care provider in an emergency.

Selected references

Abrams, R. (1988). *Electroconvulsive therapy.* New York: Oxford Press.

American Psychiatric Association (APA) (1987). *Diagnostic and statistical manual of mental disorders,* (3rd ed., rev.). Washington, DC: APA Press.

Barry, P. (1989). *Psychosocial nursing, assessment and intervention: Care of the physically ill patient* (2nd ed.). Philadelphia: Lippincott.

Beck, A.T., Rush, A.J., Shaw, B.F., and Emery, G. (1987). *Cognitive-therapy of depression.* New York: Guilford Press.

Buckwalter, K., and Abraham, I. (1987). Alleviating the discharge crisis: The effects of a cognitive-behavioral nursing intervention for depressed patients and their families. *Archives of Psychiatric Nursing,* 1(5), 350-358.

Carpenito, L. (1991). *Nursing diagnosis, Application to clinical practice* (4th ed.). Philadelphia: Lippincott.

Clarkin, J.F., and Haas, G.L. (1988). *Affective disorders and the family: Assessment & treatment.* New York: Guilford Press.

Derogatis, L.R., and Wise, T.N. (1989). *Anxiety and depressive disorders in the medical patient.* Washington, DC: APA Press.

Doenges, M.E., and Moorhouse, M.F. (1991). *Nurse's pocket guide: Nursing diagnoses with interventions* (3rd ed.). Philadelphia: Davis.

Doenges, M., Townsend, M., and Moorhouse, M. (1989). *Psychiatric care plans: Guidelines for patient care.* Philadelphia: Davis.

Dreyfus, J.K. (1988). The treatment of depression in an ambulatory care setting. *Nurse Practitioner,* 13(7), 14-33.

Fopma-Loy, J. (1988). The prevalence and phenomenology of depression in elderly women: A review of the literature. *Archives of Psychiatric Nursing,* 2(2), 74-80.

Gulesserian, B. and Warren, C. (1987). Coping resources of depressed patients. *Archives of Psychiatric Nursing,* 1(6), 392-398.

Gulledge, A., and Calabrese, J. (1988). Diagnosis of anxiety and depression. *Medical Clinics of North America,* 72(4), 753-764.

Hayes, P.E. and Kristoff, C.A. (1986). Adverse reactions to five new antidepressants. *Clinical Pharmacology,* 5(6), 471-480.

Hensley, M., and Rogers, S. (1987). Shedding light on "SAD" ness. *Archives of Psychiatric Nursing,* 1(4), 230-235.

Kerr, N.J. (1987). Signs and symptoms of depression and principles of nursing intervention. *Perspectives in Psychiatric Care,* 24(2), 48-63.

Lewis, S., Grainger, R., et al. (1990). *Manual of psychosocial nursing interventions: Promoting mental health in medical-surgical settings.* Philadelphia: Saunders.

Maurer, F.A. (1986). Acute depression: Treatment and nursing strategies for this affective disorder. *Nursing Clinics of North America,* 21(3), 413-427.

Rosenthal, N.E., and Blehar, M.C. (1989). *Seasonal affective disorders and phototherapy.* New York: Guilford Press.

Simmons-Alling, S. (1990). Genetic implications for major affective disorders. *Archives of Psychiatric Nursing,* 4(1), 67-71.

Townsend, M.C. (1990). *Drug guide for psychiatric nursing.* Philadelphia: Davis.

Turner, J., Link, S. (1991). Clients with mood disorders. In G. McFarland and M.J.B. Thomas, (Eds.), *Psychiatric mental health nursing: Application of the nursing process.* Philadelphia: Lippincott.

PSYCHOTIC DISORDERS

Schizophrenic Disorders

DSM III-R classifications
295.1x Schizophrenic disorder, disorganized type
295.2x Schizophrenic disorder, catatonic type
295.6x Schizophrenic disorder, residual type
295.9x Schizophrenic disorder, undifferentiated type

Psychiatric nursing diagnostic class
Disruption in relatedness

Introduction
Schizophrenia is a disorder, or perhaps a group of disorders, manifested by a cluster of symptoms resulting in psychotic behavior. Symptom onset usually occurs in young adulthood and can lead to one of several major schizophrenic types. This plan covers *disorganized, catatonic, residual,* and *undifferentiated schizophrenia.* These types display certain common characteristics, including delusions, looseness of association, hallucinations, functional deterioration, and a duration of symptoms of at least 6 months.

Each type of schizophrenia also has its own specific symptoms. The disorganized type is characterized by incoherence, blunted or inappropriate affect, and an absence of systematized delusions. The catatonic type includes catatonic stupor, negativism, rigidity, excitement, and posturing. The residual type is characterized by a history of previous schizophrenic episodes, blunted affect, withdrawn or eccentric behavior, and illogical thinking. In addition, individuals with residual schizophrenia are no longer psychotic after a schizophrenic episode. The undifferentiated type includes delusions, hallucinations, incoherence, and disorganized behavior, none of which resembles the corresponding symptoms of other schizophrenic disorders.

ETIOLOGY AND PRECIPITATING FACTORS
Current biological research supports a link between genetics and schizophrenia. Generally, researchers believe that individuals inherit a predisposition to the disorder; however, tracing the responsible gene through a family's history is not possible because the gene may not manifest in every generation. Other biological research indicates that structural anomalies in the brain, as well as biochemical, metabolic, and electrical alterations, may cause schizophrenia.

Psychological theories implicate dysfunctional family relationships in the occurrence of schizophrenia. Families that exhibit high conflict and anxiety are believed to foster maladaptive relationships in which parents become overly involved with their children. Such relationships inhibit a child's ability to develop trust and autonomy—both important coping skills. In other cases, parents may convey conflicting messages, creating within the child emotional ambivalence and a disturbed self-image. Psychological researchers also propose that individuals with a history of schizophrenia are more likely to suffer relapses when they come from families that are excessively critical, hostile, involved, and even supportive.

Assessment guidelines
NURSING HISTORY (Functional health pattern findings)
The client may report or exhibit one or more of the findings grouped here according to functional health patterns.

Health perception–health management pattern
• presence or severity of symptoms
• need for treatment
• poor physical health secondary to psychotic symptoms and disorganized thoughts
• weight loss
• poor hygiene and grooming

Nutritional-metabolic pattern
• fear that food is being tampered with

Elimination pattern
• constipation secondary to poor nutritional status or medication use

Activity-exercise pattern
• pacing to relieve anxiety
• hypervigilance
• decreased motivation and interest in activities
• psychomotor retardation
• restlessness secondary to adverse effects of medication or psychotic symptoms
• disorganized or bizarre behavior and posturing

Sleep-rest pattern
• insomnia secondary to hallucinations or delusions
• sedation secondary to medication

Cognitive-perceptual pattern
• hallucinations
• delusions
• decreased attention span
• difficulty concentrating
• disturbed thought processes (manifested as blocking, loose associations, flight of ideas, tangentiality, or ideas of reference)
• lack of insight or denial of illness

Self-perception–self-concept pattern
- low or exaggerated self-esteem
- feelings of persecution

Role-relationship pattern
- disturbed interpersonal relationships
- inability to assume responsibilities for parenting, employment, or relationships
- inability to trust others
- feelings of loneliness

Sexual-reproductive pattern
- sexual dysfunction secondary to medication effects
- discomfort about masturbation

Coping–stress tolerance pattern
- symptom escalation following exposure to stressors

Value-belief pattern
- paranoia or grandiose delusions
- delusions of possessing special powers or a different identity
- overreliance on or identification with religion or religious figures

PHYSICAL FINDINGS
The client may report or exhibit one or more of the following physical findings.

Cardiovascular
- excessive perspiration
- increased heart rate
- increased or decreased blood pressure
- orthostatic changes resulting from psychotropic medications

Gastrointestinal
- constipation
- dry mouth

Genitourinary
- amenorrhea
- difficulty achieving or maintaining erection

- retarded ejaculation
- diminished sex drive

Musculoskeletal
- body posture alterations
- balance disturbance
- gait disturbances
- muscle tension
- restlessness

Neurologic
- catatonia
- dilated pupils
- hyperreflexia
- parkinsonian movements (such as tremors and pill-rolling finger movements)
- sensory abnormalities (such as hyperesthesia, hypoesthesia, or paresthesia)
- sleep disturbances (such as inability to sleep or difficulty staying asleep)

Psychological
- ambivalence
- anger
- anxiety
- apathy
- argumentativeness
- delusions
- emotional lability
- lack of facial expression
- hallucinations
- paranoia

Potential complications
If left untreated, schizophrenia can lead to aggressive, violent behavior toward self or others as well as to catatonic behavior, depression, and suicide. Extrapyramidal adverse reactions to medications include muscle rigidity, tremors, drooling, shuffling gait, and restlessness. Tardive dyskinesia and neuroleptic malignant syndrome (an emergency characterized by high fever, tachycardia, muscle rigidity, stupor, tremors, incontinence, and renal failure) also can occur.

Nursing diagnosis: *Altered thought processes related to psychosis and evidenced by disruptions in thought flow, form, or content*

NURSING PRIORITY: To help the client differentiate between delusions and reality

Interventions
1. Provide the client with honest and consistent feedback.

Rationales
1. By being consistently straightforward, the nurse reinforces the client's orientation to reality and fosters trust.

2. Avoid challenging the content of the client's disturbed thoughts.

2. The client believes that such thoughts are accurate. Challenging this perceived accuracy can only increase mistrust and conflict between the nurse and client.

3. Focus interactions on the client's behavior.

3. By focusing on present behavior, the nurse minimizes the potential for conflict and misunderstanding.

4. Communicate with the client clearly, concisely, and honestly, avoiding slang and figures of speech.

4. Complex words and sentences, as well as slang and idiomatic speech, can increase client frustration and miscommunication. By speaking clearly, the nurse can prevent these problems and help the client to concentrate and communicate without anxiety.

5. Point out when you cannot understand the client's thoughts.

5. Doing so demonstrates that the nurse is listening carefully and helps to establish trust between the nurse and client.

6. Maintain objectivity when listening to the client. Do not take personally any ethnic slurs or judgmental statements.

6. The client may frequently use these types of statements to create emotional and psychological barriers between self and others because closeness increases anxiety. By not taking such statements personally, the nurse can gain the client's trust.

7. Be aware of the client's personal space, and use gestures and touch judiciously.

7. Invading the client's personal space can increase anxiety. The anxious client may misinterpret gestures as aggressive moves.

8. Administer medications as ordered, and monitor the client's response.

8. Drug therapy can reduce psychotic symptoms and promote more organized thought processes.

9. Teach the client and family about the uses, actions, and adverse effects of any prescribed medication (see *Client-family guidelines for using neuroleptics*).

9. Knowing about the prescribed medication and how to manage adverse reactions enhances compliance.

10. Do not minimize the client's subjective experience of an adverse reaction to a prescribed neuroleptic. Adverse reactions include drowsiness or sedation, dry mouth, blurred vision, photosensitivity (especially with phenothiazines), constipation or urine retention, orthostatic hypotension, general hypotension, weight gain, and altered sexual functioning. Extrapyramidal effects include parkinsonian symptoms, restlessness, acute muscle spasms, and tardive dyskinesia symptoms (including tongue protrusion, lip smacking, and grimacing).

10. Acknowledging the potentially distressing adverse reactions to neuroleptics can foster client trust and compliance.

11. Teach the client and family how to recognize and cope with relapse symptoms, such as increased hallucinations and agitation.

11. Providing the client and family with effective coping strategies will increase their sense of control in coping with the disorder.

Nursing diagnosis: *Visual alterations related to psychosis-induced hallucinations*

NURSING PRIORITY: To orient the client to reality and help alleviate hallucinations

Interventions

1. Observe the client for signs of hallucinations, such as a listening pose, laughing or talking to self, and halting in mid-sentence.

Rationales

1. Early recognition of hallucinations and subsequent intervention may help the nurse prevent an aggressive client response to command hallucinations.

CLIENT-FAMILY GUIDELINES FOR USING NEUROLEPTICS

Neuroleptics are commonly prescribed for clients with psychotic disorders. Here are some general guidelines to follow.

Prescribed medication: _____

Precautions

• Do not drink alcohol while taking this medication or during the first few days after stopping the medication.

• Expect some drowsiness from the medication. Do not drive a car, operate machinery, or perform tasks that require alertness until you have completely adjusted to taking the medication.

Drug interactions

This medication may interact with other prescribed and over-the-counter drugs. Be sure to alert all of the health care providers you see that you are taking a neuroleptic.

• Do not take this medication with an antacid or an antidiarrheal medication. Take them at least 1 hour apart.

• Avoid using alcohol.

Adverse reactions

You may experience the following problems:

• dry mouth
• constipation
• sensitivity to sunlight
• tachycardia
• hypotension.

When to call the physician

Contact your physician immediately if you experience any of these problems:

• muscle stiffness
• restlessness
• dizziness or fainting
• unsteadiness
• blurred vision
• sore throat
• fever
• mouth sores
• skin rash
• dark colored urine
• difficulty urinating
• yellow eyes or skin
• unusual movements of the face, tongue, or arms.

If you forget to take a dose

Contact your physician or pharmacist immediately if you miss a dose of this medication.

Additional instructions

_____

_____

_____

Adapted from guidelines established by Thomas Jefferson University Hospital, Philadelphia, 1992. Used with permission.

2. Ask if the client hears or sees things that others do not.

2. By doing so, the nurse acknowledges the validity of the client's perceptions without challenging them and promotes trust.

3. If possible, determine the content of hallucinations.

3. Knowing the content of the hallucinations can help the nurse determine the level of observation required for client safety. A client who hears deprecatory or hostile voices may become increasingly agitated or violent. Command hallucinations commonly contain suicidal or violent directives, which the client may act on impulsively.

4. Assess the client's response to hallucinations.

4. Hallucinations may frighten and confuse the client, who may consequently require closer supervision.

5. Acknowledge the client's feelings about any disturbing hallucinations.

5. Supportive, empathetic responses foster trust and enhance the client's sense of safety and reality. Acknowledging the client's feelings also can help prevent unnecessary agitation.

6. Provide reality-based, supportive feedback, such as "I know you see that, but I do not".

6. Acknowledging the client's perceptions while responding honestly can help the client begin to distinguish real from unreal.

7. Monitor the client's responses to the environment and make any appropriate changes, which might include providing seclusion or reducing visual stimuli (see *Assessing the schizophrenic client in the hospital environment*).

7. An overresponsiveness to environmental stimuli can increase client misperceptions, thereby increasing anxiety and, consequently, hallucinations.

8. Provide appropriate measures to ensure client safety, and explain to the client why you are doing so.

8. Implementing and explaining safety measures can promote trust and decrease anxiety while increasing the client's sense of security.

ASSESSING THE SCHIZOPHRENIC CLIENT IN THE HOSPITAL ENVIRONMENT

When evaluating the environment and assessing the client's well-being in the hospital, consider the following points:

Safety
• Is staffing adequate to allow one nurse per shift to provide consistent care and supervision for the client?
• Are dangerous objects out of the client's reach?
• Is a secluded, quiet area available if the client needs to have stimuli reduced?

Meaningful activity
• Is the client bored or inactive?
• Is the environment sufficiently stimulating?
• Are drawing, handicraft, and other materials available to help prevent the client from withdrawing into fantasy?

Socialization
• Is the client anxious in social situations?
• Can the client tolerate a one-to-one relationship with selected individuals?

• Do you have enough time to develop a one-to-one relationship with the client?
• Do you and your colleagues encourage the client to interact with more people?
• Is a supportive group available to strengthen the client's ability to interact and to provide learning opportunities?
• In a group setting, does the client behave appropriately and interact with others?

Coping skills
• Does the client have enough insight to recognize and cope with common life problems and return to the community?
• Does the community setting provide enough support in coping with anxiety, managing stress, developing social skills, training for a job, monitoring medication, and handling crises?

From *Psychosocial crises*. NurseReview. Springhouse, PA: Springhouse Corp., 1990.

9. During any interaction, encourage the client to focus on you and your voice.

9. Doing so can help the client distinguish the real from the unreal. It also can help prevent misunderstandings between the nurse and client.

10. Administer antipsychotic medications as ordered, and monitor the client's response.

10. Antipsychotics can decrease hallucinations, thereby alleviating the client's subjective discomfort and agitation.

11. Encourage the client to participate in recreational and diversionary activities.

11. Such activities can reduce the client's preoccupation with internal stimuli. They also provide opportunities for improving self-esteem and self-confidence.

12. Encourage the client to identify situations or experiences that increase or decrease hallucinations.

12. Understanding the relationship between anxiety-producing experiences and hallucinations can enhance the client's feelings of self-control. For example, the client can learn to avoid certain situations that bring on hallucinations, thus enhancing self-control.

13. Help the client and family to assess their communication patterns and emotional styles and to identify those that might be related to symptom development.

13. Research shows a relationship between certain styles of emotional expression and symptom development. Identifying aggravating, albeit unintentional, behaviors is necessary before adjustments in those behaviors can be made.

14. Provide opportunities for the client to learn adaptive social skills in a nonthreatening environment.

14. Learning new social skills can enhance the client's adjustment after discharge.

Nursing diagnosis: *Potential for violence, directed at self or others, related to delusional thinking*

NURSING PRIORITY: To ensure that the client does not harm self, others, or the environment while in the hospital

Interventions

Rationales

Note: The following interventions are arranged according to the client's escalating anxiety and propensity for violence.

Agitation
Early interventions at the initial signs of agitation can prevent symptom escalation.

1. Monitor the client for behaviors that indicate increased anxiety.

1. Early intervention can help prevent escalating anxiety, which usually precedes agitation and aggression.

2. Collaborate with the client to identify anxious behaviors as well as their probable causes.

2. Involving the client in self-examination of behavior can increase the client's sense of self-control.

3. Inform the client of available alternatives for dealing with anxiety and agitation. Such alternatives include moving to a less stimulating environment, engaging in diversionary activities, talking with the nurse, and taking prescribed medications.

3. Using such alternatives can enable the client to channel energy in more adaptive ways. Anxiolytics can be effective at this time because they provide fast relief of anxiety symptoms. Neuroleptics take longer to produce therapeutic effects, although their sedative effects can be beneficial at this point.

4. In an accepting, nonthreatening manner, encourage the client to verbalize feelings and perceptions.

4. By encouraging the client to express unacceptable feelings, the nurse can help put those feelings into perspective.

5. Tell the client that you will help maintain control.

5. By acknowledging the client's possible fear of losing control, the nurse provides reassurance and fosters trust.

6. In a supportive, nonjudgmental, yet firm manner, set limits on the client's behavior.

6. Setting limits for behavior helps the client identify boundaries and provides structure.

7. Remove all other clients and unnecessary spectators from the environment.

7. The client is more likely to cooperate with the nurse when alone.

Escalation

If the client does not respond to early intervention and the anxiety continues to escalate, the nurse must assume more control through interactions.

8. Speak in a quiet, slow, self-assured manner, using clear, concise language.

8. By speaking quietly and slowly, the nurse might prevent the interaction from getting out of control. A self-assured manner communicates a sense of control to the client.

9. To prepare for possible continued escalation, form a care team and designate one member to maintain client interaction.

9. Planning ahead gives everyone involved a sense of control and ensures teamwork. Having only one person interact with the client prevents confusion and provides the client with a single external stimulus on which to focus.

10. Give the client focused, realistic options; however, be sure you know and distinguish for the client what is optional and what is not. (For example, if you have decided that the client needs medication, this need is no longer an option. However, the client could choose the administration route. You might say, "You need medication. Would you prefer to have it by mouth or by injection?")

10. Providing options allows the client to maintain self-esteem and can foster a sense of self-control.

11. Follow through with the options you provide. (For example, you might say to the client, "I am going to ask you to go to the seclusion room; you can walk with me, or we can take you there." If the client chooses not to walk, make sure you have enough help.)

11. The client probably will respond positively to structure and a sense of control. This can make the situation safer and more predictable.

12. Provide the client with adequate interpersonal space, taking care not to enter that space without warning.

12. As anxiety and agitation increase, the client may feel the need for increased interpersonal space. If crowded or threatened, the client might assault someone.

13. Maintain eye contact, but do not stare; be aware of the client's position and posture.

13. The client might perceive staring as intrusive or challenging. If preparing to strike out, the client will glance quickly to check for a clear path. The client also may be scanning the environment for a weapon.

14. Ensure that only one person maintains verbal interaction with the client.

14. Restricted verbal interaction can keep the client focused and promotes a sense of being cared for and supported.

Aggression

If escalation continues, the nurse must take control and make decisions for the safety of the client and others. At this level of agitation, the nurse must be prepared for physical intervention. Training in safe physical interventions is essential to prevent injury.

15. Make sure that all potential weapons and obstacles are removed from the environment.

15. Removing potential weapons decreases the chance of injury and communicates to the client that everyone will be safe.

16. Inform the care team of your plan, and define each member's responsibility.

16. Doing so fosters confidence among team members and helps to ensure effective teamwork.

17. Determine the need for external controls, including seclusion or restraints. Communicate your decisions to the client.

17. This communicates to the client that the nurse is in control.

18. Once you have initiated a plan, follow through with it.

18. Interrupting a plan can create confusion and increase anxiety for all involved. If the client perceives that the nurse or other care team members are not in control, anxiety may escalate to violence, resulting in injury.

19. When agitation decreases, establish with the client a behavioral contract that identifies specific behaviors that indicate regained self-control.

19. Such a contract provides both the staff and client with criteria that indicate the client is ready and able to maintain control and tolerate frustration.

Nursing diagnosis: *Potential activity intolerance related to adverse reactions to medications*

NURSING PRIORITY: To establish an activity routine for the client

Interventions

1. Assess the client's response to any prescribed antipsychotics.

2. Teach the client and family about therapeutic effects of and adverse reactions to antipsychotics.

3. Encourage the client to report any adverse reactions to the prescribed antipsychotics.

4. Teach the client strategies that decrease adverse reactions to antipsychotics. These strategies include gradually increasing activity, rising slowly from a prone or sitting position, and dangling the feet while sitting. Monitor for signs of orthostatic hypotension, including a drop in blood pressure with a position change, increased heart rate when arising from a prone or sitting position, dizziness, light-headedness, and falls.

5. Assess the client's ability to perform activities of daily living (see *Assessing self-care in schizophrenia,* page 100). Collaborate with the client to establish a daily routine within physical limitations.

Rationales

1. Assessment data helps the nurse to plan and implement appropriate interventions.

2. Client and family knowledge of the prescribed drug helps ensure compliance.

3. By knowing the client's response to prescribed medications, the nurse can help promote optimal functioning.

4. Such strategies can help decrease the dizziness caused by orthostatic hypotension and prevent accidental falls.

5. A realistic daily routine can help the client overcome adverse reactions to antipsychotic medications. For example, the nurse can avoid scheduling activities that require alertness when the client's sedative medication achieves its peak effect.

ASSESSING SELF-CARE IN SCHIZOPHRENIA

Schizophrenia may interfere with such daily activities as maintaining proper hygiene and appearance, ensuring adequate rest, and promoting urinary and fecal elimination. Consider the following points when assessing a schizophrenic client.

Eating and drinking
- Can the client eat independently?
- Does the client act appropriately at meals?
- Is the client's fluid intake sufficient to prevent dehydration?
- Is caloric intake sufficient according to the client's size and activity level?
- Are suspicions or preoccupations preventing the client from eating or drinking enough?
- Does the client eat too much — a possible indication that neuroleptic drugs have increased the client's appetite?
- Has the client's weight changed?

Hygiene and appearance
- Can the client meet personal appearance and hygiene needs?
- Does the client dress appropriately?
- Does the client have fears or beliefs that prevent regular bathing?
- How much supervision does the client require to ensure a proper appearance?

Oxygenation
- Does the client have any adverse effects from neuroleptic drugs, such as cardiac arrhythmias, postural hypotension, or tachycardia?

Personal safety
- Does bizarre behavior or a poor grasp of reality suggest that the client might harm himself or others?
- Does the client hear threatening or accusatory voices or voices that provoke violent acts?
- Are neuroleptic drugs causing adverse effects?

Rest and activity
- Does the client get sufficient rest and physical activity?
- Does hyperactivity or suspiciousness interfere with sleep patterns?
- Do neuroleptic drugs affect motor activity?

Sensory and cognitive function
- Does the client have hallucinations, delusions, or other perceptual disturbances?
- Can the client interpret environmental stimuli and reality appropriately and respond to them?
- Do certain stimuli upset the client?

Sexuality
- Does the client have any bizarre ideas about sexual identity?
- Is the client experiencing any adverse drug effects, such as altered libido, gynecomastia, ejaculatory inhibition, menstrual irregularities, or lactation?
- Does the client feel sexually unattractive or seem to have little interest in sex?

Urinary and fecal elimination
- Is the client experiencing urine retention, a possible result of catatonic negativism or adverse drug effects (in clients with prostatic hypertrophy)?
- Is the client constipated, possibly indicating adverse effects of drugs on the autonomic nervous system, low-fiber diet, or low activity levels?
- Does the client suffer from incontinence or smear feces, both of which indicate severe regression?
- Can the client use the bathroom without being supervised?
- Does the client hide elimination products — an indication of depersonalization?

From *Psychosocial crises.* NurseReview. Springhouse, PA: Springhouse Corp., 1990.

Nursing diagnosis: *Potential anxiety related to extrapyramidal effects of antipsychotic medications*

NURSING PRIORITY: To decrease the client's anxiety over the extrapyramidal effects of antipsychotic medications

Interventions

1. Assess the client for extrapyramidal effects. Signs and symptoms include abnormal posturing; continual hand, mouth, or body movements; drooling; fatigue; mandibular movements; masklike facial expression; opisthotonos; tongue protrusion; restlessness; tremors; and arm and leg weakness.

2. Reassure the client that the extrapyramidal effects are reversible.

Rationales

1. Early identification of extrapyramidal effects can help diminish or eliminate the client's anxiety related to these symptoms.

2. Knowing that the effects are reversible can reduce anxiety caused by these frightening symptoms.

3. Teach the client about the extrapyramidal effects of antipsychotic medications. Include the signs and symptoms of akathisia, dyskinesia, dystonias, and pseudoparkinsonism.

3. Knowing about these effects can decrease the client's anxiety, help ensure early identification and treatment, and promote compliance.

4. Administer medications as ordered to reverse extrapyramidal reactions.

4. Antiparkinsonian agents can reverse extrapyramidal symptoms, thereby alleviating anxiety.

Nursing diagnosis: *Altered oral mucous membrane related to adverse reactions to antipsychotic medications*

NURSING PRIORITY: To help the client maintain a moist, intact oral mucous membrane while taking antipsychotic medications

Interventions

1. Determine the client's hydration status by assessing oral mucosa, fluid intake and output, and urine specific gravity.

2. Encourage an adequate fluid intake of 8 to 10 8-oz glasses (1,900 to 2,400 ml) of water daily, within the client's physical capabilities.

3. Monitor the client's fluid intake, and observe for signs and symptoms of water intoxication, including headaches, dizziness, vomiting, and coma.

4. Encourage good oral hygiene and lip lubrication.

5. Provide hard candy or sugarless gum.

Rationales

1. If the client's hydration status is inadequate, the nurse should implement appropriate interventions to improve it, such as offering beverages at regular intervals.

2. Adequate fluid intake can help prevent dry mucous membranes.

3. The client may periodically overhydrate while taking antipsychotic medications.

4. Practicing good oral hygiene and lubricating the lips help prevent skin breakdown and maintain normal function and structure of mucous membranes.

5. Sucking on hard candy or chewing gum increases salivation and lubrication in the oral cavity, thereby decreasing dry mouth.

Outcome criteria

As treatment progresses, the client, family, or both should be able to:
• demonstrate adaptive coping methods evidenced by decreased suspiciousness
• verbalize or demonstrate reality orientation by recognizing and clarifying possible misinterpretations
• demonstrate improved social and communication skills
• demonstrate appropriate emotional responses
• report or demonstrate a decrease in hallucinations
• report or demonstrate improved judgment and insight
• demonstrate an improved attention span and concentration ability
• interact in a goal-directed manner
• verbalize an understanding of what causes a relapse.

Discharge criteria

Nursing documentation indicates that the client:
• has demonstrated improved reality orientation
• has demonstrated an improved attention span and ability to concentrate
• can control impulses
• can use more adaptive coping skills
• has demonstrated improved social skills
• has reported a decrease in or absence of hallucinations.

Nursing documentation also indicates that the family:
• knows the signs and symptoms of relapse
• is aware of the client's aftercare needs and knows how to make the necessary arrangements
• understands the client's medication dosage and potential adverse reactions as well as how to manage those reactions
• knows who to contact should an emergency arise.

Selected references

Ambrose, J. (1989). Joining in: Therapeutic groups for chronic patients. *Journal of Psychosocial Nursing,* 27(11), 28-32.

Barrett, N., et al. (1990). Clozapine: A new drug for schizophrenia. *Journal of Psychosocial Nursing,* 28(2), 24-28.

Bostrum, A. (1988). Assessment scales for tardive dyskinesia. *Journal of Psychosocial Nursing,* 26(6), 8-12.

Buchanan, R.W., et al. (1990). Clinical correlates of the deficit syndrome of schizophrenia. *American Journal of Psychiatry,* 147(3), 290-294.

Caracci, G., et al. (1990). Subjective awareness of abnormal involuntary movements in chronic schizophrenic patients. *American Journal of Psychiatry,* 147(3), 295-298.

Chesla, C.A. (1989). Parents' illness models of schizophrenia. *Archives of Psychiatric Nursing,* 3(4), 218-225.

Conley, R., and Baker, R. (1990). Family response to improvement by a relative with schizophrenia. *Hospital and Community Psychiatry,* 41(8), 898-901.

Corrigan, P., et al. (1990). From noncompliance to collaboration in the treatment of schizophrenia. *Hospital and Community Psychiatry,* 41(11), 1203-1211.

Dauner, A., and Blair, D.T. (1990). Akathisia: When treatment creates a problem. *Journal of Psychosocial Nursing,* 28(10), 13-18.

DeCangas, J. (1990). Exploring expressed emotion: Does it contribute to chronic mental illness? *Journal of Psychosocial Nursing,* 28(2), 31-34.

DeLuca, A., et al. (1988). Neuroleptic reduction helps prevent relapse. *Journal of Psychosocial Nursing,* 26(8), 13-17.

Garza-Trevino, E., et al. (1990). Neurobiology of schizophrenic syndromes. *Hospital and Community Psychiatry,* 41(9), 971-980.

Goodwin, G., and Guze, S. (1989). *Psychiatric Diagnosis* (4th ed.). New York: Oxford University Press.

Greenberg, L., et al. (1988). An interdisciplinary psychoeducation program for schizophrenic patients and their families in an acute care setting. *Hospital and Community Psychiatry,* 39(3), 277-282.

Hamilton, D. (1990). Clozapine: A new antipsychotic drug. *Archives of Psychiatric Nursing,* 4(4), 278-281.

Lancaster, J. (1988). *Adult Psychiatric Nursing* (2nd ed.). New York: Medical Examination Publishing.

Maurin, J. (Ed.) (1989). *Chronic mental illness coping strategies.* NJ: Slack.

Michaels, R., and Mumford, K. (1989). Identifying akinesia and akathisia: The relationship between patient's self-report and nurses assessment. *Archives of Psychiatric Nursing,* 3(2), 97-101.

Mitchell, R.G. (1986). *Essential psychiatric nursing.* New York: Churchill Livingstone.

Nasrallah, H., and Weinberger, D. (1986). *Handbook of schizophrenia: Vol. 1. The neurology of schizophrenia.* New York: Elsevier.

Norris, A., et al. (1990). Carbamazepine treatment of psychosis: Implications for patient welfare and nursing practice. *Journal of Psychosocial Nursing,* 28(12), 13-18.

Plante, T. (1990). Social skills training: A program to help schizophrenic clients cope. *Journal of Psychosocial Nursing,* 27(3), 7-10.

Shives, L.R. (1990). *Basic concepts of psychiatric-mental health nursing* (2nd ed.). Philadelphia: Lippincott.

Sulliger, N. (1988). Relapse. *Journal of Psychosocial Nursing,* 26(6), 20-23.

Sullivan, G. and Lukoff, D. (1990). Sexual side effects of antipsychotic medication: Evaluation and interventions. *Hospital and Community Psychiatry,* 41(11), 1238-1241.

PSYCHOTIC DISORDERS

Delusional (Paranoid) Disorder

DSM III-R classification
297.10 Delusional (paranoid) disorder

Psychiatric nursing diagnostic class
Anger

Introduction

Delusional (paranoid) disorder is characterized by several types of persistent, nonbizarre delusional thinking, including erotomanic, grandiose, jealous, persecutory, and somatic (see *Delusional themes*). With the erotomanic type, the individual has an erotic delusion of being loved by another in a romantic and spiritual way rather than a sexual one. A person with the grandiose type believes that he possesses great, unrecognized talent or insight or has made a significant discovery. An individual with the jealous type believes that his partners are unfaithful. A person experiencing the persecutory type believes without cause that another person is trying to harm him or is slandering him. A somatic-type individual believes that he emits foul body odors, that he is infested with insects or parasites, or that certain body parts are ugly, deformed, or nonfunctional.

Whereas schizophrenia usually develops in young adulthood, delusional (paranoid) disorder tends to appear later, usually without prominent hallucinations or bizarre behavior. The client may exhibit resentment and anger, which can lead to aggressive or violent behavior.

ETIOLOGY AND PRECIPITATING FACTORS
Biological research with twins indicates that delusional (paranoid) disorder may have a genetic cause and that people whose relatives display symptoms are more likely to develop the disorder.

Psychological theories maintain that paranoia results from a maladaptive parent-child relationship characterized by a lack of warmth, attention, and trust. The individual's subsequent insecurity leads to extreme anxiety and a guarded, suspicious behavior pattern.

Psychoanalytic theory maintains that paranoid delusions result from repressed homosexual tendencies. Individuals in conflict over these tendencies perceive the world as a hostile and threatening place. They typically use projection to defend the ego against this perceived assault, attributing negative qualities to the surrounding environment and the world in general. (See *Delusional disorders: The psychoanalytic theory*, page 104)

DELUSIONAL THEMES

Some common themes appear in delusions, including erotomania, grandiosity, jealousy, persecution, and somatic complaints. See below for an explanation of each type.

Erotomanic delusions
A prevalent theme, erotomanic delusions concern romantic or spiritual love. The client believes that he or she shares in a idealized (rather than sexual) relationship with someone of higher status—a superior at work, a celebrity, or an anonymous stranger. The client may hold this delusion in secret, but more commonly will try to contact the person through calls, letters, gifts, or even spying. The client may attempt to rescue the beloved person from imagined danger. Clients with erotomanic delusions commonly harass public figures and often come to the attention of the police.

Grandiose delusions
The client with grandiose delusions believes that he or she has great unrecognized talent, special insight, or prophetic power or has made an important discovery. To achieve recognition, the client may contact government agencies, such as the U.S. Patent Office or the FBI. The client with a religiously oriented delusion may become a cult leader. Less commonly, the client believes that he or she shares a special relationship with some well-known personality, such as a rock star or a world leader. The client may assume the identity of the famous person, believing that the famous person is really an impostor.

Jealous delusions
These delusions focus on fidelity. For example, a client may believe, without cause, that a lover has acted unfaithfully and may find evidence to justify the delusion, such as finding spots on the bed sheets. The client may confront the lover, try to control the lover's movements, follow the lover, or even track down the suspected paramour. The client may physically attack the lover or, in some cases, the perceived rival.

Persecutory delusions
The most common delusionary theme, persecutory delusions cause the client to believe that he or she is being followed, harassed, plotted against, poisoned, mocked, or deliberately prevented from achieving long-term goals. The client may perceive a simple or complex persecutory scheme. The client who develops a delusional system may interpret slight offenses as part of the scheme. The client perceiving injustice may file numerous lawsuits or seek redress from government agencies (querulous paranoia). The client who becomes resentful and angry may lash out violently against the perceived injurer.

Somatic delusions
The client may perceive a foul personal odor emitting from the skin, mouth, rectum, or other body part. Other delusions involve skin-crawling insects, internal parasites, and dysfunctional body parts.

From *Psychiatric problems*. NurseReview. Springhouse, PA: Springhouse Corp., 1990.

Assessment guidelines

NURSING HISTORY (Functional health pattern findings)

The client may report or exhibit one or more of the findings grouped here according to functional health patterns.

Health perception–health management pattern

• denial of illness, problems, or stressors

Nutritional-metabolic pattern

• concern about or evidence of weight loss secondary to fear that food is tampered with, poisoned, or rotten
• dehydration evidenced by dry mucous membranes, poor skin turgor, or concentrated urine

Activity-exercise pattern

• activity changes secondary to social withdrawal
• extreme anxiety and easy agitation

Sleep-rest pattern

• concern over or evidence of sleep disturbance secondary to fear, especially fear of harm

Cognitive-perceptual pattern

• belief that others are trying or want to hurt him
• actual incidents from which delusional beliefs are derived
• hypervigilance or scanning of the environment accompanied by misperceived observations
• lack of insight or understanding
• inability to acknowledge inaccurate perceptions
• use of projection as a primary defense for managing anger, resentment, and hostility unacceptable to the ego

Self-perception–self-concept pattern

• low self-esteem
• feelings of being victimized or persecuted

Role-relationship pattern

• difficulty relating to others
• inability to trust others
• poor social skills
• avoidance of social interactions or situations

Coping–stress tolerance pattern

• difficulty coping with anxiety
• increased paranoid thinking and behavior with high stress
• agitation or violence during stressful situations

Value-belief pattern

• belief that punishment is deserved

DELUSIONAL DISORDERS: THE PSYCHOANALYTIC THEORY

Psychoanalysts from Freud to Fenichal have attempted to fathom the cause of delusional disorders.

Sigmund Freud, for instance, explained paranoia as a response to repressed homosexual wishes. According to Freud, the repressed desire ("I love him") emerged as the opposite ("I hate him") and through projection became a persecutory delusion ("He hates me"). The notion that paranoia results from repressed homosexual wishes has since fallen out of favor, but Freud's view has greatly influenced modern concepts of projection and reaction formation.

Harry Stack Sullivan proposed that the paranoid person's deep sense of inferiority, insecurity, and rejection causes unbearable feelings of loneliness and unworthiness. The paranoid gains a sense of security by projecting painful feelings onto others.

Melanie Klein focused on fixations that occur in early stages of childhood development to explain delusional thinking. The child projects aggressive impulses onto the mother and then incorporates the mother as an internal persecutor. Although many of Klein's views are controversial, her theory made an important contribution by moving away from the Freudian focus on the libido as the source of aggressive behavior.

Otto Fenichal emphasizes the role of the superego in paranoid delusions. A strict superego and unrealistic personal expectations cause internalization of guilt and feelings of inadequacy, which are projected in the form of sadistic delusions.

From *Psychiatric problems.* NurseReview. Springhouse, PA: Springhouse Corp., 1990.

PHYSICAL FINDINGS

The client may report or exhibit one or more of the following physical findings.

Cardiovascular

• excess perspiration
• increased heart rate
• increased or decreased blood pressure
• orthostatic changes with psychotropic medications

Gastrointestinal

• constipation
• dry mouth

Genitourinary

• amenorrhea
• difficulty achieving or maintaining erection
• retarded ejaculation
• diminished sex drive

Musculoskeletal
- body posture alterations
- balance disturbance
- gait disturbances
- muscle tension
- restlessness

Neurologic
- catatonia
- dilated pupils
- hyperreflexia
- parkinsonian movements (such as tremors and pill-rolling finger movements)
- sensory abnormalities (such as hyperesthesia, hypoesthesia, or paresthesia)
- sleep disturbances (such as difficulty sleeping or staying asleep)

Psychological
- ambivalence
- anger
- anxiety
- apathy
- argumentativeness
- delusions
- emotional lability
- lack of facial expression
- hallucinations
- paranoia

Potential complications
If left untreated, delusional (paranoid) disorder can cause aggressive, violent behavior and weight loss from self-imposed dietary restrictions.

Nursing diagnosis: *Social isolation related to an inability to trust others*

NURSING PRIORITY: To help the client develop and use social skills and an effective support system

Interventions

1. Encourage the client to talk about feelings, but do not expect immediate trust.

2. Encourage the client to reveal delusions without engaging in a power struggle over their content.

3. Agree to do only realistic, possible things and then follow through with the plan. For example, you might agree to allow the client to take a walk with a staff member every Wednesday morning. Inform the client in advance if you are changing the plan.

4. Use a supportive, empathic approach to focus on the client's feelings about troubling events, situations, and conflicts.

5. Minimize the number of nurses on the client's care team, establishing a primary nurse or case manager.

6. Collaborate with the client when developing the plan of care and setting goals.

7. When setting limits on client behavior, communicate care and acceptance of the client as a worthwhile person.

Rationales

1. In the initial stages of treatment, the client lacks the capacity to trust; therefore, the nurse should work to ensure a predictable, honest, and safe environment.

2. Struggling over content may cause the client to perceive the nurse as a threat. Avoiding such struggles can foster trust between the nurse and client.

3. By demonstrating consistency and reliability with the client, the nurse can help establish a trusting and therapeutic relationship.

4. A supportive approach fosters trust. Focusing on feelings may eventually help the client to identify and reveal their causes (see *Dynamics of delusional thinking,* page 106, for contributing factors and mechanisms leading to and resulting from delusional thinking).

5. Assigning a regular care team provides consistency and continuity for the client; this, in turn, decreases anxiety and promotes trust.

6. Including the client in planning can help diminish suspicion while increasing the client's self-esteem and sense of control.

7. The client should feel cared for as a person even though behavior is unacceptable.

DYNAMICS OF DELUSIONAL THINKING

The client first uses denial to cope with pain. When this defense mechanism fails, the client projects personal thoughts onto others and develops a delusional system.

Contributing factors	Defenses	Symptoms

Anxiety, loss, rejection, isolation, fear, physical illness, sensory deprivation, narcissism, stress, low self-esteem, poor coping skills

Denial → Projection → Delusional thinking →

Anger, hostility, mistrust, secretiveness, pride, aloofness, superiority, delusions, hallucinations, ideas of reference

Rationalization to support delusional thinking

From *Psychosocial problems*. NurseReview. Springhouse, PA: Springhouse Corp., 1990.

---

8. Encourage and provide opportunities for participation and socialization in groups and group activities.

8. A suspicious and paranoid client needs encouragement to engage in social activities. Reality testing in selective, supportive group activities can increase socialization success.

9. Respond positively when the client participates in social activities and interacts successfully with others.

9. Rewarding adaptive behavior can enhance self-esteem and increase the likelihood that the behavior will continue.

10. Be aware of the client's personal space, and use touch judiciously.

10. The client may feel trapped if the nurse moves in too closely. This feeling can lead to insecurity, increased anxiety, and violence. The client also might interpret attempts at touch as aggression and respond violently.

11. Recognize signs and symptoms of increased anxiety, and take appropriate measures (such as providing emotional support and decreasing environmental stimuli) to prevent its escalation.

11. Early intervention can prevent anxiety from escalating to violent levels.

12. Teach the client alternative methods of coping with increased anxiety. These methods include verbalization of feelings, diversionary activities, rest periods, and relaxation techniques.

12. Such alternative coping methods represent new and useful skills. Learning them can enhance the client's self-esteem and self-control.

13. Help the client to identify behaviors that alienate others.

13. The client needs to understand that people usually interpret guarded and suspicious behavior as threatening and that this perception causes them to behave in a wary and cautious manner. Such a pattern only serves to reinforce the client's inaccurate perceptions.

14. Teach the family ways to cope with the client's paranoid thinking, such as not challenging the client about the content of the delusions.

14. Family members may be frightened, confused, or angered by the content of the client's delusions. Teaching them effective coping methods can increase their sense of control.

15. Provide the client and family with information about aftercare options, appointments, and emergency services, and opportunities for increasing social contacts.

15. Effective discharge teaching makes the client and family aware of options, decreases discharge anxiety, and facilitates a smoother transition.

Nursing diagnosis: *Altered nutrition, less than body requirements, related to a fear of eating*

NURSING PRIORITY: To help the client maintain adequate food and fluid intake

Interventions

1. Monitor the client's food and fluid intake and weight.

2. Give the client some control over food and dining location selection. When possible, serve the food in closed or original containers.

3. Provide the client with preferred fluids frequently throughout the day.

4. Ensure that the client is taking medications as prescribed.

Rationales

1. Careful monitoring can alert the nurse that the client may be refusing to eat for fear the food has been tampered with.

2. Allowing the client to select the food and dining location can provide a sense of control and decrease fears of food tampering. Offering the food in closed or original containers may allay fears and increase food intake, thereby maintaining adequate nutrition.

3. Adequate fluid intake ensures adequate hydration.

4. The client may be reluctant to take medications. Administering them in liquid form and checking the client's mouth to see that all the medication has been swallowed can help ensure compliance.

Outcome criteria

As treatment progresses, the client, family, or both should be able to:
• demonstrate improved social skills
• report feeling less suspicious and fearful of others
• demonstrate alternative coping methods
• initiate interactions with others
• describe the signs and symptoms of increasing anxiety.

Discharge criteria

Nursing documentation indicates that the client:
• has demonstrated improved reality testing
• has demonstrated less suspicious behavior
• can use alternate coping strategies
• can identify signs and symptoms of increased anxiety
• is aware of follow-up plans and support resources.

Nursing documentation also indicates that the family:
• reports the client is exhibiting less withdrawn and isolated behavior
• has been referred to the appropriate community support resources
• has scheduled follow-up appointments
• knows how to obtain emergency help.

Selected references

Ambrose, J. (1989). Joining in: Therapeutic groups for chronic patients. *Journal of Psychosocial Nursing, 27*(11), 28-34.

American Psychiatric Association Task Force Report (1989). *Treatments of psychiatric disorders.* Washington, DC: APA Press.

DeCongas, J.P.C. (1990). Exploring expressed emotion: Does it contribute to chronic mental illness? *Journal of Psychosocial Nursing, 28*(2), 31-34.

Goodwin, G., and Guze, S. (1989). *Psychiatric diagnosis* (4th ed.). New York: Oxford University Press.

Harris, J. (1990). Self-care actions of chronic schizophrenics associated with meeting solitude and social interaction requisites. *Archives of Psychiatric Nursing, 4*(5), 298-307.

Houseman, C. (1990). The paranoid person: A biopsychosocial perspective. *Archives of Psychiatric Nursing, 4*(3), 176-181.

Kelly, K., et al. (1990). Fostering self-help on an inpatient unit. *Archives of Psychiatric Nursing, 4*(3), 161-165.

Munro, A. (1987). Paranoid (delusional) disorders: DSM-III-R and beyond. *Comprehensive Psychiatry, 28*(1), 35-39.

Plante, T. (1989). Social skills training: A program to help schizophrenic clients cope. *Journal of Psychosocial Nursing, 27*(3), 6-10.

Whitley, G. (1991). Client's with delusional (paranoid) disorder. In G.K. McFarland and M.D. Thomas (Eds.), *Psychiatric mental health nursing: Application of the nursing process.* Philadelphia: Lippincott.

Miscellaneous Psychotic Disorders

DSM III-R classifications
295.40 Schizophreniform disorder
295.70 Schizoaffective disorder
297.30 Induced psychotic disorder
298.80 Brief reactive psychosis
298.90 Psychotic disorder not otherwise specified
  (atypical psychosis)

Psychiatric nursing diagnostic class
Disruption in relatedness

Introduction
Schizophreniform disorder closely resembles schizophrenia. However, unlike schizophrenia, schizophreniform disorder has a duration of less than 6 months and the client is likely to recover.

The distinguishing characteristics of *schizoaffective disorder* include a history of manic or depressive disorder with psychotic features, remission periods without residual symptoms, and delusions or hallucinations that are not mood congruent. These symptoms usually last more than 2 weeks but less than 6 months. The similarity of schizoaffective disorder to schizophrenia and schizophreniform disorder makes definitive diagnosis difficult.

Induced psychotic disorder occurs when an individual develops delusions as a result of a close relationship with a person who already has a psychotic disorder with prominent delusions. The content of the delusions is often based on the common experiences of the two individuals, who generally have lived together in isolation for a long time and who rarely seek treatment.

Brief reactive psychosis is characterized by a sudden onset of psychotic symptoms that occurs shortly after a stressful event. The individual experiences emotional conflict and turmoil, manifested by rapid, inappropriate changes in affect, overwhelming perplexity, and confusion. Transient hallucinations and delusions also can occur. Symptoms last at least 2 hours but no more than 1 month, and the individual eventually returns to the premorbid functioning state.

Psychotic disorders not otherwise specified (or *atypical psychosis*) describes disorders with psychotic symptoms that include delusions, incoherence, hallucinations, loose associations, disorganized behavior, and catatonic excitement or stupor. This classification is used only when symptoms do not meet the criteria for other nonorganic psychotic disorders.

ETIOLOGY AND PRECIPITATING FACTORS
Current biological research supports a link between genetics and the various miscellaneous psychotic disorders. Generally, researchers believe that individuals inherit a predisposition to the disorders; however, tracing the responsible gene is impossible because it may not manifest itself in every generation. Other research indicates that structural anomalies in the brain, as well as biochemical, metabolic, and electrical alterations, may cause these disorders.

Psychological theories implicate dysfunctional family relationships in schizophrenia-related disorders. Families that exhibit high conflict and anxiety are believed to foster maladaptive relationships in which parents become overly involved with their children. Such a relationship inhibits a child's ability to develop trust and autonomy—both important coping skills. In other cases, parents may convey conflicting messages, creating within the child emotional ambivalence and a disturbed self-image. Psychological researchers also propose that individuals with a history of schizophrenia-related disorders are more likely to suffer relapses when they come from families that are excessively critical, hostile, involved, and even supportive.

Assessment guidelines
NURSING HISTORY (Functional health pattern findings)
The client may report or exhibit one or more of the findings grouped here according to functional health patterns.

Health-perception–health-management pattern
• concern about abrupt symptom onset
• denial of symptoms or illness
• lack of concern about symptoms
• history of noncompliance with previous treatment or aftercare
• presence or severity of symptoms
• need for treatment
• poor physical health secondary to psychotic symptoms and disorganized thoughts
• weight loss
• poor hygiene and grooming

Nutritional-metabolic pattern
• weight loss secondary to apathy and lack of appetite or hyperactivity and distractibility
• fear that food is being tampered with

Elimination pattern
• constipation secondary to poor nutritional status or medication use

Activity-exercise pattern
• psychomotor agitation or retardation
• concern over symptoms interfering with ability to carry out normal daily activities or with usual functional level
• pacing to relieve anxiety
• hypervigilance
• decreased motivation and interest in activities
• restlessness secondary to adverse reactions to medication or psychotic symptoms
• disorganized or bizarre behavior and posturing

Sleep-rest pattern
• increased sleeping
• decreased sleeping caused by early morning awakening or insomnia
• insomnia secondary to hallucinations or delusions
• sedation secondary to medication

Cognitive-perceptual pattern
• concern about disturbed thinking
• hallucinations
• delusions
• decreased attention span
• difficulty concentrating
• disturbed thought processes (such as blocking, loose associations, flight of ideas, tangentiality, and ideas of reference)
• lack of insight or denial of illness

Self-perception–self-concept pattern
• grandiose thoughts
• feelings of powerlessness
• inability to meet expectations
• low or exaggerated self-esteem
• feelings of persecution

Role-relationship pattern
• disturbed interpersonal relationships secondary to symptom development
• altered ability to perform role of spouse, parent, or worker
• inability to trust others
• feelings of loneliness

Sexual-reproductive pattern
• hypersexuality
• decreased libido
• sexual dysfunction
• discomfort about masturbation

Coping–stress tolerance pattern
• feelings of being overwhelmed
• symptom exacerbation during stressful times
• escalation of symptoms from exposure to specific stressors

Value-belief pattern
• feelings of worthlessness, hopelessness, or helplessness
• paranoia or grandiose delusions
• delusions of having a different identity
• overreliance on or identification with religion or religious figures

PHYSICAL FINDINGS
The client may report or exhibit one or more of the following physical findings.

Cardiovascular
• excessive perspiration
• increased heart rate
• increased or decreased blood pressure
• orthostatic changes with psychotropic medications

Gastrointestinal
• constipation
• dry mouth

Genitourinary
• amenorrhea
• difficulty achieving or maintaining erection
• retarded ejaculation
• diminished sex drive

Musculoskeletal
• altered body posture
• balance disturbance
• gait disturbances
• muscle tension
• restlessness

Neurologic
• catatonia
• dilated pupils
• hyperreflexia
• parkinsonian movements (such as tremors and pill-rolling finger movements)
• sensory abnormalities (such as hyperesthesia, hypoesthesia, or paresthesia)
• sleep disturbances (such as inability to sleep or difficulty staying asleep)

Psychological
- ambivalence
- anger
- anxiety
- apathy
- argumentativeness
- delusions
- emotional lability
- absence of facial expression
- hallucinations
- paranoia

Potential complications

If left untreated, the client's condition may progress to aggressive, violent behavior, posing an immediate danger to the client and others.

The nurse should be aware that some disorders cause signs and symptoms similar to those of psychosis. An undiagnosed medical condition can lead to serious, even life-threatening problems. For a list of disorders that can produce similar signs and symptoms, see *Physical disorders that may mimic psychosis.*

PHYSICAL DISORDERS THAT MAY MIMIC PSYCHOSIS

The disorders listed below can produce signs and symptoms similar to those of psychosis:

Drug toxicity (corticosteroids, digitalis, disulfiram [Antabuse], isoniazid [Laniazid], levodopa [Dopar], and methyldopa [Aldomet])

Endocrine disorders (Addison's disease, Cushing's syndrome, hyperparathyroidism, hypoparathyroidism, and hypothyroidism)

Heavy metal poisoning (lead, manganese, mercury, and thallium)

Infections (bacterial meningitis, cerebrovascular syphilis, delirium related to cerebral infection, and postencephalitic syndrome)

Neurologic disorders (brain tumors, complex partial temporal lobe seizures, degenerative central nervous system diseases, hydrocephalus, and multiple sclerosis)

Substance abuse disorders (alcohol intoxication or withdrawal, amphetamine intoxication, barbiturate withdrawal, drug-induced mania, and phencyclidine intoxication)

Vitamin deficiencies (niacin, pyridoxine, and thiamine deficiencies and pernicious anemia)

Other disorders (atropine psychosis, general paresis, insecticide poisoning, pheochromocytoma, porphyria, Schilder's disease, systemic lupus erythematosus, tubercular meningitis, and Wilson's disease).

From *Psychosocial crises*. Clinical Skillbuilders. Springhouse, PA: Springhouse Corp., 1992.

Nursing diagnosis: *Ineffective individual coping related to misinterpretation of environment and impaired communication style*

NURSING PRIORITY: To help the client develop and use adaptive coping skills

Interventions

1. Provide the client with information and realistic feedback about symptoms.

2. In a nonjudgmental manner, encourage the client to verbalize feelings.

3. Encourage the client to explore adaptive behaviors that help in socializing and accomplishing normal daily activities.

4. Administer medication as ordered, and monitor the client's response.

5. Teach the client and family about the illness and treatment.

Rationales

1. By speaking frankly and accurately about the disorder, the nurse can develop trust and a therapeutic alliance with the client.

2. Talking about feelings can develop the client's awareness and understanding of emotional reactions.

3. Developing useful adaptive behaviors can enhance the client's self-esteem.

4. Medications can help diminish psychotic symptoms.

5. An informed client and family are more likely to comply with the treatment plan.

6. Ensure the safety of the client and others.

6. Because any psychotic client can become aggressive toward self and others, the nurse must implement interventions to ensure safety. Providing a safe, secure environment also increases client trust.

7. Collaborate with the client to establish a balanced daily schedule of activity and rest.

7. Because the client may exhibit disrupted sleep and activity patterns, establishing a balanced schedule can help restore optimal functioning.

Nursing diagnosis: *Altered health maintenance related to an inability to meet basic health needs consistently*

NURSING PRIORITY: To teach the client strategies for assuming health maintenance responsibilities

Interventions

1. Assess the client's health maintenance knowledge and capacity for self-care.

2. Teach and rehearse with the client behavior modification strategies, including cuing, behavioral contracting, anticipatory guidance, positive reinforcement, and keeping a daily journal.

3. Collaborate with the client to determine appropriate community support referrals, such as a local mental health center or the National Alliance for the Mentally Ill.

Rationales

1. Such assessment can help the nurse and client plan for the cognitive and perceptual restructuring necessary to change client behavior.

2. Such concrete problem-solving and cognitive strategies can help the client control inappropriate health-related behaviors.

3. External support systems can help the client maintain changes that promote health.

Outcome criteria

As treatment progresses, the client, family, or both should be able to:
• identify signs and symptoms of illness exacerbation
• demonstrate or verbalize improved judgment and insight
• display emotions that are appropriate and congruent
• demonstrate psychomotor behavior within the expected range
• verbalize or demonstrate appropriate reality testing
• demonstrate improved grooming and hygiene
• verbalize the need to plan for aftercare and emergency care.

• has demonstrated improved psychomotor behavior within acceptable limits
• is able to use alternative coping methods and socialization skills
• is aware of aftercare needs and plans.

Nursing documentation also indicates that the family:
• can identify symptoms of illness exacerbation
• has been referred to the appropriate community resources
• can cope with the client's illness
• has scheduled necessary follow-up appointments
• knows how to obtain emergency assistance if needed.

Discharge criteria

Nursing documentation indicates that the client:
• has demonstrated improved reality orientation
• has demonstrated an improved ability to perform normal daily activities
• has demonstrated a decline in or absence of violence directed at self and others

Selected references

Atwood, N. (1990). Integrating individual and family treatment for outpatients vulnerable to psychosis. *American Journal of Psychotherapy,* 44(2), 247-255.

Bardenstein, K.K., and McGlashan, T.H. (1990). Gender differences in affective, schizoaffective, and schizophrenic disorders: A review. *Schizophrenia Research,* 3(3), 159-172.

Bellack, A.S., Morrison, R.L., Mueser, K.T., and Wade, J. (1989). Social competence in schizoaffective disorder, bipolar disorder, and negative and non-negative schizophrenia. *Schizophrenia Research,* 2 (4-5), 391-401.

Buchanan, R.W., et al. (1990). Clinical correlates of the deficit syndrome of schizophrenia. *American Journal of Psychiatry,* 147(3), 290-294.

Fadden, G., Bebbington, P., and Kuiper, L. (1987). The burden of care: The impact of functional psychiatric illness on the patient's family. *British Journal of Psychiatry,* 150, 285-292.

Goodwin, G., and Guze, S. (1989). *Psychiatric diagnosis* (4th ed.). New York: Oxford University Press.

Greenfeld, D., Strauss, J.S., Bowers, M.B., and Mandelkern, M. (1989). Insight and interpretation of illness in recovery from psychosis. *Schizophrenia Bulletin,* 15(2), 245-252.

Marneros, A., and Tsuang, M.T. (1986). *Schizoaffective Psychoses.* New York: Springer-Verlag.

Romme, M.A.J., and Escher, A. (1989). Hearing voices. *Schizophrenia Bulletin,* 15(2), 209-216.

Salliger, N. (1988). Relapse. *Journal of Psychosocial Nursing,* 26(6), 20-23.

Samson, J.A., Simpson, J.C., and Tsuang, M.T. (1988). Outcome studies of schizoaffective disorders. *Schizophrenia Bulletin,* 14(4), 543-554.

Cluster A Personality Disorders

DSM III-R classifications
301.00 Paranoid personality disorder
301.20 Schizoid personality disorder
301.22 Schizotypal personality disorder

Psychiatric nursing diagnostic class
Relatedness disruptions

Introduction

Cluster A personality disorders, which generally begin in early adulthood, share certain characteristics, including eccentric behavior, suspicious ideation, and social isolation. In addition, the personality disorders discussed in this plan have their own peculiar features. For an overview of the major types (clusters) of personality disorders and their various subclassifications, see *Classifying personality disorders,* page 114.

Clients with *paranoid personality disorder* have a pervasive and unwarranted perception that others are deliberately demeaning or threatening them. Paranoid individuals usually are secretive, hypervigilant, and argumentative. They have difficulty confiding in others and search for any evidence of an impending attack. They generally do not seek psychiatric assistance on their own and rarely require hospitalization.

Schizoid personality disorder is characterized by a pervasive indifference to social relationships and a stable but restricted emotional range. Individuals with this disorder are typically "loners" who have no close friends and are not close to their family. They usually engage in solitary activities and display little if any desire for sexual relations. They may, however, perform adequately in the workplace if the occupation promotes social isolation (for example, a night security guard) and makes few demands on their abilities.

The distinguishing characteristics of *schizotypal personality disorder* include peculiar ideas (such as superstitious beliefs) and eccentric appearance and behavior. These deviations, however, are not severe enough to meet schizophrenia criteria. Under extreme stress, schizotypal individuals may experience psychotic symptoms, including paranoid ideation, suspicion, ideas of reference (belief that certain events are directly related to an individual, such as that Christmas is celebrated each year because the individual was born on December 25), odd beliefs, and magical thinking, as well as digressive, vague, and inappropriately abstract speech.

ETIOLOGY AND PRECIPITATING FACTORS

A higher incidence of personality disorders in identical twins than in fraternal twins seems to indicate that the disorders are genetically linked and transmitted. Further clinical research is required, however, before a biological theory can be formulated.

The object-relations theory suggests that age-appropriate ego development is arrested and that specific character types result, depending on the developmental stage involved. Consequently, the individual becomes unable to modify preconceived ideas and perceptions about how things should be, and immature behavior, feeling, and thinking ensue. For example, a 24-year-old client who became an alcoholic at age 12 will probably act more like an adolescent than a young adult.

Psychodynamic theorists suggest that the schizoid and schizotypal personality disorders result from disturbed mother-child relationships. The infant or child develops a primary defense mechanism and shuns relationships because of a perceived inability to give or receive love. Such a child grows into an adult who is unable to experience love and intimacy.

According to psychoanalytic theory, paranoid personality disorder develops from a child's projection of unacceptable feelings, thoughts, ideas, and impulses onto other people. Such projection enables the individual to avoid personal guilt or shame as well as internal conflict.

Family theorists believe that disrupted relationships and communications within the family lead to personality disorders. These theorists suggest that individuals raised with inconsistent or nonexistent parenting experience emotional deprivation that produces feelings of inadequacy and leads to inappropriate behaviors.

Assessment guidelines
NURSING HISTORY (Functional health pattern findings)
The client may report or exhibit one or more of the findings grouped here according to functional health patterns

Health perception–health management pattern
• minimal concern about general health
• no history of psychiatric disturbance
• no perceived need or desire for psychiatric intervention
• inability or reluctance to follow up on health care recommendations

CLASSIFYING PERSONALITY DISORDERS

Type and disorder		Characteristics
CLUSTER A: ODD, ECCENTRIC	**Paranoid**	• Pervasive, unwarranted mistrust of others, manifested by jealousy, envy, and guardedness • Hypersensitivity, frequent feelings of being mistreated and misjudged • Restricted affect, evidenced by lack of tenderness and poor sense of humor
	Schizoid	• Inability to form social relationships, absence of warm and tender feeling for others • Indifference to praise, criticism, and feelings of others • Apparently little or no desire for social involvement; few, if any, close friends • Generally reserved, withdrawn, and seclusive; preference for solitary interests or hobbies • Dull or flat affect, appears cold or aloof
	Schizotypal	• Various oddities of thought, perception, speech, and behavior • Possible magical thinking, ideas of reference, paranoid ideation, illusions, depersonalization, peculiarities in word choice, social isolation, and inappropriate affect
CLUSTER B: DRAMATIC, EMOTIONAL, ERRATIC, IMPULSIVE	**Histrionic**	• Lively, dramatic, attention-seeking behavior • Tantrums and angry outbursts • Demanding, egocentric, inconsiderate behavior • Manipulation and divisiveness • Seductive or charming behavior, superficial personal attachments
	Antisocial	• General disregard for others' rights and feelings • History of persistent antisocial behavior. • Poor school or job performance record • Inability to maintain close interpersonal relationships, especially a sexually intimate one • Superficial charm, often with manipulative and seductive behavior
	Narcissistic	• Exaggerated sense of self-importance, manifested by extreme self-centeredness • Preoccupation with fantasies involving power, success, wealth, beauty, or love • No capacity for empathy • Need for constant admiration and attention • Manipulative behavior
	Borderline	• Instability in interpersonal behavior, marked by intense and unstable relationships • Impulsive and unpredictable behavior • Profound, inappropriate shifts in mood and affect • Poor identity with uncertainty in such areas as self-image, sexual preference, and values
CLUSTER C: ANXIOUS, FEARFUL	**Obsessive-compulsive**	• Inability to express affection • Overly cold and rigid demeanor • Preoccupation with rules, trivial details, and other expressions of conformity • Superior attitude, need to control • Tendency toward perfection, valuing work more than pleasure or relationships
	Dependent	• Extreme self-consciousness, accompanied by feelings of inadequacy and helplessness • Dependency in relationships, subordinating own needs and leaving major decisions to others • Overly passive and compliant
	Avoidant	• Anxiety and fearfulness • Low self-esteem, hypersensitivity to potential humiliation, rejection, or shame • Social withdrawal accompanied by longing for close relationships
	Passive-aggressive	• Intentional inefficiency in social and occupational function • Resentment, sullenness, and stubbornness unaccompanied by overt hostility • Fear of authority

From *Psychiatric problems*. NurseReview. Springhouse, PA: Springhouse Corp., 1990.

Nutritional-metabolic pattern
• concern about using food to soothe self
• peculiar eating rituals or patterns (such as eating particular foods in a set order)

Elimination pattern
• constipation secondary to medication use

Activity-exercise pattern
• hypervigilance
• inability to relax
• significant self-restriction of daily activity

Sleep-rest pattern
• sleep disruption during times of stress
• excessive sleeping to avoid conflict

Cognitive-perceptual pattern
• transient ideas of reference
• absentmindedness
• magical thinking
• unusual perceptual experiences, such as clairvoyance and telepathy
• illusions
• indecisiveness
• poor decision-making abilities

Self-perception–self-concept pattern
• perception of self as a "loner"
• desire to be left alone
• self-centeredness
• guardedness
• secretiveness
• belief that others are to blame for personal mistakes
• eccentric behaviors (such as wearing a black cape and a straw hat when going out)

Role-relationship pattern
• need for rigid routines to function in occupation
• difficulties functioning at work
• fear of intimacy
• fear or suspicion of others
• anxiety in social settings
• avoidance of family gatherings
• no significant personal relationships

Sexual-reproductive pattern
• little or no desire to have sexual relations

Coping–stress tolerance pattern
• anger when stressed
• fear of losing control
• indifference to criticism
• psychotic symptoms when stressed

Value-belief pattern
• belief that others are threatening or trying to inflict harm
• belief in clairvoyance, telepathy, or a sixth sense

• belief that others are capable of "eavesdropping" on the client's thoughts and feelings

PHYSICAL FINDINGS
The client may report or exhibit one or more of the following physical findings.

Cardiovascular
• increased heart rate
• increased blood pressure

Respiratory
• increased respiratory rate when stressed and if psychotic symptoms develop

Gastrointestinal
• dry oral mucous membranes secondary to psychotropic medication use
• increased gastric acidity
• increased salivation

Genitourinary
• frequent urination

Integumentary
• bruises resulting from banging or hitting things

Musculoskeletal
• clenched fists
• muscle tension

Neurologic
• hypervigilance

Psychological
• aloofness
• anger
• anxiety in social settings
• unusual perceptual experiences (such as sensing that someone who is not present is actually in the room)
• feelings of constriction
• eccentric behavior or appearance
• digressive, vague, or overly abstract speech
• jealousy
• odd beliefs (such as belief in the ability to predict the future)
• paranoid ideation
• desire for social isolation
• suspicion of others
• little or no desire to forgive others

Potential complications
Certain features of paranoid personality disorder, such as suspicion and hypersensitivity, can predispose the client to delusional (paranoid) disorder or schizophrenia (paranoid type).

Nursing diagnosis: *Impaired social interaction related to disorganized thinking*

NURSING PRIORITY: To help the client identify feelings that inhibit social interaction

Interventions

1. Establish a good working relationship by listening and responding to the client and showing respect for thoughts and feelings.

2. Collaborate with the client to develop a schedule of specific social interactions and activities.

3. Review with the client the family's social behaviors as well as the ways family members relate among themselves. Identify any behavioral rules or expectations that the client may have learned from the family.

4. Encourage the client to participate in social interactions and provide objective feedback on individual behavior and its effects on others.

5. Encourage the client to identify personal behaviors that cause discomfort in social situations, thereby inhibiting socialization.

6. Teach the client strategies for changing undesirable social behaviors, such as teaching the client how and when to ask others for help. Allow the client to rehearse these strategies by role playing specific social situations. This can be done alone with the client or, if appropriate, in a group setting.

7. Help the client to assume responsibility for personal behavior. Suggest keeping a daily journal and making entries describing social situations, related feelings, socializing strategies, and degrees of success achieved.

8. Refer the client to appropriate community programs, support groups, and self-help lectures and programs. Encourage participation in these programs.

9. Encourage the client and family to participate in ongoing psychotherapy.

Rationales

1. A trusting relationship between the nurse and client helps to establish a safe environment in which the client can practice social interaction skills and prepare for future socialization.

2. Such a schedule can reduce the client's anxiety about social interactions and activities; it also helps to ensure participation in such activities.

3. Examining family behavior can help the nurse identify and understand the client's dysfunctional social behaviors.

4. The client who begins to comprehend how others perceive types of behaviors may feel more comfortable interacting socially.

5. Identifying factors that impair the client's social interactions can help the nurse develop appropriate interventions and help the client understand and overcome a desire for social isolation.

6. Rehearsing socializing strategies in a safe environment provides the client with immediate feedback, including praise for successes and recommendations for changing or revising behaviors.

7. Keeping a journal can help the client identify behavioral patterns and their causes. The journal also enables the client to evaluate the success of implemented socializing strategies.

8. Participation in such programs can reinforce positive behaviors, expand the client's social support network, and decrease opportunities for social isolation.

9. Ongoing psychotherapy can promote and maintain positive change for the client and family.

Nursing diagnosis: *Ineffective individual coping related to the client's inability to trust others, self-absorption, or unusual perceptions and communication patterns*

NURSING PRIORITY: To help the client cope with the current situation and feel safe and comfortable about changing behaviors

Interventions

1. Inform the client about the norms and rules of therapy and hospitalization, if appropriate.

Rationales

1. Explaining procedures and rules can help foster a trusting relationship between the nurse and client. Such a relationship can make the client feel more secure and help prevent unnecessary surprises.

2. Introduce the hospitalized client to the psychiatric unit or mental health center personnel, providing each person's name, title, and expected role or duties.

2. Knowing involved staff members can decrease the client's anxiety about uncertainty.

3. During the client's hospital stay, establish daily meetings and meet all scheduled commitments on time.

3. Establishing and maintaining a daily schedule helps to create a secure, predictable environment for the client and fosters trust.

4. Communicate clearly and concisely with the client.

4. Direct, unambiguous communication helps prevent misunderstanding and misinterpretation, which in turn enhances social interaction.

5. During interactions with the client, keep in mind that any client resistance to recommended changes is symptomatic of the condition and not a personal challenge.

5. Responding to client resistance in an unchallenging and unthreatening way can foster a trusting relationship.

6. Collaborate with the client and multidisciplinary team to establish a reward system for compliance with clearly defined expectations.

6. Tangible reinforcement for meeting expectations can strengthen the client's positive behaviors.

Outcome criteria

As treatment progresses, the client, family, or both should be able to:
• verbalize factors that cause impaired social interactions
• identify feelings that inhibit social interactions
• attend and participate willingly and actively in group and social activities
• verbalize and demonstrate decreased suspicion and increased security
• demonstrate the ability to establish new relationships.

Discharge criteria

Nursing documentation indicates that the client:
• has demonstrated the ability to engage in social exchanges
• has demonstrated an ability to receive and use constructive criticism
• can use newly acquired coping strategies in social situations
• is aware of available community and family resources
• has demonstrated a willingness to participate in follow-up therapy.

Nursing documentation also indicates that the family:
• understands the client's diagnosis, treatment, and expected outcomes
• can use new coping strategies to handle the client's condition
• has agreed to participate in a follow-up therapy program
• has been referred to the appropriate community resources.

Selected references

Akhtar, S. (1987). Schizoid personality disorder: A synthesis of developmental, dynamic, and descriptive features. *American Journal of Psychotherapy,* 41(4), 499-518.

Akhtar, S. (1990). Paranoid personality disorder: A synthesis of developmental, dynamic, and descriptive features. *American Journal of Psychotherapy,* 44(1), 5-25.

American Psychiatric Association (APA) (1987). *Diagnostic and statistical manual of mental disorders* (3rd ed. rev.). Washington, DC: APA Press.

Caplan, G. (1990). Loss, stress and mental health. *Community Mental Health Journal,* 26(1), 27-47.

Carr, A.C., Schwartz, F., and Fishler, P. (1989). The diagnosis of schizotypal personality disorder by use of psychological tests. *Journal of Personality Disorders,* 3(1), 36-44.

Cook, J.S., and Fontaine, K.L. (1991). *Essentials of mental health nursing* (2nd ed.). Redwood City, CA: Addison-Wesley.

Doenges, M.E., and Moorhouse, M.F. (1991). *Nursing diagnoses with interventions* (3rd ed.). Philadelphia: F.A. Davis.

Glantz, K., and Goisman, R.M. (1990). Relaxation and merging in the treatment of personality disorders. *American Journal of Psychotherapy,* 44(3), 405-13.

Greenberg, D., and Stravynski, A. (1985). Patients who complain of social dysfunction as their main problem: I: Clinical and demographic features. *Canadian Journal of Psychiatry,* 30(3), 206-211.

Hymowitz, P., Frances, A., Jacobsberg, L.B., Sickles, M., and Hoyt, R. (1986). Neuroleptic treatment of schizotypal personality disorders. *Comprehensive Psychiatry,* 27(4), 267-671.

Jenike, M.A., Baer, L., Minichiello, W.E., Schwartz, C.E., and Carey, R.J., Jr. (1986). Concomitant obsessive-compulsive disorder and schizotypal personality disorder. *American Journal of Psychiatry*, 143(4), 530-532.

Lieberz, K. (1989). Children at risk for schizoid disorders. *Journal of Personality Nursing Disorders*, 3(4), 329-337.

Livesley, W.J., and Schroeder, M.L. (1990). Dimensions of personality disorder: The DSM III-R Cluster A Diagnoses. *Journal of Nervous and Mental Disease*, 178(10), 627-635.

McLemore, C., and Brokaw, D. (1987). Personality disorders as dysfunctional interpersonal behavior. *Journal of Personality Disorders*, 1(3), 270-285.

Rosenfarb, I.S., Hayes, S.C., and Linehan, M.M. (1989). Instructions and experiential feedback in the treatment of social skills deficits in adults. *Psychotherapy*, 26(2), 242-251.

Schulz, S.C., Schulz, P.M., and Wilson, W.H. (1988). Medication treatment of schizotypal personality disorder. *Journal of Personality Disorders*, 2(1), 1-13.

Thompson-Pope, S.K., and Turkat, I.D. (1990). Reactions to ambiguous stimuli among paranoid personalities. *Journal of Psychopathology and Behavioral Assessment*, 10(1), 21-32.

Trull, T.J., Widiger, T.A., and Frances, A. (1987). Covariation of criteria sets for avoidant, schizoid, and dependent personality disorders. *American Journal of Psychiatry*, 144(6), 767-771.

Turkat, I.D., and Banks, D.S. (1987). Paranoid personality and its disorder. *Journal of Psychopathology and Behavioral Assessment*, 9(3), 295-304.

Turner, S.M. (1987). The effects of personality disorder diagnosis on the outcome of social anxiety symptom reduction. *Journal of Personality Disorder*, 1(2), 136-143.

Williams, J.G. (1988). Cognitive intervention for a paranoid personality disorder. *Psychotherapy*, 25(4), 570-575.

Cluster B Personality Disorders

DSM III-R classifications
301.50 Histrionic personality disorder
301.70 Antisocial personality disorder
301.81 Narcissistic personality disorder
301.83 Borderline personality disorder

Psychiatric nursing diagnostic class
Altered self-concept

Introduction

Cluster B personality disorders are referred to as ego-syntonic, meaning that the client does not believe the symptoms to be disturbing. Consequently, the client rarely seeks treatment unless related difficulties, such as substance abuse or court-ordered treatment, necessitate it.

Histrionic personality disorder, characterized by overly dramatic and controlling behavior, commonly affects attractive and quite seductive people. That this disorder has traditionally been noted more frequently in women than in men may be related more to social and cultural conventions than to actual incidence.

Antisocial personality disorder is characterized by a complete lack of empathy toward and total disregard of others' thoughts and feelings. Clients with this disorder project murderous rage and libidinous impulses onto everyone and may boast without remorse of physically or emotionally hurting others. In addition, those with antisocial personality have little or no ability to postpone gratification and, as a result, reject routines, compromises, and anything that may involve authority figures. They frequently change jobs or schools, habitats, and relationships. Risk taking and an accident history are prevalent among such individuals.

Persons with *narcissistic personality disorder* may seem socially engaging on the surface but cold or empty inside. When involved in a relationship, they may be exploitative and even overdependent, oscillating between idealizing and disdaining their loved one. Though commonly described as dependent individuals, those with narcissistic personalities usually have a derogatory view of others and are in fact unable to depend on or trust anyone else.

The client with *borderline personality disorder* typically exhibits extreme instability commonly accompanied by self-mutilation, intense fear of being alone, and complaints of being easily bored. Those with borderline personality disorder tend to make mean, satiric comments and frequently display an uncanny talent for identifying and dwelling on another's insecurities.

See *Classifying personality disorders,* page 114, for additional information on these disorders.

ETIOLOGY AND PRECIPITATING FACTORS

Psychodynamic explanations of cluster B personality disorders emphasize the presence and interrelation of several concepts, which are defined below:

• *Denial* represents an unconscious attempt to avoid unacceptable or threatening feelings. The individual using denial cannot express feelings adequately and therefore may act out in unacceptable, sometimes self-destructive ways.

• *Splitting,* which normally develops soon after birth, is an anxiety-reducing defense mechanism by which an infant differentiates between self-images and object-images and perceives good as coming from one object and bad from another object. As ego integration occurs and the child learns to distinguish good traits from bad and their ability to coexist in one person, a unified, stable identity develops, and splitting becomes unnecessary. When ego integration does not occur, the individual continues to separate the self and others into good and bad categories; thus, the boundaries between the self and objects remain blurred and splitting continues.

• *Projection* refers to the act of attributing an aspect of the self to someone else. The individual who uses projection does not experience the projected aspect as a part of the self but only as belonging to the other person.

• *Projective identification* is a mechanism by which an individual projects an unwanted aspect onto another person but continues to experience it as a part of the self.

• *Symbiosis* describes the normal interrelationship between an infant and mother or primary caregiver. At the toddler stage, the child normally begins to depend less and less on the symbiotic relationship and to assert individuality. The client with a personality disorder, however, may maintain this symbiotic relationship with the parent or develop one with an idealized parent figure. Separation from the parent or parent figure can cause frustration, fear, and self-destructive feelings.

• *Narcissism* refers to the practice of seeing another person as an idealized extension of the self. The idealized person is usually manipulated and treated possessively. *Omnipotence* is a similar concept in which the individual feels a sense of unlimited power and authority over others.

Behavioral theorists believe that personality disorders reflect several complex behaviors linked in repetitive patterns. The first is a conditioned response to fear. Classically conditioned fear responses are automatic physiological responses to external cues, such as loud voices, perceived criticism, and touching. Such responses result in the arousal of the sympathetic nervous system and release of epinephrine and norepinephrine. As a result, pulse rate, blood pressure, respiratory rate, and sweating increase. Other conditioned responses are more complex. To a person who has become used to crises and fear, even a seemingly innocuous cue can trigger hostile or withdrawn behavior. For example, a nurse trying to increase the client's comfort may be met with such a remark as "My, aren't we being helpful today."

According to behavioral theorists, another behavior represents a response to inconsistencies between behaviors and responses. For example, when a laboratory animal is given a food pellet followed randomly by a shock or nothing, it will begin to display signs of fear. The animal may quiver and behave tentatively, unsure of whether or not to respond, let alone which response to try. Likewise, a person will eventually perceive an unpredictable environment as hostile and will engage in manipulative behaviors that elicit predictable responses from others. Even behaviors that evoke consistently negative responses are preferable if they decrease randomness.

Behavioralist research also indicates that when positive behavior elicits no response or only random praise while negative or dramatic behavior consistently elicits attention, a person will begin to view the negative attention as positive. A negative response, such as punishment, may be perceived as an expression of attention, even of love.

Family systems theories indicate that children in dysfunctional families eventually believe that their family is typical and that if anything hurtful or wrong occurs, they are to blame. Trying to act as adults without the corresponding coping strategies, these children typically become accustomed to crises and have difficulty differentiating emotionally between themselves and others. They also have difficulty saying "No" and rarely feel good about themselves. Even when such children are grown and physically distant, they may continue to use coping strategies from childhood. For example, a boy who responded to parental conflict by climbing out of his bedroom window and running away may as an adult respond to conflict with a loved one by leaving the house.

Other family systems research indicates that physical and sexual abuse plays an important part in personality disorder development. Chronic abuse can lead to a diminished sense of self-worth and a decreased ability to trust others. The abused person may describe the resultant low self-esteem and dissociation as "hollowness" or "emptiness" and perceive the world as hostile.

Cognitive theories maintain that a person who is abused verbally with words such as "bad," "crazy," "stupid," or "ugly," eventually feels victimized and inferior. The person ends up thinking that the bad things are happening because the person is bad and deserves what occurs. Therefore, such a person will probably not ask for help.

Assessment guidelines
NURSING HISTORY (Functional health pattern findings)
The client may report or exhibit one or more of the findings grouped here according to functional health patterns.

Health perception–health management pattern
• real or perceived crises
• substance abuse
• fear of losing control, "going crazy," or being abandoned
• anxiety
• restlessness or irritability
• tendency to attribute difficulties to anyone else but self
• frustration with not being understood by health care providers
• denial of the extent of drug or alcohol use

Nutritional-metabolic pattern
• finickiness about or lack of interest in food
• weight gain or loss
• anorexia, bulimia, or bulimarexia

Elimination pattern
• frequent use of laxatives or cathartics
• diarrhea, flatulence, or irritable bowel
• excessive focus on elimination patterns
• frequent urination

Activity-exercise pattern
• decreased energy
• excessive exercise
• exhaustively detailed descriptions of activities
• withdrawn or seclusive feelings
• difficulties relaxing and engaging in leisure activities

Sleep-rest pattern
• insomnia, early morning awakening, nightmares, or unusually vivid dreams
• substance use or abuse to aid sleep
• fears related to going to bed, including hypervigilance, difficulty sleeping alone, sleeping on couch or floor, or needing a nightlight
• expectation of being exempt from hospital unit schedule

Cognitive-perceptual pattern
• disturbed body image
• difficulty concentrating
• difficulty with recent memory
• suspicion or paranoia about interview with nurse or physician
• vague somatic complaints such as generalized muscle aches
• impaired social judgment

Self-perception–self-concept pattern
- poor self-esteem and feelings of worthlessness or emptiness
- poor frustration tolerance
- increased irritability
- increased anxiety
- feelings of powerlessness, helplessness, or hopelessness
- exaggerated sense of abilities
- distorted body image
- ambivalence regarding self and decision-making and task-completion abilities
- confusion about gender, gender role, or sexual orientation

Role-relationship pattern
- feelings of not being understood or supported by loved ones
- detachment from loved ones
- tendency to deny or minimize relationship's importance
- history of multiple relationships
- history of physical or sexual abuse
- being overinvolved with or estranged from family
- being overwhelmed by work or school
- history of multiple jobs
- feeling adequate or competent only at work or school
- social withdrawal and increased sense of isolation
- suspicious, guarded, seductive, irritable, controlling, or condescending behaviors
- being victimized in abusive relationships
- frequent crises in relationships

Sexual-reproductive pattern
- difficulties with intimacy
- engaging in indiscriminate sex, sometimes with multiple partners at one time or when the risk of "getting caught" is high
- sporadic or no use of contraception
- little or no satisfaction with sexual relationships

Coping–stress tolerance pattern
- chronic or acute muscle tension in back, neck, or back of head
- poor frustration tolerance
- chronic irritability
- impulsive engagement in high-risk activities (such as mountain climbing or hang gliding)
- chemical substance use for stress relief
- self-mutilation as means of stress relief
- inability to identify stress or how to cope with it
- frequent suicidal thoughts
- alternating social withdrawal and overinvolvement

Value-belief system
- religious fanaticism or magical thinking
- perception of self as superior to or having no need for religion
- hopelessness
- spiritual distress
- rage concerning spiritual issues
- guilt caused by spiritual distress

PHYSICAL FINDINGS
The client may report or exhibit one or more of the following physical findings.

Cardiovascular
- cold, clammy skin
- elevated blood pressure
- hot and cold flashes
- increased heart rate
- palpitations
- sweating
- tingling sensation

Respiratory
- increased respiratory rate
- shortness of breath
- smothering sensation
- choking sensation

Gastrointestinal
- dry mouth
- abdominal distress
- nausea
- vomiting
- diarrhea
- difficulty swallowing

Genitourinary
- frequent urination

Musculoskeletal
- increased fatigue
- muscle aches, pains, or soreness
- muscle tension
- restlessness
- shakiness
- trembling
- twitching

Neurologic
- dilated pupils
- dizziness or faintness
- light-headedness
- paresthesia
- restlessness

Psychological
- feeling keyed up or on edge
- inability to concentrate
- irritability
- blank mind
- sleep disturbance (such as insomnia or early awakening)

Potential complications

Undiagnosed medical reasons for anxiety symptoms may lead to the exaggeration of previously problematic yet adaptive behaviors. Furthermore, explosiveness, dramatic behavior, social withdrawal, and self-absorption may indicate cranial changes associated with such conditions as tumors or aneurysms.

Nursing diagnosis: *Potential for violence, self-directed or directed at others, related to depression or low self-esteem*

NURSING PRIORITY: To ensure that the client will not harm self or others

Interventions

1. Establish a contract by which the client agrees to inform the staff when the client feels out of control.

2. Search the client's belongings and remove sharp objects, belts, and medications that can be used harmfully.

3. Clearly define for the client treatment expectations and rules as well as the consequences of noncompliance.

4. Document and communicate the plan of care to all staff and enlist their cooperation.

5. Use an appropriate degree of observation, seclusion, or restraints and prescribed medications to prevent the client from harming self or others.

6. Observe the client for verbal and nonverbal cues indicating increased agitation.

7. Work with the client to establish a meeting schedule. Be sure to arrive promptly for any scheduled meeting.

8. Work with the calm client, preferably during a planned meeting, to identify events that trigger harmful behavior.

Rationales

1. Such an agreement can increase the client's self-control and understanding that behavioral choices are available.

2. Removing potentially harmful objects provides a safe environment for the client and others and communicates to the client that the staff is concerned about personal safety.

3. Communicating directly and clearly helps the client understand that external controls will ensure safety even when personal controls are collapsing. This, in turn, can make the client feel more secure.

4. Communication among the members of the treatment team helps to ensure consistency and increases predictability during treatment.

5. Providing external controls and structure reduces the client's potential for impulsive harm.

6. If the nurse intervenes early to prevent violent and harmful behavior, the client will probably be permitted to remain in a less restrictive environment.

7. Collaboration between the nurse and client can increase predictability and reinforce normal behavior by decreasing the client's need for attention.

8. Identifying internal triggers that lead to harmful behaviors can enhance the client's sense of self-control and decrease feelings of powerlessness.

Nursing diagnosis: *Fear related to impulsiveness, poor judgment, or feelings of hopelessness, helplessness, powerlessness, or low self-esteem*

NURSING PRIORITY: To help diminish incapacitating anxiety and allow the client to feel safe

Interventions

1. When interacting with the client, use a candid, calm, steady approach.

Rationales

1. The nurse must guard against becoming upset by the client's behavior to ensure the client's sense of safety and security.

2. Use a formal, not overly familiar, approach, and respect the client's sense of personal space.

2. Formal, respectful nursing behavior, both physical and verbal, helps to decrease the client's confusion about boundaries. It also helps to decrease client suspicion while increasing trust.

3. Define expected client behaviors, and explain why they are desired.

3. By clearly defining expected behaviors, the nurse increases predictability for the client.

4. Consistently maintain the limits set for client behaviors, and expect the client to test these limits frequently.

4. Maintaining behavioral limits increases predictability and communicates to the client that the nurse is in control.

5. Avoid unnecessary confrontations and power struggles by establishing clear expectations for client behavior in various settings.

5. The client may attempt to involve the nurse in many power struggles. The nurse must decide which ones are important and require follow-up interventions.

6. Hold the client responsible for behaviors.

6. Insisting on such responsibility can help the nurse develop a collaborative as opposed to an adversarial relationship with the client. Doing so also gives the client a sense of self-control.

7. Work with the client to schedule meetings. Avoid meeting when the client is acting out.

7. Regularly scheduled meetings increase predictability; refusing to meet with a client who is acting out reinforces normal behavior.

Nursing diagnosis: *Impaired social interaction related to behaviors that produce hostility in others, low self-esteem, or poor social skills*

NURSING PRIORITY: To help the client learn more appropriate behaviors

Interventions

1. Identify nonverbal behaviors that the client uses when acting out or manipulating others, such as throwing hands up in the air, winking, or smiling.

2. Set appropriate expectations for social interaction, being careful not to fall short of or tax the client's abilities.

3. Teach the client more appropriate behaviors through role playing, suggestions, and written assignments (such as listing desired objects or activities and the means to acquire them).

4. Avoid forming unrealistic expectations about the client's ability to stop using splitting as a defense mechanism. Expect a decrease in this behavior instead.

5. Provide a structured setting in which the client and family can talk calmly with each other about the disorder and its ramifications.

Rationales

1. By recognizing these behaviors and not responding positively to them, the nurse can avoid unintentionally reinforcing the client's dysfunctional behaviors.

2. The client will quickly interpret low expectations as demeaning. Expectations exceeding the client's abilities will frustrate both the nurse and client.

3. The client needs to learn new, more appropriate behaviors to replace those that are being discarded.

4. Years of therapy are required before splitting, a core element of personality disorders, can be brought under control, if at all.

5. A supportive environment, both before and after discharge, can promote client progress.

Nursing diagnosis: *Ineffective individual coping related to feelings of loneliness, emptiness, boredom, poor impulse control, poor frustration tolerance, or fear of abandonment*

NURSING PRIORITY: To help the client make connections among thoughts, feelings, and behaviors

Interventions	Rationales
1. Collaborate with the client to schedule meetings. Avoid meeting when the client is acting out.	1. Regularly scheduled meetings increase predictability; refusing to meet with a client who is acting out can reinforce normal behavior.
2. Use a formal, not overly familiar, approach, and respect the client's sense of personal space.	2. Formal, respectful nursing behavior, both physical and verbal, helps decrease the client's confusion about boundaries. It also decreases suspiciousness while increasing trust.
3. Discuss with the client the consequences of behavior, such as keeping others at a distance; during calm periods, suggest some effective alternatives. Keep in mind that you may have to identify some effects on others because the client will probably be incapable of emphathizing with others and understanding their feelings.	3. Frank but supportive conversations provide the client with objective responses to behavior and may encourage some behavioral risks. Such conversations also may provide the client with evidence that not all interactions result in rejection.
4. Encourage the client to use the words "I" and "me" when referring to self.	4. Using the words "I" and "me" helps reverse the dissociative process and forces the client to assume responsibility for personal feelings.
5. Work with the client, preferably during planned meeting times, to identify events that trigger acting-out behaviors.	5. Identifying behavioral triggers can help the client to see relationships between internal and external events and behaviors. This new understanding helps increase the client's sense of self-control.
6. Help the client to identify manipulative behaviors, focusing on observable behaviors.	6. Helping the client to view behavior more objectively can decrease the perception of others as extensions of the self.
7. Be aware of your reactions to the client's behaviors. Tell the client how the behaviors make you feel.	7. If the client can understand that the nurse is a separate person with feelings, the client's perception of others as extensions of the self should decrease.
8. Limit interactions with the client to a few consistent staff members.	8. Limited interactions can increase the client's sense of predictability, which in turn promotes trust.

Outcome criteria

As treatment progresses, the client, family, or both should be able to:
• demonstrate adherence to an agreed upon plan not to harm self or others.
• verbalize when feeling out of control and seek assistance from appropriate persons
• demonstrate reduced manipulative behaviors and make consistent statements to different staff members
• refer to the self as "I" or "me"
• arrive punctually for therapy sessions
• demonstrate acceptance of some responsibility for present difficulties
• identify some connections among thoughts, feelings, and behaviors
• talk to other family members calmly.

Discharge criteria

Nursing documentation indicates that the client:
• has regularly exhibited nonviolent behavior
• has demonstrated ability to seek help from staff as an alternative to self-destructive behaviors
• has demonstrated a desire not to harm self or others and to learn other coping behaviors
• has demonstrated an ability to make some connections among thoughts, feelings, and behaviors
• consistently refers to self as "I" and "me"
• is aware of available appropriate community resources.

Nursing documentation also indicates that the family:
• has demonstrated the ability to identify sources of internal and external support
• verbalizes an understanding of the client's diagnosis, treatment, and expected outcomes
• verbalizes an understanding of usual and unusual responses to any prescribed medication
• understands when, why, and how to contact the appropriate health care professional in case of an emergency
• has been referred to the appropriate community and family support groups
• demonstrates a willingness to participate in follow-up therapy.

Selected references

American Psychiatric Association (APA) (1987). *Diagnostic and statistical manual of mental disorders* (3rd ed. rev.). Washington, DC: APA Press.

Barry, P.D. (1989). *Psychosocial nursing assessment and intervention: The care of the physically ill person*, (2nd ed.). Philadelphia: Lippincott.

Blume, S.B. (1989). Dual diagnosis: Psychoactive substance dependence and the personality disorders. *Journal of Psychoactive Drugs*, 21(2), 139-144.

Cook, J.S., and Fontaine, K.L. (1991). Personality disorders. In J.S. Cook and K.L. Fontaine (Eds.), *Essentials of mental health nursing* (2nd ed.). Redwood City, CA: Addison-Wesley.

Doenges, M.E., Townsend, M.C., and Moorhouse, M.F. (1989). *Psychiatric care plans: Guidelines for client care*. Philadelphia: Davis.

Feldman, T.B. (1990). Patients with other personality disorders. In S. Lewis, R.D. Grainger, W.A. McDowell, R.J. Gregory, and R.L. Messner (Eds.). *Manual of psychosocial nursing interventions: Promoting mental health in medical-surgical settings*. Philadelphia: Saunders.

Fine, M.A., and Sansone, R.A. (1990). Dilemmas in the management of suicidal behavior in individuals with borderline personality disorder. *American Journal of Psychotherapy*, 44(2), 160-171.

Freeman, S.K. (1988). Inpatient management of a patient with borderline personality disorder: A case study. *Archives of Psychiatric Nursing*, 2(6), 360-365.

Gallop, R. (1988). Escaping borderline stereotypes: Working through the maze of staff-patient interactions. *Journal of Psychosocial Nursing and Mental Health Services*, 26(2), 16-20.

Glantz, K., and Goisman, R.M. (1990). Relaxation and merging in the treatment of personality disorders. *American Journal of Psychotherapy*, 44(3), 405-413.

Goldstein, W.N. (1991). Clarification of projective identification. *American Journal of Psychiatry*, 148(2), 153-161.

Gordon, M. (1987). *Nursing diagnosis: Process and application* (2nd ed.). New York: McGraw-Hill.

Greene, J.A. (1989). Maladaptation: The personality disorders. In B.S. Johnson (Ed.). *Adaptation and growth: Psychiatric-mental health nursing* (2nd ed.). Philadelphia: Lippincott.

Griese, A.A., Leibenluft, E., Filson, C.R., Zimmerman, E.A., and Gardner, D.L. (1990). The effect of borderline personality disorder on the hospital course of affective illness. *Hospital and Community Psychiatry*, 41(9), 988-992.

Kay, S.R., Wolkenfeld, F., and Murrill, L.M. (1988). Profiles of aggression among psychiatric patients. *Journal of Nervous and Mental Disease*, 176(9), 539-545.

Kroessler, D. (1990). Personality disorder in the elderly. *Hospital and Community Psychiatry*, 41(12), 1325-1329.

Meisner, W.W. (1980). A note on projective identification. *Journal of the American Psychoanalytic Association*, 28(1), 43-67.

Morton, G.B. (1990). The patient with an antisocial personality disorder. In S. Lewis, R.D. Grainger, W.A. McDowell, R.J. Gregory, and R.L. Messner (Eds.). *Manual of psychosocial nursing interventions: Promoting mental health in medical-surgical settings*. Philadelphia: Saunders.

Piccinino, S. (1990). The nursing care challenge: Borderline patients. *Journal of Psychosocial Nursing and Mental Health Services*, 28(4), 23-27, 40-41.

Steele, K. (1989). Looking for answers: Understanding multiple personality disorder. *Journal of Psychosocial Nursing and Mental Health Services*, 27(8), 5, 33-34.

Cluster C Personality Disorders

DSM III-R classifications
301.40 Obsessive-compulsive personality disorder
301.60 Dependent personality disorder
301.82 Avoidant personality disorder
301.84 Passive-aggressive personality disorder
301.90 Personality disorder not otherwise specified

Psychiatric nursing diagnostic class
Relatedness disruption

Introduction

Cluster C personality disorders typically begin in adolescence or earlier and continue throughout adulthood, diminishing in middle age. These disorders share certain common characteristics, including fearfulness and high anxiety. They also have their own specific features. See *Classifying personality disorders*, page 114, for more information.

Individuals with *obsessive-compulsive personality disorder* typically are rigid, inflexible, indecisive, ruminative, perfectionistic, moralistic, emotionally and cognitively blocked, and highly judgmental of themselves and others. They generally are unable to express emotions and use rituals and rules to maintain control and manage feelings of helplessness and powerlessness.

Dependent personality disorder is characterized by dependent and submissive behavior. Individuals with this disorder experience significant difficulty making everyday decisions and require excessive advice, direction, and reassurance from others. They have difficulty initiating projects, experience devastation and helplessness when close relationships end, and are preoccupied with the fear of being abandoned.

Individuals with *avoidant personality disorder* generally develop in early adulthood a fear of negative evaluation and timidity. They usually expect rejection and are self-deprecating, easily hurt by criticism, and devastated by disapproval. Typically, they have few or no close friends other than first-degree relatives and are unwilling to become involved unless they can be certain of being liked by the other person. Once a relationship is established, however, they tend to be very clinging and fearful of losing it.

Passive-aggressive personality disorder is characterized by passive resistance to others' requests and demands and other manipulative interpersonal behavior. Characteristic behaviors include procrastination, poor work performance, and forgetfulness of obligations. Individuals with this disorder typically fear conflict and overt expressions of anger and consequently manage these feelings with underlying hostility and sabotage.

A diagnosis of *personality disorder not otherwise specified* is used when features of the disorder do not meet the full criteria of any one personality disorder type but significantly interfere with social or occupational functioning. Such disorders include *immature personality disorder*, *impulsive personality disorder*, *sadistic personality disorder*, and *self-defeating personality disorder*. For a comparison of the characteristics displayed in *sadistic personality disorder* and *self-defeating personality disorder*, see *Comparing sadistic and self-defeating personality disorders*.

ETIOLOGY AND PRECIPITATING FACTORS

Cluster C personality disorders, like Cluster A disorders, are more prevalent in identical twins than in fraternal twins. This finding points to a genetic link, but further clinical research is needed before a biological theory can be formulated.

The object-relations theory suggests that when age-appropriate ego development is arrested, specific character types result, depending on the developmental stage involved. As a result, the individual becomes unable to modify preconceived ideas and perceptions about how things should be, and immature behavior, feelings, and thinking develop.

Family theorists maintain that individuals raised with inconsistent or nonexistent parenting are emotionally deprived and never learn appropriate behaviors; the consequent feelings of inadequacy lead to personality disorders. Family theorists also believe that passive-aggressive personality disorder is more likely to develop in families that do not tolerate overt expressions of feelings, especially anger. The children of such families learn to express hostility and anger through subtle, rebellious behaviors.

Assessment guidelines

NURSING HISTORY (Functional health pattern findings)
The client may report or exhibit one or more of the findings grouped here according to functional health patterns.

Health perception–health management pattern
• anxiety
• numerous minor, chronic physical complaints or illnesses
• fatigue from compulsive working
• inability to assume responsibility for behavior
• history of physical or sexual abuse

COMPARING SADISTIC AND SELF-DEFEATING PERSONALITY DISORDERS

Compared with each other, sadistic and self-defeating personality disorders represent the opposite ends of the spectrum of personality problems.

Sadistic personality disorder

The client with sadistic personality disorder may humiliate others in private or in public, enforce overly harsh discipline on individuals under the client's control, take pleasure in the psychological or physical suffering of others (including animals), or commit acts of violence, aggression, exploitation, or even terror. Such a client does not use violence to achieve some impersonal goal, but views cruelty and domination as an end in itself.

The client is likely to dominate friends and family and may restrict their movements—for example, by refusing to allow them to attend social functions outside the home. The client may collect weapons, martial arts paraphernalia, and books or videotapes with violent themes. This behavior is directed toward more than one individual and is not solely for the purpose of sexual arousal.

Self-defeating personality disorder

In this disorder, the affected client is resigned to failure, suffering, and exploitation. The client believes the misfortunes are justified and willingly develops harmful relationships with others.

The client typically rejects or ignores efforts of those who offer help. Following success, the client experiences depression and guilt and reverts to self-defeating behavior. Despite demonstrated ability, the client often fails to accomplish his objectives. The client also may deliberately provoke anger from an acquaintance and later feel rejected and hurt. Such a client refuses to acknowledge the few occasions that provide enjoyment and acts submissive and self-sacrificing, regardless of whether others want or expect such acquiescence.

From *Psychiatric problems*. NurseReview. Springhouse, PA: Springhouse Corp., 1990.

Nutritional-metabolic pattern
• dietary deficiencies and imbalances
• concern about weight
• skin problems, such as rashes or hives

Elimination pattern
• concern over gastrointestinal disturbances
• frequent or urgent urination
• difficulty controlling urination
• excessive perspiration

Activity-exercise pattern
• restlessness
• withdrawn behavior
• desire for isolation
• inability to engage in leisure activities
• compulsive work habits excluding leisure activities and family life
• apathy

Sleep-rest pattern
• inability to sleep restfully
• sleeping to avoid conflict
• reliance on sleeping medications

Cognitive-perceptual pattern
• inability to concentrate because of overwhelming problems
• forgetfulness
• preoccupation with work

Self-perception–self-concept pattern
• dependency and indecisiveness
• excessively ordered, rigid, or controlling behavior
• concern over perfectionistic behavior
• feeling overly conscientious and loyal
• perception of self as incompetent and powerless
• inflexibility
• perception of self as overly sensitive to criticism
• perception of self as a procrastinator

Role-relationship pattern
• fear of developing relationships
• family-taught traits, such as an inability to talk about feelings
• avoidance of social situations and close relationships
• devastation when close relationships end
• dependence on and fear of being abandoned by family or friends
• desire to obstruct the efforts of family members, friends, or co-workers by failing to perform tasks or work duties

Sexual-reproductive pattern
• difficulty expressing affection
• difficulty with intimacy
• concern about involvement in high-risk sexual behavior, such as unprotected sex or promiscuity
• history of sexual or physical abuse

Coping–stress tolerance pattern
• exhaustion by the mere effort of getting to a social event
• exaggerated concern over potential difficulties
• frequent perception of events as catastrophies
• feelings of helplessness when alone
• preoccupation with details, rules, lists, order, or schedules to cope with uncertainty and anxiety
• inability to refuse the requests of others
• extreme criticism of others
• concern about doing things for others to obtain approval and acceptance

Value-belief pattern
• inability to discard worn-out or worthless objects, even those without sentimental value
• feeling powerless to achieve life goals
• lack of self-regard
• avoidance of job promotions that require increased social demands
• inability to believe in anything or anyone
• intolerance of others' beliefs
• exaggerated involvement in religion

PHYSICAL FINDINGS
The client may report or exhibit one of more of the following physical findings.

Cardiovascular
• elevated blood pressure
• flushed face
• increased heart rate
• palpitations
• sweating

Respiratory
• increased respiratory rate
• increased respiratory infections

Gastrointestinal
• abdominal pain
• diarrhea
• increased salivation
• nausea
• ulcerative colitis

Genitourinary
• frequent urination
• infections
• sexually transmitted diseases

Musculoskeletal
• frequent falls and bruising
• clenched fists
• exhaustion
• increased fatigue
• muscle aches, pains, or soreness
• muscle tension
• jaw tension

Neurologic
• dizziness or faintness
• headaches
• restlessness
• sleep disturbance (such as insomnia and early morning awakening)

Psychological
• annoyance
• anxiety
• argumentativeness
• decreased self-esteem
• forgetfulness
• irritability
• loneliness
• disbelief about diagnostic study findings
• obsessive thinking
• overachievement
• restricted interests and knowledge
• ruminative thinking
• scornfulness

Potential complications
If untreated, cluster C personality disorders can lead to impaired occupational functioning. In addition, social phobia may result from avoidant personality disorder. Major depression is a common complication of dependent personality disorder. Obsessive-compulsive disorder can lead to hypochondriasis and major depression and, in conjunction with cluster A personality disorders, may be linked with cardiac disease, myocardial infarction, or sudden cardiac death. Possible complications associated with passive-aggressive personality disorder include major depression, dysthymia, and substance abuse.

Nursing diagnosis: *Altered family process related to rigidity in functions, roles, and rules*

NURSING PRIORITY: To help the client and family challenge family rules and learn to use new strategies to increase role flexibility

Interventions

1. Work with the client and family to identify specific roles and behavioral rules that they have established for one another. Concentrate on behaviors that supposedly protect the family from emotional outbursts.

2. Explore with the client and family the effects of rigid and inflexible behaviors on family, friends, and co-workers. Use concrete examples and role playing to make these effects more vivid.

3. Work with the client and family to plan role and function changes and to develop healthful family rules.

Rationales

1. Identifying roles and behaviors that might be causing family dysfunction is necessary before the client and family members can affect changes.

2. Explanations and dramatizations can clarify how dependency and rigid adherence to constricted role behaviors produce rigidity and a lack of spontaneity within the family.

3. By working together to renegotiate their relationships with one another, family members can gain a sense of control over their situation. Working together also provides family members with opportunities to interact in an effective and balanced manner.

Nursing diagnosis: *Altered thought processes related to indecision or doubt over decisions*

NURSING PRIORITY: To help the client learn and use a problem-solving approach to decision making

Interventions

1. Encourage the client to make decisions.

2. Examine how the client avoids or makes decisions, and discuss the negative consequences of indecision with the client.

3. Teach, model, and rehearse with the client problem-solving processes and decision-making behaviors.

4. Respond clearly and directly to the client's efforts to learn new coping strategies.

5. Help the client to identify anxiety related to the need for perfection or for knowing everything, as well as the origin of this behavior (possibly a parent or other family role model).

6. Explain to the client how ritualistic behaviors (such as creating laundry lists or schedules and compulsive reading) are implemented to decrease anxiety about being imperfect and inadequate.

Rationales

1. Encouraging self-determination can help dispel the client's perception of being inadequate and a failure.

2. Understanding how the client avoids decisions and where the coping strategies were learned can help the nurse develop effective and appropriate interventions for managing client anxiety.

3. Learning how to conceptualize a problem, develop options, select the most reasonable one, and evaluate and revise the plan if necessary can decrease the anxiety that fosters avoidance. Modeling behaviors and role playing can provide the client with immediate evidence that these strategies can work.

4. Responding to the client's efforts and to positive behavioral change can increase and reinforce client self-awareness and confidence.

5. Finding causes for seemingly inexplicable behaviors or needs not only increases client awareness but also helps the client to make connections between feelings and certain behaviors or beliefs.

6. Knowing the rationale behind certain behaviors can help the client begin to understand an underlying fear of being exposed as incompetent or inadequate.

Nursing diagnosis: *Ineffective individual coping related to the inability to ask for help, the need always to be right and perfect, verbal manipulation, and the need to use rules and routines to maintain a secure environment*

NURSING PRIORITY: To teach the client new adaptive coping strategies

Interventions

1. Discuss any fears the client has about seeking help. Teach and rehearse ways of asking for help.

2. Discuss past instances in which the client asked for help. Evaluate the client's behavior and feelings as well as responses from others and the outcome of these incidents.

3. Avoid any power struggles with the client.

4. Encourage the client to accept responsibility for behavior and to explore how behavior affects others. Also encourage the client to monitor or check behaviors with trusted family members or loved ones.

5. Discuss what exactly the client thinks will happen if one is wrong about something. Work with the client to identify realistic and unrealistic outcomes. Encourage the client to discuss what the family has taught its members about being right or wrong.

6. Help the client to develop a sense of humor about the use of perfectionism to cope with tension and anxiety. Point out that being able to regard oneself with humor is a valuable trait.

7. Accept the client's self-image and respect personal rights.

8. Maintain established routines, and keep scheduled appointments with the client.

9. Give positive reinforcement of the client's diminishing use of rules and routines and eventual use of healthier coping strategies.

Rationales

1. The client should realize that fear of rejection may make seeking help impossible. Learning adaptive strategies for seeking help can progressively decrease any related anxiety.

2. Self-appraisal of behaviors and feelings as well as appraisal of others' responses help the client look at fears more realistically.

3. Power struggles are unresolvable and reinforce the client's maladaptive behavior pattern.

4. The client may develop a more realistic view of how individual behavior affects others, and this may support self-initiated behavioral changes.

5. Such discussion allows the client to explore and challenge dysfunctional messages learned in the family. The client also may begin to understand that perfectionism can be destructive.

6. Humor and laughter can be therapeutic, providing pleasurable physical sensations that reduce tension and anxiety. Humor also can decrease a person's emotional distance from others, while enhancing a general sense of well-being.

7. Through acceptance and respect, the nurse can enhance the client's self-worth and promote feelings of adequacy.

8. Consistency and predictability create a secure environment for the client and consequently decrease anxiety.

9. When abandoning old rules and routines, the client may fear rejection and experience anxiety and guilt. To allay such fears, the nurse should maintain a supportive, secure relationship with the client.

Nursing diagnosis: *Powerlessness related to perfectionistic behavior that protects against inferiority feelings, or to intellectualization or denial of feelings as a means to gain self-control*

NURSING PRIORITY: To decrease the client's use of perfectionistic behaviors, intellectualization, or denial to manage anxiety and gain self-control

Interventions

1. Encourage the client to identify perfectionistic behaviors and to consider how these behaviors suppress anxiety and feelings of helplessness and powerlessness. Slowly and deliberately encourage the client to consider the feelings associated with these behaviors.

2. Assign and review home or group exercises that require the client to experience a mistake or imperfect behavior and to describe in a journal anticipated consequences and what actually occurred.

3. Collaborate with the client to establish realistic, attainable goals and a definitive, achievable plan for managing stress.

4. Refer the client to appropriate support groups and activities, including a comprehensive stress management program, an intensive program for the children of alcoholics or members of dysfunctional families, and other support groups, such as Adult Children of Alcoholics (ACOA) and Codependents Anonymous (CODA).

Rationales

1. The client needs to experience a safe environment and relationship with the nurse before beginning the anxiety-producing process of linking behaviors and feelings.

2. Such exercises can help the client realize that the consequences of imperfect behavior are not usually as dire as expected and are commonly mild or neutral. Recording observations in a journal enables the client to review and revise distorted thinking.

3. Attainable goals and a structured anxiety management plan can help the client to perceive capabilities and limitations more realistically and to learn concrete skills for managing stress.

4. Knowing about appropriate support groups and activities can decrease the client's sense of loneliness, uniqueness, and isolation.

Nursing diagnosis: *Social isolation related to an inability to establish and maintain relationships*

NURSING PRIORITY: To help the client develop skills for establishing and maintaining at least one new relationship

Interventions

1. Assess the client's present socialization pattern, and encourage the client to relate to you.

2. After establishing a mutually agreed upon time to meet, begin at the client's interaction level and do not prematurely move to a higher level.

3. Cautiously invite the client to interact with you and another carefully selected person. Initially invite participation in a neutral, nonthreatening, and noncompetitive activity, such as watching television or going for a walk.

Rationales

1. Assessing the client's socialization pattern can help the nurse determine both the duration of the disturbance as well as the probable time needed for treatment. As an objective, trustworthy, nonthreatening person, the nurse can promote a successful personal interaction.

2. Building a trusting relationship with the client requires the nurse's consistency and reliability. Forcing or pursuing complex interactions prematurely will heighten the client's fear of failure and produce social withdrawal and avoidance.

3. The nurse's support and activity planning provide the client opportunities for gradually expanding interaction to a social group. Nonthreatening activities allow the client to practice socialization skills.

Outcome criteria

As treatment progresses, the client, family, or both should be able to:
• verbalize and share fears and anxieties
• identify rigid family rules and explain how these rules affect each member
• identify specific areas requiring change
• demonstrate a willingness to participate in ongoing therapy
• use problem-solving and decision-making skills to manage anxiety previously managed by avoidance, dependency, passivity, or perfectionism
• identify and express feelings as they occur
• demonstrate realistic self-appraisal and use others for feedback and validation of feelings
• demonstrate beginning attempts to establish a new relationship.

Discharge criteria

Nursing documentation indicates that the client:
• has demonstrated an increased ability to distinguish between thoughts and actions
• has demonstrated a decreased reliance on ritualistic behaviors and activities
• understands the diagnosis, treatment, and expected outcomes
• is aware of available community and family resources
• can use alternative coping skills.

Nursing documentation also indicates that the family:
• understands how family rules affect the client
• can identify appropriate internal and external support resources
• demonstrates an ability to use alternative coping skills
• has demonstrated a willingness to participate in an ongoing therapy program.
• has been referred to the appropriate community and family resources
• has scheduled necessary follow-up appointments
• understands when, why, and how to contact appropriate health care professionals in case of an emergency.

Selected references

Ackerman, R.J. (1989). *Perfect daughters: Adult daughters of alcoholics.* Deerfield Beach, FL: Health Communications.

Adderholdt-Elliott, M. (1987). *Perfectionism: What's bad about being too good.* Minneapolis: Free Spirit Publishing.

Beck, A.T., and Freeman, A. (1990). *Cognitive therapy of personality disorders.* New York: Guilford Press.

Bloom-Feshback, J., and Bloom-Feshback, S. (1987). *The psychology of separation and loss.* San Francisco: Jossey-Bass.

Brown, S., Beletsis, S., and Cermak, T. (1989). *Adult children of alcoholics in treatment.* Deerfield Beach, FL: Health Communications.

Cermak, T.L. (1986). *Diagnosing and treating co-dependence.* Minneapolis: Johnson Institute Books.

Flett, G.L., Hewitt, P.L., et al. (1991). Perfectionism and learned resourcefulness in depression and self-esteem. *Personality and Individual Differences,* 12(1), 61-68.

Fossum, M.A., and Mason, M.J. (1989). *Facing shame: families in recovery.* New York: W.W. Norton.

Gorton, G., and Akhtar, S. (1990). The literature on personality disorders, 1985-1988. Trends, Issues, and controversies. *Hospital and Community Psychiatry,* 41(1), 39-51.

Greenberg, R.P., and Bornstein, R.F. (1988). The dependent personality: I. Risk for physical disorders. *Journal of Personality Disorders,* 2(2), 126-135.

Greenberg, R.P., and Bornstein, R.F. (1988). The dependent personality: II. Risk for psychological disorders. *Journal of Personality Disorders,* 2(2), 136-143.

Hill, C.A. (1991). Seeking emotional support: The influence of affiliative need and partner warmth. *Journal of Personality and Social Psychology,* 60(1), 112-121.

Kaye, Y. (1991). *The child that never was: Grieving your past to grow into the future.* Deerfield Beach, FL: Health Communications.

Lego, S. (1990). The fear of moving beyond one's parents. *Perspectives in Psychiatric Care,* 26(1), 28-31.

Livesley, W.J., Schroeder, M.L., and Jackson, D.N. (1990). Dependent personality disorder and attachment problems. *Journal of Personality Disorders,* 4(2), 131-140.

McCann, J.T. (1988). Passive-aggressive personality disorder: A review. *Journal of Personality Disorders,* 2(2), 170-179.

Nergaard, M., and Silberschatz, G. (1989). The effects of shame, guilt and the negative reaction in brief dynamic psychotherapy. *Psychotherapy,* 26(3), 330-337.

Pilkonis, P.A. (1988). Personality prototypes among depressives: Themes of dependency and autonomy. *Journal of Personality Disorders,* 2(2), 144152.

Pollak, J. (1987). Obsessive-compulsive personality: Theoretical and clinical perspectives and recent research findings. *Journal of Personality Disorders,* 1(3), 248-262.

Reich, J., Noyes, R., and Troughton, E. (1987). Dependent personality disorder associated with phobic avoidance in patients with panic disorder. *American Journal of Psychiatry,* 144(3), 323-326.

Roskies, E. (1987). *Stress management for the healthy type A: Theory and practice.* New York: Guilford Press.

Sayre, J. (1990). Psychodynamics revisited: An object-relations framework for psychiatric nursing. *Perspectives in Psychiatric Care,* 26(1), 7-12.

Silberschatz, G., Curtis, J.T., and Nathans, S. (1989). Using the patient's plan to assess progress in psychotherapy. *Psychotherapy,* 26(1), 40-46.

Smith, A.W. (1990). *Overcoming perfectionism: The superhuman syndrome.* Deerfield Beach, FL: Health Communications.

Smith, T.W., O'Keeffe, J.L., and Jenkins, M. (1988). Dependency and self-criticism correlates of depression or moderators of the effects of stressful events. *Journal of Personality Disorders,* 2(2), 160-169.

Trull, T.J., Widiger, T.A., and Frances, A. (1987). Covariation of criteria sets for avoidant, schizoid and dependent personality disorders. *American Journal of Psychiatry,* 144(6), 767-771.

West, M., and Sheldon, A.E.R. (1988). Classification of pathological attachment patterns in adults. *Journal of Personality Disorders,* 2(2), 153-159.

Dissociative Disorders

DSM III-R classifications
300.12 Psychogenic amnesia
300.13 Psychogenic fugue
300.14 Multiple personality disorder
300.15 Dissociative disorder not otherwise specified
300.60 Depersonalization disorder

Psychiatric nursing diagnostic class
Identity disturbance

Introduction

Dissociative disorders range in severity from psychogenic amnesia to multiple personality disorder, depending on the amount of dissociated memory or consciousness produced by an event stressful beyond the client's coping abilities. The nature and frequency of the stressful event and the degree of the client's intolerance influence the degree of dissociation.

Psychogenic amnesia, usually related to a traumatic event and not to an organic problem, has four distinct types. The most common type is localized amnesia, characterized by a defined period of memory loss related to a traumatic event. A second type, selective amnesia, also is characterized by a defined period of memory loss; however, within that period, the client may have a partial memory of events. A client with generalized amnesia typically exhibits a complete memory loss of the past, whereas one with continuous amnesia experiences a memory loss that begins at a particular time and continues to the present. These last two are the least prevalent forms.

The client with *psychogenic fugue,* a rare dissociative disorder, wanders or travels and assumes modified identities, usually in response to a painful circumstance or acute stress. The fugue state may last from several hours to days, during which time the client may appear normal or disoriented and may behave in ways inconsistent with personal beliefs and values. The state may end abruptly, and the client may experience partial or complete memory loss of the time period.

The client with *multiple personality disorder* exhibits two or more distinct personalities. Each personality manifests a separate memory, value and belief system, behavioral pattern, attitudes, and self-image. The primary or "host" personality may display partial awareness of the other personalities. This chronic type of dissociative disorder also is characterized by identity and memory disturbances.

Dissociative disorder not otherwise specified is one in which the exhibited dissociative symptoms do not meet the criteria for the other dissociative disorders.

One example is a trance state, characterized by an altered consciousness with diminished responsiveness to stimuli.

Depersonalization disorder is characterized by feelings of detachment from one's mental processes or body. Other symptoms include sensory anesthesia and a sense of not being in control of one's actions.

ETIOLOGY AND PRECIPITATING FACTORS
Researchers generally believe that dissociative disorders, though not diagnosed until adulthood, result from traumatic events experienced in childhood. Almost all clients report a history of emotional, physical, or sexual abuse in childhood.

Though no research or literature supports a genetic basis for dissociative disorder, a significant incidence of other psychiatric disorders, especially substance abuse, in client families suggests some genetic relationship.

Assessment guidelines
NURSING HISTORY (Functional health pattern findings)
The client may report or exhibit one or more of the findings grouped here according to functional health patterns.

Health perception–health management pattern
• history of headaches
• palpitations
• loss of consciousness
• anxiety or panic symptoms
• substance abuse

Nutritional-metabolic pattern
• weight loss secondary to appetite loss

Activity-exercise pattern
• lethargy
• loss of interest in usual activities

Cognitive-perceptual pattern
• impaired recall
• amnesia
• hearing own thoughts spoken aloud
• hearing others talking in head
• sudden awareness of being in strange surroundings with no memory of getting there
• feeling of being outside the body

Self-perception–self-concept pattern
• perception of the self as "we"
• awareness of "other parts" of self
• feeling like a different person at times
• low self-esteem

Role-relationship pattern
• incidents of being approached by strangers who seem or claim to be acquaintances or friends
• difficulty maintaining relationships
• difficulty functioning at work

Coping–stress tolerance pattern
• memory lapses when stressed or anxious
• sudden trips away from familiar surroundings

Value-belief pattern
• hearing from others about allegedly engaging in behaviors that would conflict with personal values or beliefs
• inability to accomplish life goals

PHYSICAL FINDINGS
The client may report or exhibit one or more of the following physical findings.

Cardiovascular
• cold, clammy skin
• elevated blood pressure
• hot and cold flashes
• increased heart rate
• palpitations
• sweating
• tingling sensation

Respiratory
• increased respiratory rate
• shortness of breath
• smothering sensation
• choking sensation

Gastrointestinal
• dry mouth
• abdominal distress
• nausea
• vomiting
• diarrhea
• difficulty swallowing

Genitourinary
• frequent urination

Musculoskeletal
• increased fatigue
• muscle aches, pains, or soreness
• muscle tension
• restlessness
• shakiness
• trembling
• twitching

Neurologic
• dilated pupils
• dizziness or faintness
• light-headedness
• paresthesia
• restlessness

Psychological
• feeling keyed up or on edge
• inability to concentrate
• irritability
• blank mind
• sleep disturbance (such as insomnia or early morning awakening)

Potential complications
If left untreated, dissociative disorders can cause aggressive behavior toward the self or others. Such behavior might include assaults, depression, hypochondriasis, post-traumatic stress disorder, psychoactive substance abuse disorder, rape, self-mutilation, and suicide attempts.

Nursing diagnosis: *Personal identity disturbance related to underdeveloped ego, threat to self-concept, or childhood abuse or trauma*

NURSING PRIORITY: To help the client understand the relationship between anxiety and dissociation and to learn to use adaptive coping skills

Interventions

1. Develop an honest, nonjudgmental relationship with the client.

Rationales

1. A client with a dissociative disorder typically exhibits extreme difficulty establishing trusting relationships, especially with authority figures. This difficulty is probably the result of having been betrayed in the past by a parent or loved one.

2. Assess the client for memory loss.

3. Assess the client for homicidal or suicidal thoughts or impulses.

4. Assess the client for auditory hallucinations.

5. Share and analyze findings with all members of the treatment team.

6. Discuss the diagnosis and treatment plan with the client.

7. Explain to the client with multiple personality disorder that the treatment goal is the integration of subpersonalities, and establish a contract with the client to work toward that goal.

8. Establish contact with the client's subpersonalities, and work with them toward integration. If possible, include the subpersonalities in any treatment contract.

9. Develop a contract with the client that identifies the treatment team members and client subpersonalities that are to participate in treatment, the treatment expectations, and limits on aggressive behavior toward self or others.

10. Obtain a client history that includes when and why each subpersonality was created, where each fits chronologically in the client's life, what function each serves, and when and how each is triggered.

11. Try to establish communication between or among the client's subpersonalities, taking care not to overwhelm the client with information or memories.

12. Avoid focusing on the communication barriers between subpersonalities. Instead, explore the reasons why such barriers exist.

13. Help the client to incorporate the dissociated material into conscious memories by encouraging the sharing of painful, repressed memories. Usually, abreaction (verbal disclosure of repressed thoughts or emotions) of painful memories effectively leads to this incorporation.

2. The client probably will be amnesic about periods when a modified or distinct personality is dominant.

3. Aggressive behavior, especially toward the self, and self-mutilation commonly occur during dissociative states.

4. Unlike schizophrenics, who usually hear voices as if they were in the external world, clients with dissociative disorder typically perceive voices arguing inside their own heads. Full-blown auditory hallucinations would suggest another problem, such as schizophrenia.

5. Strong, consistent teamwork can help ensure successful treatment.

6. An open and honest discussion of the diagnosis and treatment helps establish trust between the nurse and client. Such trust can induce the client to cooperate in the treatment.

7. The integration process is usually lengthy, and active client participation increases the chances for success.

8. Communicating with and eliciting the cooperation of the client's subpersonalities is essential to integration.

9. A contract can promote safety when angry, hostile, or aggressive subpersonalities dominate the client.

10. Developing a history that includes subpersonalities helps to fill in any gaps in the client's conscious history and may subsequently reveal the traumatic events that caused the dissociative state.

11. The client's subpersonalities are shields from painful memories. To maintain client trust and cooperation, the nurse must take care to reveal these dissociated memories in a nonthreatening, supportive manner and environment.

12. Focusing on why barriers between subpersonalities exist can make crossing them less threatening for the client.

13. After the memory is identified, the client needs to verbalize the memory and repressed emotions. This time-consuming process must occur with each subpersonality and for each dissociated event.

Nursing diagnosis: *Ineffective individual coping related to a severe level of repressed anxiety*

NURSING PRIORITY: To help the client learn and use new coping skills

Interventions	Rationales
1. Remain with the client, and reassure him that he is safe and secure.	1. The presence of a trusted individual, such as the nurse, can help create a secure environment and alleviate the client's fear of a dissociative event.
2. Identify stressors that caused the client's severe anxiety and explore feelings related to the stressors.	2. The nurse must obtain information about stressors to develop a relevant plan of care. Explaining that others experience similar feelings in similar situations can reinforce the client's self-esteem.
3. Collaborate with the client to identify alternative methods of coping with identified stressors. Identify which responses are adaptive and which are dissociative.	3. When extremely anxious, the client may be unable to evaluate the appropriateness of behavior and may require assistance with solving problems and making decisions. By providing such information, the nurse helps the client to change inappropriate behavior and adopt new coping strategies.
4. Help the client to learn and use new coping strategies (such as talking with someone or practicing relaxation techniques) for managing stressful events.	4. The client must replace dissociation with new, more constructive coping strategies to prevent regression.
5. Acknowledge and reinforce the client's attempts at change.	5. Positive reinforcement can enhance the client's self-esteem and encourage him to continue desired behaviors.
6. Provide information, education, and support to the client's family or loved ones during treatment.	6. Family members and loved ones should know about the disorder and how to cope with it because they probably will be the ones confronted by the client's subpersonalities. Furthermore, the more family and loved ones know about the disorder, the more likely they will support treatment.
7. Inform and educate the client about the need for long-term follow-up therapy.	7. Because the client is going to be facing previously avoided issues, such as relationships, sexuality, and work, he will need ongoing support to cope effectively.

Outcome criteria

As treatment progresses, the client, family, or both should be able to:
• demonstrate a decrease or absence of amnesia
• verbalize an awareness of previously dissociated material
• demonstrate that no subpersonalities are dominant
• verbalize feelings of improved self-esteem
• demonstrate adaptive coping skills
• verbalize an understanding of dissociation as a way of coping
• report an absence of voices.

Discharge criteria

Nursing documentation indicates that the client:
• has demonstrated a decrease in or absence of control by subpersonalities

• understands that dissociation is a way of coping
• has demonstrated an absence of aggressive or self-destructive thinking and behavior
• can identify and describe the signs and symptoms of relapse
• has demonstrated improved self-esteem
• understands the need for long-term follow-up treatment
• is aware of available community and family resources.

Nursing documentation also indicates that the family:
• has verbalized an understanding of the client's diagnosis, treatment, and expected outcomes
• can use alternative coping skills in dealing with the client's subpersonalities

• understands the long-term nature of the integration process
• know when, why, and how to contact the appropriate health care professional in case of an emergency
• has been referred to the appropriate community and family resources
• has demonstrated a willingness to participate in a follow-up therapy program.

Selected references

Anderson, G. (1988). Understanding multiple personality disorder. *Journal of Psychosocial Nursing and Mental Health Services*, 26(7), 26-30, 36-37.

Anderson, G., and Ross, C.A. (1988). Strategies for working with a patient who has multiple personality disorder. *Archives of Psychiatric Nursing*, 2(4), 236-243.

Bliss, E.L. (1986). *Multiple personality: Allied disorders and hypnosis.* London: Oxford University Press.

Braun, B.G. (1989). Psychotherapy of the survivor of incest with a dissociative disorder. *Psychiatric Clinics of North America*, 12(2), 307-324.

Chu, J., and Dill, D. (1990). Dissociative symptoms in relation to childhood physical and sexual abuse. *American Journal of Psychiatry*, 147(7), 887-892.

Coons, P.M., and Milstein, V. (1990). Self-mutilation associated with dissociative disorders. *Dissociation*, 3(2), 81-87.

Drew, B. (1988). Multiple personality disorder: An historical perspective. *Archives of Psychiatric Nursing*, 2(4), 227-230.

Dunn, R. (1985). Issues of self-concept deficit in psychotherapy. *Psychotherapy*, 22(4), 747-751.

Frankel, F.H. (1990). Hypnotizability and dissociation. *American Journal of Psychiatry*, 147(7), 823-829.

Franklin, J. (1990). The diagnosis of multiple personality disorder based on subtle dissociative signs. *Journal of Nervous and Mental Disease*, 178(1), 4-14.

Franklin, J. (1990). Dreamlike thought and dream mode processes in the formation of personalities in MPD. *Dissociation*, 3(2), 70-80.

Kemp, K., Gilberson, A., and Torem-Moshe, S. (1988). The differential diagnosis of multiple personality disorder from borderline personality disorder. *Dissociation*, 1(4), 41-46.

Kluft, R.P. (1987). An update on multiple personality disorder. *Hospital and Community Psychiatry*, 38(4), 363-373.

Lego, S. (1988). Multiple personality disorder: An interpersonal approach to etiology, treatment, and nursing care. *Archives of Psychiatric Nursing*, 2(4), 231-235.

Middleton-Moz, J. (1989). *Children of trauma: Rediscovering your discarded self.* Deerfield Beach, FL: Health Communications.

Putnam, F. (1989). *Diagnosis and treatment of multiple personality disorder.* New York: Guilford Press.

Rew, L. (1990). Childhood sexual abuse: Toward a self-care framework for nursing intervention and research. *Archives of Psychiatric Nursing*, 4(3), 147-153.

Ross, C.A. (1989). *Multiple Personality Disorder: Diagnosis, Clinical Features, and Treatment.* New York: Wiley.

Ross, C.A. (1990). Twelve cognitive errors about multiple personality disorder. *American Journal of Psychotherapy*, 44(3), 348-356.

Ross, C.A., and Gahan, P. (1988). Techniques in the treatment of multiple personality disorder. *American Journal of Psychotherapy*, 42(1), 40-52.

Ross, C.A., Joshi, S., and Currie, R. (1991). Dissociative experiences in the general population: A factor analysis. *Hospital and Community Psychiatry*, 42(3), 297-301.

Sanders, S. (1986). The perceptual alteration scale: A scale measuring dissociation. *American Journal of Clinical Hypnosis*, 29(2), 95-102.

Sanders, B., and Giolas, M. (1991). Dissociation and childhood trauma in psychologically disturbed adolescents. *American Journal of Psychiatry*, 148(1), 50-54.

Steele, K. (1989). Looking for answers: Understanding multiple personality disorder. *Journal of Psychosocial Nursing*, 27(8), 5-10.

Torem, M.S. (1990). Covert multiple personality underlying eating disorders. *American Journal of Psychotherapy*, 44(3), 357-368.

Adjustment Disorders

DSM III-R classifications

309.00 Adjustment disorder with depressed mood
309.23 Adjustment disorder with work (or academic) inhibition
309.24 Adjustment disorder with anxious mood
309.28 Adjustment disorder with mixed emotional features
309.30 Adjustment disorder with disturbance of conduct
309.40 Adjustment disorder with mixed disturbance of emotions and conduct
309.82 Adjustment disorder with physical complaints
309.83 Adjustment disorder with withdrawal
309.90 Adjustment disorder not otherwise specified

Psychiatric nursing diagnostic class

Altered self-concept

Introduction

Adjustment disorders are generally characterized by maladaptive reactions to identifiable psychosocial stressors. Such stressors may include job loss, relationship termination, academic problems, and family or work problems. The intensity of the individual's reaction, which typically occurs within 3 months of stressor onset and persists no longer than 6 months, is not always proportionate to the intensity of the stressor.

Adjustment disorder with depressed mood includes feelings of hopelessness and tearfulness. Individuals with *adjustment disorder with work (or academic) inhibition* exhibit a significant decrease in and inhibition of their former capabilities. Anxiety and depression symptoms are common. *Adjustment disorder with anxious mood* is predominantly characterized by nervousness, worrying, and jitteriness.

Adjustment disorder with mixed emotional features represents a combination of anxiety and depression or other emotional responses. *Adjustment disorder with disturbance of conduct* is characterized by conduct that violates the rights of others or age-appropriate societal norms and rules. Behaviors include truancy, vandalism, fighting, defaulting on legal obligations, and reckless driving. *Adjustment disorder with mixed disturbance of emotions and conduct* has both emotional symptoms (such as anxiety and depression) and conduct disturbances (such as truancy and fighting).

Major features of *adjustment disorder with physical complaints* include fatigue, aches and pains, headache, or backache. *Adjustment disorder with withdrawal* is characterized by social withdrawal specifically without depression or anxiety symptoms.

Adjustment disorder not otherwise specified involves maladaptive reactions to psychosocial stressors. For example, an individual's intense reaction to a medical diagnosis could produce pathological denial or noncompliance.

ETIOLOGY AND PRECIPITATING FACTORS

Many factors can inhibit an individual's ability to adjust to life changes, thereby causing an adjustment disorder. One person may have difficulty trusting friends or family; another may perceive change as a threat to the self or family. Other factors include inadequate communication, inability to use health care resources, lack of family support, satisfaction with current situation, lack of motivation, and unrealistic or incongruent goals. Unmet dependency needs, retarded ego development, fixation in an earlier developmental stage, and low self-esteem also can contribute to adjustment disorder development.

Other factors related to the family may play a part in the development of these disorders. As children, individuals with adjustment difficulties may have received inadequate or nonexistent role modeling in dysfunctional or shame-based families. Such experiences inhibit the development of self-esteem, adequate coping skills, and self-regulation skills.

Assessment guidelines

NURSING HISTORY (Functional health pattern findings)

The client may report or exhibit one or more of the findings grouped here according to functional health patterns.

Health perception–health management pattern

• concern over acute or chronic illness or disability
• numerous somatic complaints (such as headaches, backaches, or stomachaches) with or without diagnostic validation
• numerous illnesses, colds, flu, or general fatigue
• aches and pains

Nutritional-metabolic pattern

• concern over eating behaviors
• appetite changes
• weight loss or gain
• healing difficulties secondary to a chronic health problem
• skin problems secondary to a chronic health problem

Elimination pattern

• bowel and urinary elimination problems

Activity-exercise pattern
• concern about being easily fatigued
• difficulty performing normal daily activities
• withdrawn or apathetic behavior
• diminished interest or ability to participate in leisure activities

Sleep-rest pattern
• fatigue after sleep
• difficulty falling or staying asleep
• early morning awakening

Cognitive-perceptual pattern
• learning difficulties that inhibit work or academic performance
• concentration difficulties that inhibit work or academic performance
• impaired memory
• vision or hearing dysfunction
• acute or chronic pain

Self-perception–self-concept pattern
• perception of self as dependent and indecisive
• perception of self as inadequate and anxious
• perception of self as angry and hostile
• concerns about body image, self-esteem, and self-worth
• fear, anxiety, resentment, or general disappointment

Role-relationship pattern
• concern over relationships with family and loved ones
• manipulative or limit-testing behavior or behavior that plays family members or friends against one another
• concern over the lack of support for necessary lifestyle changes from family and friends
• refusal to interact with others or a preference for isolation
• intense need to be independent and self-reliant

Sexual-reproductive pattern
• difficulty with intimacy
• dissatisfaction with sexual relations
• concern about involvement in high-risk sexual behavior, such as promiscuity
• concern about involvement with high-risk partners, including I.V. drug users and homosexual or bisexual partners

Coping–stress tolerance pattern
• inappropriate expressions of anger
• difficulties in academic or work performance
• depressed, tense, jittery, or tearful appearance
• inability to identify persons or measures that would help the condition
• presence of one or several psychosocial stressors in the past year
• substance use or abuse

Value-belief pattern
• feeling unable to achieve life goals
• disbelief about present situation

PHYSICAL FINDINGS
The client may report or exhibit one or more of the following physical findings.

Cardiovascular
• cold, clammy skin
• elevated blood pressure
• hot and cold flashes
• increased heart rate
• palpitations
• sweating
• tingling sensation

Respiratory
• increased respiratory rate
• shortness of breath
• smothering sensation
• choking sensation

Gastrointestinal
• dry mouth
• abdominal distress
• nausea
• vomiting
• diarrhea
• difficulty swallowing

Genitourinary
• frequent urination

Musculoskeletal
• backache
• fatigue
• muscle aches and pains

Neurologic
• headaches
• nervousness

Psychological
• ambivalence
• anger
• depression
• hopelessness
• tearfulness
• worrying

Potential complications
An undiagnosed physical problem can sometimes closely resemble an adjustment disorder, thereby delaying appropriate treatment and leading to more serious physical deterioration.

Nursing diagnosis: *Impaired adjustment related to inadequate support systems, disability requiring life-style changes, unresolved grieving, or impaired cognition*

NURSING PRIORITY: To help the client develop new strategies for coping with limitations or losses

Interventions

1. Assess the client's physical and psychosocial status to determine the degree of impaired function.

2. Encourage the client to explore feelings and to talk about perceived inabilities to adapt to the present situation.

3. Have the client identify significant past stressors and coping methods used. Acknowledge the client's efforts to cope and adjust.

4. Teach and rehearse with the client this problem-solving approach: Identify and isolate the problem, seek out alternatives and resources, determine pros and cons of each alternative, make an appropriate decision, and reevaluate it. Encourage the client to select another solution if the first option does not succeed.

5. Collaborate with the client to identify available and appropriate support systems.

6. With the client and family, develop and implement a plan for meeting immediate and future needs. Also, encourage them to anticipate future changes and to develop a preventive plan.

7. Help the client to become aware of appropriate additional resources, such as occupational therapy, vocational rehabilitation training, and physical therapy.

Rationales

1. An accurate assessment can help the nurse develop a more appropriate plan of care and can make the client more aware of how the condition affects life-style.

2. Helping the client to express feelings and perceptions can foster trust between the client and nurse. Doing so also helps the nurse more clearly understand the client's condition.

3. Recalling previous successes with coping and adjusting can improve the client's confidence and ability to manage present situations.

4. The client may need specific education about solving problems logically and systematically. Supporting the client in problem-solving efforts, including unsuccessful attempts, can build self-confidence and give the client a more realistic perspective on behavior.

5. The client may feel more relaxed and therefore benefit more when working from within a supportive family or community network.

6. Working together to solve problems and make appropriate adjustments can give the client and family an increased sense of control over the immediate situation and the future.

7. Knowing about support resources and how to obtain referrals provides the client with new skills and strategies for managing life-style and health status changes and for making realistic plans.

Nursing diagnosis: *Dysfunctional grieving related to a real and perceived but uncertain loss, multiple losses and bereavement processes, or inhibited grieving*

NURSING PRIORITY: To help the client verbalize feelings associated with the usual stages of grief

Interventions

1. Determine the client's stage of grief, and identify specific behaviors associated with it.

2. Speak clearly and honestly when communicating with the client, and keep any commitments made.

3. Encourage the client to discuss feelings about the loss or losses. Allow the client to direct the discussion, and accept unconditionally any emotional responses, unless expressed aggression or violence requires intervention.

Rationales

1. An accurate baseline assessment enables the nurse to form an effective plan of care.

2. These strategies form the basis of a trusting and therapeutic relationship.

3. Verbalizing feelings, especially anger, in a nonthreatening and supportive environment can help the client understand that responses to the loss are legitimate. Doing so also can help the client resolve unfinished issues.

4. Arrange for and monitor physical activities that allow the client to vent anger, such as walking, jogging, exercising, biking, playing volleyball or basketball, and using a punching bag.

5. Encourage the client to examine and discuss realistically the lost person or object.

6. Collaborate with the client to identify appropriate strategies for coping with loss. Provide reinforcement and feedback when the client tries new strategies.

7. Collaborate with the client and family to develop a plan that incorporates cultural and religious beliefs that might help the client cope with loss. Involve a religious leader if this is appropriate.

8. Explain to the client that loss can have physiologic effects, and stress the importance of maintaining physical well-being through good nutrition, rest, exercise within limits, proper hydration, regular elimination patterns, and regular physical examinations.

4. Physical exercise can provide a safe, effective outlet for relieving stored-up muscle tension and anger.

5. Relinquishing idealized perceptions while acknowledging and accepting both negative and positive aspects of the lost person or object can help the client resolve the grief.

6. Reinforcing efforts and successes can enhance self-esteem, confidence, and self-reliance and encourage the client to incorporate positive behaviors.

7. A culturally sensitive plan of care may facilitate grief resolution, especially if the client gains strength from spiritual support.

8. Instituting health practices to correct any adverse physiologic effects of stress and grief can help prevent physical illness.

Nursing diagnosis: *Defensive coping related to inadequate support systems, work overload, unmet expectations, or personal vulnerability*

NURSING PRIORITY: To help the client reduce the sense of distress

Interventions

1. Assess the client's anxiety and functional levels and ability to comprehend the present situation. Determine what is stressful or threatening to the client.

2. Identify the client's usual coping mechanisms (such as blaming, projection, or rationalization) and in which circumstances they are used. Observe the client's interactions with others, and discuss these observations, using role playing when necessary to clarify meaning.

3. Provide safe outlets and opportunities for the client to socialize with others. Encourage involvement in activities and classes in which new skills, especially assertiveness skills, can be learned and practiced.

4. Collaborate with the client to set realistic, attainable, and concrete goals. Acknowledge accomplishments toward defined goals.

Rationales

1. This assessment can help the nurse to evaluate the client's capacity to learn new coping strategies and to make appropriate suggestions for change.

2. Clear and honest communication about the nurse's observations can give a more realistic perspective on the client's behavior and help him appraise behaviors and situations more realistically.

3. Participating in classes and social activities can help the client acquire knowledge and new skills, adjust distorted thinking, and improve self-esteem.

4. Encouraging realistic goals and conveying a belief in the client's ability to achieve these goals enhances confidence and self-esteem.

Nursing diagnosis: *Impaired social interaction related to decreased perception of appropriate social behavior*

NURSING PRIORITY: To help the client learn an effective social interaction style

Interventions

1. Encourage the client to verbalize feelings rather than acting them out or internalizing them.

2. Set limits on client behaviors that adversely affect social interaction with peers, family members, or visitors, such as making embarrassing comments or ridiculing others.

3. Encourage the client to engage in support, psychoeducation, or activity groups (such as group games or crafts).

Rationales

1. Verbalizing feelings represents straightforward behavior, which can allow for appropriate social interactions.

2. Inappropriate behavior can alienate the client from peers and family and may result in frustration, hostile outbursts, or social withdrawal.

3. Attending and participating in group activities can decrease the client's sense of isolation and reinforce behavioral change.

Outcome criteria

As treatment progresses, the client, family, or both should be able to:
• identify stressful situations that lead to impaired adjustment and articulate specific actions for dealing with them
• initiate necessary life-style changes appropriate to the disorder
• report or demonstrate progress in coping with grief
• participate in activities of daily living
• demonstrate active self-care
• verbalize hope for the future
• assume responsibility for actions, achievements, and failures
• establish and maintain relationships
• identify factors and feelings that lead to impaired social interactions
• report or demonstrate a decreased manipulation of others for personal gratification
• describe appropriate alternative coping strategies.

Discharge criteria

Nursing documentation indicates that the client:
• can use newly learned skills to manage adjustment problems
• has verbalized an understanding of the loss and grief
• understands the diagnosis, treatment, and expected outcome
• is willing to participate in an ongoing follow-up psychotherapy program
• can use alternative coping skills
• is aware of available community and family resources.

Nursing documentation also indicates that the family:
• understands the client's diagnosis, treatment, and expected outcome
• has developed a realistic plan for adjusting to the client's present and future condition
• demonstrates a willingness to participate in an ongoing psychotherapy program
• verbalizes an understanding of the potential psychophysiologic responses to bereavement
• can use alternative coping skills
• has been referred to the appropriate community and support resources
• has scheduled the necessary follow-up appointments
• knows when, why, and how to contact appropriate emergency health care.

Selected references

Badger, T.A. (1990). Men with cardiovascular disease and their spouses: Coping, health, and marital adjustment. *Archives of Psychiatric Nursing, 4*(5), 319-324.

Bednar, R.L., Wells, M.G., and Vanden Bos, G.R. (1991). Self-esteem: A concept of renewed clinical relevance. *Hospital and Community Psychiatry, 4*(2), 123-125.

Bernstein, N.R., Breslau, A.J., and Graham, J.A. (1988). *Coping strategies for burn survivors and their families.* New York: Praeger.

Caroselli-Karinja, M.F. (1990). Asthma and adaptation: Exploring the family system. *Journal of Psychosocial Nursing, 28*(4), 34-41.

Cowen, E.L., Pedro-Carroll, J.L., and Alpert-Gillis, L.J. (1990). Relationships between support and adjustment among children of divorce. *Journal of Child Psychology and Psychiatry and Allied Disciplines, 31*(5), 727-735.

Deits, B. (1988). *Life after loss: A personal guide dealing with death, divorce, job change and relocation.* Tucson: Fisher Books.

Doka, K.J. (1989). *Disenfranchised grief: Recognizing hidden sorrow.* New York: Free Press.

Gorman, L.M., Sultan, D., and Luna-Railes, M. (1989). *Psychosocial nursing handbook for the nonpsychiatric nurse.* Baltimore: Williams & Wilkins.

Hedges, S.M., Krantz, D.S., Contrada, R.J., and Rozanski, A.R. (1990). Development of a diary for use with ambulatory monitoring of mood, activities and physiological function. *Journal of Psychopathology and Behavioral Assessment,* 12(3), 203-217.

Klagsburn, S.C., and Goldberg, I.K. (1988). *Psychiatric aspects of terminal illness.* Philadelphia: Charles Press.

Levy, R.S., Tendler, C., Van Devanter, N., and Cleary, P.D. (1990). A group intervention model made for individuals testing positive for HIV antibody. *American Journal of Orthopsychiatry,* 60(3), 452-59.

Lewis, S., Knowles-Grainger, R.D., et al. (1989). *Manual of psychosocial nursing interventions: Promoting mental health in medical-surgical settings.* Philadelphia: Saunders.

Lubkin, I.M. (1990). *Chronic illness: Impact and interventions* (2nd ed.). Boston: Jones & Bartlett.

Mishel, M. (1988). Uncertainty in illness. *Image: Journal of Nursing Scholarship,* 20(4), 225-232.

Noshpitz, J.D., and Coddington, R.D. (1990). *Stressors and the adjustment disorders.* New York: Wiley.

Pollock, S.E., Christian, B.J., and Sands, D. (1990). Responses to chronic illness: Analysis of psychological and physiological adaptation. *Nursing Research,* 39(5), 300-304.

Popkin, M.K., Callies, A.L., Colon, E.A., and Stiebel, V. (1990). Adjustment disorders in medically ill inpatients referred for consultation in a university hospital. *Psychosomatics,* 31(4), 410-44.

Razavi, D., Delvaux, N., Farvacques, C., and Robaye, E. (1990). Screening for adjustment disorders and major depressive disorders in cancer inpatients. *British Journal of Psychiatry,* 156, 79-83.

Sholevar, G.P., and Perkel, R. (1990). Family systems intervention and physical illness. *General Hospital Psychiatry,* 12(6), 363-372.

Stein, D., Troudart, T., Hymowitz, Z., et al. (1990). Psychosocial adjustment before and after coronary artery bypass surgery. *International Journal of Psychiatry in Medicine,* 20(2), 181-192.

Strauss, D.H., Spitzer, R.L., and Muskin, P.R. (1990). Maladaptive denial of physical illness: A proposal for DSM-IV. *American Journal of Psychiatry,* 147(9), 1168-1172.

Thomas, S.P. (1991). Toward a new conceptualization of women's anger. *Issues in Mental Health Nursing,* 12(1), 31-49.

Watson, W.L., and Bell, J. (1990). Who are we?: Low self-esteem and marital identity. *Journal of Psychosocial Nursing,* 28(4), 15-20, 40-41.

White, W., and Handal, P.J. (1990). The relationship between death anxiety and mental health/distress. *Omega: Journal of Death and Dying,* 22(1), 13-24.

Wills-Brandon, C. (1990). *Learning to say no: Establishing healthy boundaries.* Deerfield Beach, FL: Health Communications.

Attention Deficit Disorder

DSM III-R classification
314.01 Attention deficit hyperactivity disorder

Psychiatric nursing diagnostic class
Altered attention

Introduction

Identified in the 1950s, *attention deficit hyperactivity disorder* (ADHD) was successively referred to as *hyperactivity, hyperkinesis, minimal brain damage,* and *minimal brain dysfunction.* In the 1980s, the diagnostic category *attention deficit disorder* was introduced to emphasize inattention as the core symptom. Other symptoms of this disruptive behavioral disorder include impulsive behavior, hyperactivity, and consequent social and emotional problems. A client with ADHD, however, may not exhibit all of these symptoms.

Originally considered a childhood disorder, ADHD is now generally believed to persist into adolescence and adulthood, causing myriad psychosocial problems. The concept of a "residual state" refers to this persistence from childhood into adulthood.

ETIOLOGY AND PRECIPITATING FACTORS

Current biological theory concerning the etiology of ADHD focuses on neurotransmitter dysfunction in the noradrenergic and dopaminergic systems, anatomic and physiologic disturbances of the frontal lobe, and disturbances of subcortical structures, including the reticular activating system and hippocampus. Researchers believe that these dysfunctions and disturbances are related to genetic transmission, perinatal injury, or central nervous system (CNS) infection. Because ADHD is diagnosed more commonly in boys than girls, some researchers also believe that sex-linked transmission may be involved.

Neuropsychological research points to disruptions involving the behavioral inhibition system. Other evidence suggests that the pleasure or reward response usually associated with the completion of socially sanctioned tasks (such as the completion of homework assignments) is diminished in ADHD.

Psychodynamic and psychoanalytic theories center on the intrapsychic and relational dynamics underlying impulsive behaviors and inattention. In Freudian terms, ADHD symptoms are caused by an inadequate ego and superego formation that results in marginal control of id forces.

Family systems theorists express little doubt that ADHD symptoms are exacerbated by family relating problems. Adoption studies point to the prevalence of alcoholic, histrionic, and antisocial behaviors in the biological parents of ADHD-diagnosed children. Research also indicates that the ADHD client exhibiting obvious and, in many cases, disruptive symptoms tends to be seen by family members as the source of all family problems.

Assessment guidelines

NURSING HISTORY (Functional health pattern findings)

The client may report or exhibit one or more of the findings grouped here according to functional health patterns.

Health-perception–health-management pattern

• disproportionate concern about general health
• lack of concern about a significant health problem
• inordinate use of legal stimulants, such as caffeine, nicotine, and diet medication, to feel more focused
• no effect or a calming effect derived from stimulants
• inconsistent approach toward health maintenance activities
• inability to follow through on prescribed treatments

Elimination pattern

• gastrointestinal irritability secondary to caffeine or nicotine intake

Activity-exercise pattern

• constant activity or restlessness
• poor coordination dating from childhood
• irritability or anxiety when faced with unstructured time

Sleep-rest pattern

• daytime sleeping
• trouble making the transition from sleep to a conscious state
• excessive movement during sleep (usually reported by the client's partner)

Cognitive-perceptual pattern

• problems concentrating and sustaining attention dating from childhood
• excessive shifting from one activity to the next
• easy distractibility
• history of poor school performance secondary to dyslexia
• diminished response to pleasurable or painful emotional experiences

Self-perception–self-concept pattern
• perception of self as moody, difficult, irritable, short-tempered, impulsive, immature, lazy, or demanding
• perception of self as an "underachiever"
• inability to follow through on identified goals and tasks
• fear of losing self-control
• poor self-esteem
• an external locus of control

Role-relationship pattern
• history of being the family troublemaker
• history of stormy interpersonal relationships
• history of erratic school and work performance
• difficulty entertaining another person's point of view
• history of trouble with the law

Coping–stress tolerance pattern
• being tense or "wired" most of the time
• low stress tolerance and a restricted range of problem-solving skills or coping mechanisms
• alcohol or illicit substance use to ease stress

Value-belief pattern
• chronic dissatisfaction with life
• feelings of powerlessness

PHYSICAL FINDINGS
The client may report or exhibit one or more of the following physical findings.

Gastrointestinal
• abdominal distress secondary to caffeine or nicotine intake

Musculoskeletal
• muscular tension
• restlessness
• increased motor activity
• minor physical anomalies, such as curved fifth digit or elongated middle toe

Neurologic
• posturing of upper extremities when walking with a heel-to-toe gait
• diadochokinesis (ability to make antagonistic movements, such as pronation and supination of hands, in quick succession)
• poor hand-eye coordination

Psychological
• irritability
• impulsiveness
• hyperactivity
• inattentiveness
• low frustration tolerance

Potential complications
If undetected or left untreated, attention deficit disorder can lead to possible physical injury from failure to control impulses or to failing grades in school.

Nursing diagnosis: *Knowledge deficit related to misinterpretation of information about the client's disorder and treatment plan*

NURSING PRIORITY: To inform the client and family about the usual treatment plan for a client with ADHD and to alleviate any misconceptions

Interventions

1. Establish and maintain a trusting relationship with the client and family by actively listening and showing empathy and respect.

2. Assess the client's knowledge of ADHD as well as of appropriate diagnostic measures and interventions.

3. Create an educational plan that includes one-on-one sessions with the client as well as group sessions with family and loved ones.

4. Include in the client's educational plan information about the biological and psychodynamic theories of ADHD, the use of psychostimulants and antidepressants, and individual and family coping mechanisms that address psychophysiologic symptoms.

Rationales

1. These strategies can decrease the client's and family's anxiety level and help to create an optimum learning environment.

2. Assessing the client's knowledge of ADHD enables the nurse to construct an individualized educational plan.

3. The ADHD client typically learns more effectively in an individualized, low-stimulus setting. Group sessions, however, can promote consensual understanding, enhance the client's sense of control, and minimize the use of scapegoating.

4. A comprehensive teaching plan best addresses the complex nature of ADHD. Furthermore, knowledge about the disorder can increase the client's sense of control.

Nursing diagnosis: *Ineffective individual coping related to ADHD as evidenced by distracted or impulsive behavior, inability to delay gratification, inability to complete tasks, conflict-ridden relationships, and outbursts of rage*

NURSING PRIORITY: To help the client identify ADHD sequelae and learn effective coping mechanisms that diminish them

Interventions

1. Acknowledge and manage any personal feelings about the client's behaviors while avoiding judgmental responses.

2. Provide the client with structured time and a low-stimulus atmosphere for tasks and interactions.

3. Encourage the client to identify previous adaptive and maladaptive coping strategies.

4. Help the client set realistic, short-term goals.

5. Respond positively to the client's goal setting as well as to any goal achievement.

6. Administer prescribed medications, such as psychostimulants and antidepressants; monitor their effects on target symptoms, including inattention, impulsivity, and hyperactivity.

7. Develop with the client a system for self-administering medications, and have the client rehearse this system before discharge.

Rationales

1. In response to the client's behavior, the nurse may experience frustration and anger, feelings that may mirror those of the client or family. If not managed, these feelings can lead to power struggles with the client. Avoiding power struggles as well as judgmental responses enables the nurse to develop a direct, nonjudgmental, and supportive relationship with the client and promotes positive behavioral change.

2. A well-structured environment and decreased stimulation enhance the client's concentration ability.

3. Identifying both successful and unsuccessful coping strategies can help increase self-awareness and make the client feel more responsible for changing behavior.

4. Realistic, short-term goals can enhance the client's chances for success. Such success can in turn reinforce positive behaviors.

5. Positive reinforcement can promote behavioral change by enhancing the client's self-esteem and sense of control.

6. Close observation enables the nurse to provide the physician as well as the client and family with information about medication efficacy.

7. The ADHD client's usual inability to attend to details can cause significant problems with medication administration. Consequently, the nurse may have to work creatively with the client and family to ensure medication compliance.

Nursing diagnosis: *Self-esteem disturbance related to the client's condition as evidenced by excessive criticism of self and others, performance of scapegoat or clown role in family and social situations, and self-defeating behavior*

NURSING PRIORITY: To help the client identify and address causes of diminished self-esteem

Interventions

1. Acknowledge the client's struggle with ADHD sequelae.

Rationales

1. Such acknowledgment can promote the self-regard necessary for behavioral changes.

2. Help the client identify relating behaviors that diminish self-esteem and prevent growth. Such behaviors may include taking the role of scapegoat at school or work or within the family and community.

2. Recognizing such behaviors can enhance the client's sense of control and promote self-awareness, a prerequisite for lasting change.

3. Encourage the client to identify personal strengths, including personality traits and behaviors.

3. Identifying personal strengths can help the client adjust certain distorted self-perceptions. Correcting self-perceptions can enhance the client's feelings of worth and power.

4. Offer encouragement and support as the client addresses problem behaviors.

4. By being supportive during therapy, the nurse can help the client realize that behaviors, not people, are unacceptable and that such behaviors can be changed.

5. Encourage and help the client to set realistic daily goals that provide opportunities for interaction and task completion.

5. Successful experiences will refute the client's self-perceptions of worthlessness and powerlessness.

Nursing diagnosis: *Altered family processes related to the client's inattention or disruptive behaviors as evidenced by a history of unresolved conflict and by family members' attempts to blame each other for problems and their inability to acknowledge each others' contributions or limitations.*

NURSING PRIORITY: To promote the family's participation in therapy that helps to establish positive behaviors

Interventions

1. Provide or arrange for family therapy sessions in which members identify their own contributions—both adaptive and maladaptive—to current family interactions.

2. Encourage family members to credit one another and to hold one another accountable for change.

3. Help family members to explore and pursue behavioral options that can help make family life a vehicle for personal growth, mutual support, and enjoyment.

Rationales

1. Identifying adaptive as well as maladaptive contributions can help family members accept both credit and responsibility for their role in family relating. Such therapy can diminish scapegoating and help to establish trust.

2. Giving credit and demanding that family members be responsible for their behavior helps to create a trusting environment and improve family relations.

3. Given the long-standing patterns of blame, conflict, and disengagement commonly associated with ADHD, family members may require the nurse's guidance in imagining new ways of relating.

Outcome criteria

As treatment progresses, the client, family, or both should be able to:
• identify behavioral symptoms related to ADHD
• identify and use coping methods that diminish ADHD behavioral symptoms
• identify and use health care interventions (medication and follow-up therapy) aimed at reducing ADHD sequelae
• identify maladaptive coping mechanisms and behaviors that exacerbate ADHD symptoms
• engage in family relationships and behaviors that facilitate personal growth, mutual support, goal achievement, and enjoyment.

Discharge criteria

Nursing documentation indicates that the client:
• can recognize ADHD symptoms
• has demonstrated an ability to use adaptive coping skills to diminish ADHD sequelae
• understands the diagnosis, treatment, and expected outcome
• is aware of available family and community resources
• has demonstrated a willingness to pursue follow-up therapy.

Nursing documentation also indicates that the family:
• understand the client's disorder, treatment, and expected outcome
• can use appropriate coping mechanisms and newly acquired relating behaviors to diminish ADHD sequelae
• has been referred to the appropriate community resources for families of ADHD clients.
• has scheduled the necessary follow-up appointments
• understands when, why, and how to contact the appropriate health care professional in case of an emergency.

Selected references

Barkley, R.A. (1990). *ADHD: A handbook for diagnosis and treatment.* New York: Guilford Press.

Doenges, M.E., Townsend, M.C., and Moorhouse, M.F. (1989). *Psychiatric care plans: Guidelines for client care.* Philadelphia: Davis.

Haber, J., Hoskins, P.L., and Sidelau, B. (1987). *Comprehensive Psychiatric Nursing* (3rd ed.). New York: McGraw-Hill.

Hechtman, L., Weiss, G., and Perlman, T. (1984). Hyperactives as young adults: Past and current substance abuse and antisocial behavior. *American Journal of Orthopsychiatry*, 54(3), 415-425.

Morrison, J. (1980). Adult psychiatric disorders in parents of hyperactive children. *American Journal of Psychiatry*, 137(7), 825-827.

Weiss, L. (1992). *Attention deficit disorder in adults: Practical help for sufferers and their spouses.* Dallas: Taylor Publishing.

Wiener, J.M. (Ed.) (1989). Attention Deficit Hyperactivity Disorder. *Psychiatric Annals*, 19(11), 574-575.

AGE-SPECIFIC DISORDERS

Conduct Disorder

DSM III-R classification
312.90 Conduct disorder, undifferentiated type

Psychiatric nursing diagnostic class
Anger

Introduction

Disruptive behavior disorders are characterized by socially disruptive and problematic behaviors that are generally more troublesome to others than to the client exhibiting them. *Conduct disorder* — a form of disruptive behavior disorder — typically manifests before or during adolescence and is characterized by behaviors that violate others' rights and that are more firmly entrenched and destructive than normal adolescent disruptions. For example, the adolescent might continually start fights with classmates or disrupt classroom discussions.

The conduct pattern usually occurs with family members and friends as well as at school and lasts at least 6 months. Commonly, an adolescent with conduct disorder is identified and diagnosed with the problem when referred by school officials to the city or county health care or juvenile system. Persistence of conduct disorder beyond adolescence, especially when the onset was early in life, may lead to adult antisocial personality disorder.

ETIOLOGY AND PRECIPITATING FACTORS

Family systems theorists believe that the adolescent with conduct disorder usually reflects larger family problems or family dysfunction. Theorists cite certain family characteristics as contributing factors, including marital problems, drug or alcohol use, antisocial behaviors, inconsistent parenting, parental rejection, harsh discipline, and general chaos or disorganization within the family. Research further indicates that the child from such a family, in an attempt to develop an identity in a context of minimal positive regard and caring, commonly affiliates with a delinquent peer group to make up for family deficits.

Psychodynamic theorists maintain that conduct disorder may result from inadequate and inappropriate ego functioning. Lack of impulse control, trouble forming relationships, and little or no problem solving skills are characteristics of both children with ego deficits and adolescents with conduct disorder.

Assessment guidelines

NURSING HISTORY (Functional health pattern findings)
The client may report or exhibit one or more of the findings grouped here according to functional health patterns.

Health perception–health management pattern
- anger toward and blame of others for own behavior
- inability to control feelings and impulses
- general malaise
- angry, hostile, or depressed manner

Nutritional-metabolic pattern
- weight gain or loss
- eating large quantities of food
- drug or alcohol use

Activity-exercise pattern
- infrequent participation in physical and social activities
- initiating fights with other children
- hostility, physical aggression, disobedience, and defiance of authority when engaging in group activities
- poor school performance

Sleep-rest pattern
- inconsistent sleep patterns

Cognitive-perceptual pattern
- treating others as family treats self
- little or no remorse for own behavior
- denial of own behavior
- difficulty focusing and concentrating

Self-perception–self-concept pattern
- perception of self as victim of external forces
- nervousness
- self-hatred
- difficulty articulating personal strengths

Role-relationship pattern
- little to no relationships with family and peers
- behaviors that violate others' rights, including stealing, lying, setting fires, destroying property, cruelty to animals, and forced sexual acts
- runaway or truant behaviors
- disruptive and socially unacceptable behaviors with peers, including initiating fights and cheating
- dysfunctional family patterns, such as harsh discipline and cruelty
- isolation from peers
- lack of social skills

Sexual-reproductive pattern
• history of sexual abuse
• sexual abuse of others
• promiscuity

Coping–stress tolerance pattern
• lack of impulse control
• jittery feelings
• aggressive behavior toward others with little or no provocation

Value-belief pattern
• feelings that events are beyond personal control

PHYSICAL FINDINGS
The client may report or exhibit one or more of the following physical findings.

Musculoskeletal
• above- or below-average physical growth

Reproductive
• early sexual experimentation
• sexual aggressiveness

Psychological
• anxiety symptoms, such as irritability, during interactions
• difficulty concentrating
• feeling and appearance of being "wired"
• cruelty to animals
• low self-esteem
• low frustration tolerance
• lying
• anxiety and depression
• lack of remorse for misdeeds
• drug abuse

Potential complications
Without accurate assessment and intervention, adolescents with conduct disorder typically become involved in crime and end up in jail where they may not receive appropriate and necessary treatment. They also may develop a psychoactive substance abuse disorder.

Nursing diagnosis: *Potential for violence, self-directed or directed at others, related to dysfunctional family relationships manifested by overt hostility, poor impulse control, overt aggressive acts, and self-destructive behavior*

NURSING PRIORITY: To provide a safe environment that protects the client and others from harm

Interventions

1. Assess the client for past and present suicide attempts or suicidal ideation. Implement suicide precautions if the client appears to be at high risk.

2. Work with the client to identify situations or events that have triggered past aggressive acts. Assess behaviors that indicate increased anxiety or anger, such as pacing and verbal threats.

3. Provide the client with other outlets for stress and anxiety, such as exercising, listening to music, sitting quietly in a room, or playing baseball with a foam-rubber ball and bat.

4. Respond positively to the client's effective use of stress-relieving outlets.

5. If the client suddenly becomes physically aggressive or violent, use appropriate means to control the behavior. Use seclusion or restraints if the client cannot be controlled by other means.

Rationales

1. Suicide assessment gives the nurse an idea of the client's stress tolerance and coping capabilities. Suicide precautions, such as removing objects that the client could use to harm self or others and frequent observation, decrease the chances of a successful suicide attempt.

2. Recognition and intervention before an aggressive outbreak can help to break the client's behavioral cycle and to maintain a safe environment.

3. Such outlets can enable the client to decrease anxiety and stress by channeling aggressions appropriately.

4. A positive response reinforces the client's use of appropriate behavior.

5. Typically, the client's narrowed cognition and perception renders verbal and other interventions ineffective. The nurse must use external controls until the client regains internal control.

6. Use activities and projects (such as crafts and games) to begin to establish a trusting relationship with the client. Encourage the staff to interact with the client when the client's behavior is not disruptive.

6. Such strategies can help the nurse avoid developing a negative view of the client and can provide the client with opportunities for relating to others more effectively.

7. Approach the client in a consistent manner to establish a trusting relationship.

7. A level of trust between the client and nurse is necessary before the client can begin to articulate feelings and inner conflicts.

8. Work with the client to set reasonable, realistic limits on the client's most problematic behaviors. Emphasize to the client that you are setting limits on specific behaviors not feelings. For instance, you might say, "It's okay to be angry, but you may not scream." Expect the client to test these limits.

8. Setting behavioral limits is not punitive and communicates expectations for positive behavior while helping to create a secure environment. Involving the client can enhance self-control.

Nursing diagnosis: *Self-esteem disturbance related to dysfunctional family system, parental rejection, or family disruption caused by separation, death, or other events*

NURSING PRIORITY: To help the client develop strategies that can improve self-esteem

Interventions

1. Structure the client's routine to include activities that can be performed successfully. Such activities might include crafts, unit parties, sports, and individual tutoring. Encourage the client to help choose activities.

2. Spend a designated amount of time (perhaps 20 minutes per shift) with the client.

3. Work with the client to gradually explore feelings. Have the client describe events and situations that previously have led to disruptive behaviors. Ask the client to describe what he was thinking while acting out and how others might have viewed such behavior. Suggest that the client keep a daily journal in which to record these impressions.

4. Help the client to identify personal strengths. Encourage the client to identify a new strength or positive trait each day.

Rationales

1. Success can enhance self-esteem and enable the client to relate to the staff and peers in less disruptive ways. Participation in decision making can improve the client's sense of self-control.

2. Routine visits can help the nurse to avoid interacting with the client only in response to negative behaviors. Such visits also allow the client to view people less negatively and enhance feelings of self-worth.

3. An adolescent with conduct disorder probably will have difficulty articulating feelings. Having the client describe events or situations can help to establish a more objective basis from which to examine and discuss feelings. Ultimately, identifying and expressing feelings decreases the client's need to act out.

4. Identifying personal strengths and positive traits can enhance the client's self-esteem.

Nursing diagnosis: *Impaired social interaction related to a lack of role models or a dysfunctional family system*

NURSING PRIORITY: To help the client learn and participate in more productive relationships with family and peers

Interventions

1. Encourage the client to interact with the staff and peers by scheduling participation in supervised activities, such as walks, team sports, and jogging.

Rationales

1. Providing safe, structured settings for activities can improve the client's socialization skills. Participation in peer group activities promotes feelings of normalcy.

2. Assess the ways in which family members relate to one another and solve problems.

2. Examining family relationships and the family's ability to solve problems can help the nurse to understand the client's social background and suggest ways to improve social development.

3. Help identify situations that make the client uncomfortable and cause stress.

3. Identifying stressful situations can help the client know when to take appropriate stress-reducing actions.

4. Explore with the client how others perceive him.

4. Recognizing how others perceive him is among the client's first steps toward changing behavior.

5. Use role playing to help the client develop alternative behaviors for handling stressful situations.

5. Role playing gives the client opportunities to learn and rehearse alternative ways of relating to others.

6. Set behavior limits, provide feedback, and encourage the client to assume responsibility for appropriate social behavior.

6. These interventions can enhance the client's personal identity and self-esteem, which in turn can lead to improved social interactions.

Outcome criteria

As treatment progresses, the client, family, or both should be able to:
• engage in less disruptive interactions with peers and family
• engage in social activities
• report or display an absence of suicidal thinking
• report or display an absence of aggression toward others
• use alternative strategies to cope with stress
• identify feelings, events, or situations that trigger disruptive behavior
• use coping strategies that improve self-esteem
• identify personal strengths.

Discharge criteria

Nursing documentation indicates that the client:
• has demonstrated the ability to recognize triggering events and causes of disruptive behavior
• has verbalized an understanding of the need to control disruptive behaviors
• has demonstrated the ability to express anger and frustration in productive ways
• has demonstrated the ability to participate positively in peer activities
• has demonstrated the ability to use alternative ways to express anger and frustration
• is aware of appropriate family and community resources.

Nursing documentation also indicates that the family:
• understands the client's diagnosis, treatment, and expected outcome
• has demonstrated a willingness to participate in an appropriate therapy program

• has been referred to the appropriate community resources, such as parenting effectiveness classes and parent management training
• is willing to participate in a follow-up therapy program
• understands when, why, and how to contact the appropriate health care professional in case of a crisis.

Selected references

Burchard, J., and Burchard, S. (1987). *Prevention of delinquent behavior.* Newbury Park, CA: Sage Publications.

Carpenito, L.J. (1991). *Nursing diagnosis: Application to clinical practice* (4th ed.). Philadelphia: Lippincott.

Chitty, K.K., and Maynard, C.K. (1986). Managing manipulation. *Journal of Psychosocial Nursing and Mental Health Services,* 24(6), 8-13.

Doenges, M.E., Townsend, M.C., and Moorhouse, M.F. (1989). *Psychiatric care plans: Guidelines for client care.* Philadelphia: Davis.

Elliot, D., et al. (1985). *Explaining delinquency and drug use.* Newbury Park, CA: Sage Publications.

Farley, G. (1986). *Handbook of child and adolescent psychiatric emergencies and crises* (2nd ed.). Medical Exam.

Faulstich, M.E., Moore, J.R., Roberts, R.W., and Collier, J.B. (1988). A behavioral perspective on conduct disorders. *Psychiatry,* 51(4), 398-413.

Husain, S., and Vandiver, T. (1984). *Suicide in children and adolescents.* New York: Spectrum Publications.

Kazdin, A. (1987). *Conduct disorders in childhood and adolescence,* vol 9. Newbury Park, CA: Sage Publications.

Kessler, J.W. (1988). *Psychopathology of childhood.* Englewood Cliffs, NJ: Prentice-Hall.

McFarland, G. (1986). *Nursing diagnoses and process in psychiatric–mental health nursing.* Philadelphia: Lippincott.

Pasquali, E., et al. (1989). *Mental health nursing: A holistic approach.* St. Louis: Mosby-Year Book.

Popper, C. (1988). Disorders usually first evident in infancy, childhood or adolescence. In J. Talbott, et al. (Eds.) *Textbook of psychiatry.* Washington, DC: APA Press.

Spitzer, et al. (1989). *DSM-III-R case book* (3rd ed, rev.). Washington, DC: APA Press.

Taylor, C. (1990). *Mereness' essentials in psychiatric nursing.* St. Louis: Mosby-Year Book.

Organic Mental Disorders

DSM III-R classifications

290.xx Primary degenerative dementia of the Alzheimer type, senile onset (after age 65)

290.00 Primary degenerative dementia of the Alzheimer type, senile onset, uncomplicated

290.1x Primary degenerative dementia of the Alzheimer type, presenile onset (age 65 and below)

290.10 Primary degenerative dementia of the Alzheimer type, presenile onset, uncomplicated

290.11 Primary degenerative dementia of the Alzheimer type, presenile onset, with delirium

290.12 Primary degenerative dementia of the Alzheimer type, presenile onset, with delusions

290.13 Primary degenerative dementia of the Alzheimer type, presenile onset, with depression

290.20 Primary degenerative dementia of the Alzheimer type, senile onset, with delusions

290.21 Primary degenerative dementia of the Alzheimer type, senile onset, with depression

290.30 Primary degenerative dementia of the Alzheimer type, senile onset, with delirium

290.4x Multi-infarct dementia

290.40 Multi-infarct dementia, uncomplicated

290.41 Multi-infarct dementia, with delirium

290.42 Multi-infarct dementia, with delusions

290.43 Multi-infarct dementia, with depression

Psychiatric nursing diagnostic class

Impaired cognition

Introduction

Organic mental disorders represent a constellation of psychological and behavioral changes caused by brain function abnormalities, which may be structural, chemical, or electrical and which can have a rapid or insidious onset. Such brain function abnormalities may stem from a specific organic condition (see *Causes of organic mental disorders,* page 156). Although the brain abnormalities are progressive in most cases, they can sometimes be reversed, halted, or stabilized at a particular level. This plan of care addresses two main categories of organic mental disorders: *primary degenerative dementia of the Alzheimer type, senile onset* and *multi-infarct dementia.*

Dementia is characterized primarily by orientation, memory, and cognition impairments and their effects on personality and behavior. The most common form of dementia—*primary degenerative dementia of the Alzheimer type*—can manifest before age 65 (presenile onset) or after age 65 (senile onset). Typically, this dementia has an insidious onset and gradually progresses from mild to severe impairment. In the early stage, work and social activity are significantly impaired but self-care capacity is preserved. The client experiences memory loss and is prone to depression. In the second stage, more severe cognitive impairment with motor and language deficits occurs. Disorientation and confusion may lead to agitation, wandering, pacing, sleep disturbances, and disruptive behaviors. Independent living becomes dangerous, and supervision is necessary. In the terminal stage, the client is incapable of self-care; speech is severely impaired, and mobility is compromised. Also, bowel and bladder incontinence occurs.

Multi-infarct dementia results from progressive deterioration of intellectual functioning caused by cardiovascular disease. Onset is typically abrupt, but progression occurs in uneven spurts. Common characteristics include memory disturbances, impaired judgment, poor impulse control, and impaired abstract thinking.

In some cases, clients with dementia also experience delirium, delusions, depression, and activity disturbances.

Activity disturbances may manifest as overactivity or underactivity—both potentially problematic for demented clients. Overactive clients are characterized by continuous wandering, pacing, confusion, and transient agitation. Wandering is described as a tendency to move around in an unfocused, seemingly aimless way. The triad symptoms of wandering, confusion, and agitation may be directly related to the effects of brain tissue alterations.

Current research indicates that the use of restraints for confused clients may increase the risk of injury rather than minimize it. In most cases, confused or wandering clients are elderly; use of restraints puts them at high risk for strangulation, fractures, dislocations, and impaired circulation and increases their level of agitation, withdrawal, and depression.

ETIOLOGY AND PRECIPITATING FACTORS

The etiology of primary degenerative dementia of the Alzheimer type remains unknown; however, several studies support a genetic transmission theory. Researchers have found that in families with a history of primary degenerative dementia of the Alzheimer type, usually more than one family member is afflicted. Furthermore, autopsies have revealed physiologic changes in the brains of clients with primary degenerative dementia of the Alzheimer type similar to the changes seen in those with Down's syndrome; also, data indicates a higher incidence of Down's syndrome in families also afflicted with primary degenerative dementia

CAUSES OF ORGANIC MENTAL DISORDERS

Organic mental disorders can result from extrapyramidal conditions, central nervous system (CNS) disturbances, systemic illnesses, endocrine disturbances, and deficiency states.

Extrapyramidal conditions
• Huntington's disease
• Parkinson's disease

CNS disturbances
• Alzheimer's disease
• Cerebrovascular disease
• Epilepsy
• Meningitis
• Multiple sclerosis
• Neoplasms
• Syphilis
• Viral encephalitis

Systemic illness
• Anoxia
• Hepatic encephalopathy
• Hypercalcemia
• Hypoglycemia
• Hyponatremia
• Pancreatic encephalopathy
• Subacute bacterial endocarditis
• Uremia

Endocrine diseases
• Addison's disease
• Cushing's disease
• Diabetic ketoacidosis
• Hyperthyroidism
• Hypothyroidism

Deficiency states
• Folate
• Niacin
• Thiamine
• Vitamin B_{12}

From *Psychiatric problems*. NurseReview. Springhouse, PA: Springhouse Corp., 1990.

Assessment guidelines
NURSING HISTORY (Functional health pattern findings)
The client may report or exhibit one or more of the findings grouped here according to functional health patterns.

Health perception–health management pattern
• vague physical and emotional complaints
• worry and frustration over inability to remember things
• fear of losing mental faculties
• fear of being institutionalized
• worry about inability to follow medical regimen
• concern about decline in overall functioning level
• neglect of preventive medical care
• inability to identify when difficulties first began

Nutritional-metabolic pattern
• change in usual appetite
• weight gain or loss
• difficulty eating because of dental problems, such as ill-fitting dentures or lack of dental care
• lack of normal thirst
• bruises and cuts from bumping into objects
• slow healing
• concern about physical appearance

Elimination pattern
• loss of bladder or bowel continence
• constipation or diarrhea
• urinary tract infection symptoms, such as frequent or painful urination
• body odor

Activity-exercise pattern
• fatigue
• difficulty performing normal daily activities
• loss of interest in recreational and leisure activities
• difficulty going up and down steps
• difficulty maintaining balance
• coordination difficulty
• restlessness
• repeating the same action or movement

Sleep-rest pattern
• early morning awakening or insomnia
• concern about disrupted sleep patterns
• using sleep disturbances as a reason for decreased participation in daily activities
• reversed sleep-awake cycle

of the Alzheimer type. Despite the data, support for a genetic transmission theory remains inconclusive.

Other research focuses on the role of aluminum and viral agents as causes of primary degenerative dementia of the Alzheimer type, but evidence remains at best inconclusive.

Although little is known about multi-infarct dementia, researchers believe that arterial hypertension, extracranial vascular disease, and valvular disease of the heart contribute to the formation of emboli, which lead to cardiovascular dysfunctioning.

Cognitive-perceptual pattern

- hearing difficulty
- difficulty using hearing aid
- visual disturbances (such as double-vision and visual field disturbances)
- difficulty remembering to wear glasses
- difficulty remembering places, names, and situations
- difficulty concentrating
- becoming lost frequently
- repeating questions and statements
- inability to understand written language
- difficulty selecting words when speaking
- inability to grasp abstract ideas
- difficulty learning new things
- difficulty following verbal commands
- difficulty initiating and focusing on tasks
- difficulty perceiving direction, distance, and spatial relationships
- inability to recognize familiar symbols and objects

Self-perception–self-concept pattern

- perception of self as useless and powerless
- feeling like a family burden
- sadness and anger over diminished cognitive and physical functioning
- annoyance, fear, or anxiety when needs are not met promptly

Role-relationship pattern

- concern or annoyance with family's increased responsibilities and vigilance
- feeling ignored, neglected, or forgotten by family
- sadness or embarrassment over role-reversal with children
- loneliness
- longing for family or friends
- concern over financial responsibilities
- concern over not "fitting in"

Sexual-reproductive pattern

- inappropriate flirting
- inappropriate sexual behavior, such as disrobing or masturbating in public
- difficulty with intimacy

Coping–stress tolerance pattern

- tension or anxiety in new situations
- agitation in response to internal or external stimuli
- feeling out of control
- anxiety, restlessness, or frustration if unable to follow directions
- inability to solve problems

Value-belief pattern

- feeling that life goals are unattainable
- loss of interest in religious affiliations
- concern over changes in religious beliefs and practices

PHYSICAL FINDINGS

The client may report or exhibit one or more of the following physical findings.

Cardiovascular

- poor circulation
- arrhythmias
- high or low blood pressure
- increased or decreased heart rate

Gastrointestinal

- constipation
- diarrhea
- difficulty chewing and swallowing
- impactions
- incontinence

Genitourinary

- decreased urination
- incontinence
- urinary tract infections

Musculoskeletal

- muscle aches and pains
- decreased range of motion
- easy fatigability
- muscle rigidity and tension
- muscle atrophy
- pacing
- shakiness
- weakness

Neurological

- balance difficulty
- dizziness
- gait disturbance
- restlessness
- seizures
- sleep disturbances, such as frequent waking or insomnia

ASSESSING DEMENTIA: TAKING A CLIENT HISTORY

When assessing a client for dementia, you'll need to determine the answers to these questions.

• Does the client complain of memory loss or memory deficit?

• Does the client complain of forgetting the location of familiar objects or forgetting familiar names?

• How concerned is the client about memory loss?

• Are others, such as family members and employers, aware of the client's memory lapses?

• Has the client lost the ability to recall the content of a story, either read or heard?

• Does the client try to hide signs of impaired mentation?

• Do neuropsychiatric examination results show evidence of memory and concentration deficits?

• Can the client manage complex tasks?

• Has the client exhibited lability of affect?

• Does the client remember telephone numbers, dates of important events, and names of close family members?

• Has the client become disoriented to time, person, and place?

• Have the client's sleep and wake cycles changed?

• Can the client hold a conversation or utter meaningful sounds?

• Can the client perform psychomotor tasks?

• Is the client incontinent?

From *Psychiatric problems*. NurseReview. Springhouse, PA: Springhouse Corp., 1990.

Psychological
• agitation
• confusion
• decreased ability to think abstractly
• decreased concentration
• irritability
• language deficits
• memory loss

Respiratory
• cough
• increased respiratory rate
• increased susceptibility to upper respiratory tract infections
• shortness of breath
• increased sputum production

Potential complications
Without accurate diagnosis, reversible dementias can be missed, and the disease can continue unchecked and become a persistent state. In addition, falls, self-inflicted injuries, and violence can occur.

Nursing diagnosis: *Potential for injury related to cognitive deficits, debilitated state, impaired mobility, wandering behavior, balance and perceptual impairment, and depressed mood*

NURSING PRIORITY: To provide a safe environment in which the client can maintain optimum independence and safety

Interventions

1. Assess the client's physical and cognitive impairment levels (see *Assessing dementia: Taking a client history*). Obtain information from both the client and family about the client's prior habits, activities, hobbies, and usual ways of coping with stress.

2. Facilitate the client's access to personal belongings by removing obstacles and hazardous objects from the client's path. Use reflective tape on steps.

Rationales

1. Establishing a performance baseline can help the nurse develop appropriate strategies that allow the client to function at optimum levels.

2. A hazard-free environment can decrease the risk of falls and injury.

3. Avoid rushing the client with activities of daily living (ADLs) and ambulation.

3. Because the client's ability to follow directions may be significantly reduced, rushing to complete tasks can increase anxiety and frustration. A slower pace and patience on the nurse's part will make the client more comfortable and facilitate ADLs.

4. Provide adequate lighting in the client's room, and keep a bathroom light on at night. At night, help the client to the toilet every 4 hours or as needed.

4. Adequate nighttime lighting can help reduce confusion. Helping the client to the toilet can help prevent falls that might occur when the client is trying to get out of bed or is looking for the bathroom.

5. Provide the client with an identification bracelet, and keep a photograph of the client in the chart. Introduce the client to the staff. Provide other environmental cues, such as clocks and calendars as well as large signs with the client's name next to his bedroom and on the door and signs with arrows pointing to his room.

5. An identification bracelet and photograph in the chart as well as familiarity with the staff can help ensure the client's safety. Providing environmental cues can improve the client's orientation and reduce confusion.

6. Provide the client with stimulating, supervised activities requiring physical activity as well as a safe, controlled environment in which the client can wander.

6. The client may wander to release tension or decrease boredom, in response to psychotropic medications, or in search of security. Providing safe opportunities for wandering can help relieve the client's tension or frustration.

7. Provide the client with appropriate sensory or mobility aids, such as glasses, a hearing aid, or a walker.

7. By improving the client's ability to see, hear, and walk, the nurse can help prevent dangerous situations and injury. Doing so also can increase the client's potential to be physically and socially active.

8. Ensure that the client avoids complex tasks and activities involving the use of toxic materials or sharp implements that could accidentally cause injury. Encourage the client's participation in a music or exercise program.

8. Providing simple, safe tasks helps to ensure success and avoids frustrating the client. Most clients find music and simple exercise programs enjoyable and physically stimulating.

9. Carefully monitor the client's mood and assess for suicidal feelings.

9. Depression and suicidal feelings can occur with dementia.

10. Avoid using restraints. Alternatives to restraints include bean bag cushions and foam cushion wedges.

10. Restraints impair mobility and promote skin breakdown. They also can increase client agitation and confusion, which may result in an injury.

Nursing diagnosis: *Personal identity disturbance related to cognitive deficits*

NURSING PRIORITY: To ensure the client's safety and the safety of others while continuing to meet the client's needs

Interventions

1. Make sure that the client is wearing an identification bracelet or name tag with the unit location and the client's home address at all times.

Rationales

1. This ensures that the client will be returned to the proper location if the client should begin to wander.

2. Place a sign with the client's name in bold letters outside the client's room, preferably in a highly visible area, such as on the wall opposite where the door swings open.

2. Signs serve to remind the wandering or confused client where to return.

3. Check on the client frequently throughout the day. If possible, perform checks at 15-minute intervals.

3. Frequent contact decreases the client's need to seek assistance and provides the client with a sense of security and consistency. It also ensures the client's safety.

4. When communicating with the client, make a point of reorienting the client to person, place, and time.

4. Reorienting the client serves as a reality test and helps decrease confusion.

5. Have the client who is prone to wandering sit in a hallway or near the nurses' station, and provide the client with diversional activities.

5. Placing the client in a highly visible area enables more people to directly observe and interact with the client, ensuring the client's safety and decreasing the client's isolation. Diversional activities help to structure the client's time and distract the client from wandering.

6. Teach the client to check clocks, calendars, and watches frequently throughout the day.

6. This helps to keep the client oriented to time.

7. Remind the client about mealtimes, bedtime, and group activities.

7. Some clients need to be reminded to attend to activities of daily living. Frequent reminders also help keep the client oriented and more responsive to structure.

8. Ask family members to bring in recent pictures of the client. Keep one picture in the client's chart, and display any others in the client's room.

8. A recent picture can be used by staff or police to help identify a wandering client. Displaying the client's pictures keeps the client oriented to person.

Nursing diagnosis: *Potential for violence, self-directed or directed at others, related to delusional beliefs, suspicion, inability to recognize persons and places, increased stress, or decreased coping skills*

NURSING PRIORITY: To help prevent violence by minimizing sources of stress

Interventions

1. Assess the client's delusional beliefs in a supportive manner. Do not contradict or challenge the client with rational explanations.

2. Always approach the client frontally, using a slow, consistent, and calm manner. Remember to introduce yourself, and offer reassurance while you attempt to identify the client's needs. Respond nondefensively to any of the client's accusations, and avoid touching or crowding the agitated client.

3. Avoid taking the client into elevators, dining rooms, and other gathering areas.

4. Avoid talking to staff members about the client while in his presence. Do not tease or ridicule the client.

5. Should the client become verbally abusive, protect others from possible attack by having the client either calm down alone in his room or work alone or with a staff member until the behavior subsides.

6. Administer psychotropic medications as prescribed to decrease agitation. Monitor the client's vital signs and behavior closely for positive and negative changes.

7. Avoid restraining the agitated client.

Rationales

1. Assessing the client's state of mind enables the nurse to implement appropriate interventions. Trying to convince the client that delusional beliefs are unfounded will only increase agitation.

2. The client may interpret any gesture as an assault and may perceive large numbers of staff as an attack force. Both misconceptions can lead to violence. A calm, slow approach by the nurse can help prevent such an outbreak.

3. The client may feel as though personal space is being violated and become agitated.

4. The client may perceive whispers and information that he cannot decode because of brain dysfunction as a plot against him. Teasing decreases client self-esteem and may trigger emotional outbursts.

5. The demented client usually exhibits diminished impulse control. Verbal attacks may represent a response to internal sensations or to the situation rather than to any one person or thing in the environment. Calming the client usually relieves the situation.

6. Small doses of neuroleptics can help alleviate paranoid, belligerent behavior. Anxiolytics may reduce anxiety symptoms. Because drug metabolism is significantly altered in elderly persons, the client probably will require a smaller than usual dose.

7. Using restraints to control agitation can escalate violent behavior and result in increased isolation, sensory deprivation, and decreased mobility.

Nursing diagnosis: *Impaired physical mobility related to use of restraints and problems with expressing anger*

NURSING PRIORITY: To ensure the safety of the client and others while continuing to meet the client's need for food, fluids, toileting, and contact with others

Interventions

1. If the client must be restrained, make sure that adequate staff and the proper equipment are on hand to carry out the plan.

2. Make sure that the team leader communicates the plan of action and the specific roles of each staff member before attempting to restrain the client.

3. If the client is to be restrained in bed, make sure the client is placed face up on the bed with all four extremities attached securely to the bed frame. Secure one arm above the head and one arm at the client's side.

4. Assess circulation to all extremities immediately after applying restraints, then at least hourly until the restraints are removed. Make sure the client maintains good body alignment while restrained.

5. After the client has been restrained, check the fit of the cuffs. For a good fit, you should be able to insert only a fingertip between the cuff and the client's skin.

6. Provide the client with basic needs, including food, fluids, toileting, range-of-motion exercises, and proper skin care, during the duration of restraint.

7. Offer the client emotional support and prescribed medications during the restraint period.

8. Establish clear behavioral expectations that the client must meet before the restraints can be removed.

9. Include several team members in the discussion to remove restraints, and reintegrate the client into the milieu.

10. When the client meets all the established behavioral criteria and the decision to remove the restraints has been made, remove all the restraints at once.

Rationales

1. Adequate numbers of trained staff are required to preserve the therapeutic value of using restraints and to minimize the risk of injuring the client and others. If locking restraints are used, the nurse must ensure that the key is readily available in case of an emergency.

2. Poor communication or a poorly planned approach will increase the risk of injury to all involved.

3. Restraining the client in this position helps to lessen the client's fear and vulnerability and prevents the risk of suffocation. It also prevents the client from sitting up in bed. The client should be restrained only to the bed frame, never to the side rails, which could cause injury.

4. Restraints applied too tightly will impede the client's bloodflow. Proper body alignment is necessary to prevent contractures and injury.

5. The client's cuffs may have been secured too tightly or loosely at first and may need to be adjusted.

6. A restrained client should never be denied the necessities of food, fluid, and toileting. Range-of-motion exercises and skin care are necessary to prevent injury and skin breakdown.

7. Support and contact with staff are important to help the client realize that restraints are therapeutic and not a punitive measure. Medication, particularly anxiolytics, can reduce the client's agitation and anxiety associated with being restrained.

8. Setting expectations gives the client a sense of control and established clear, measurable criteria necessary for restraint removal.

9. This provides an opportunity for the staff to verbalize concerns and observations about the client's behavior. Staff members not included in decision-making processes may feel unsafe and unconsciously sabotage the client's freedom from restraint.

10. Removing only some of the restraints poses a serious danger to the client. For instance, the client who is partially restrained might attempt to get out of bed and fall. Also, removing only some of the restraints communicates lack of trust to the client.

Nursing diagnosis: *Altered thought processes related to memory loss, brain dysfunction, sleep deprivation, and conscious or unconscious conflicts*

NURSING PRIORITY: To facilitate clear communication and provide a structured environment with reduced stimuli

Interventions

1. Using assessment tools and family reports, assess the client's cognitive impairment.

2. Help the client to maintain a consistent daily routine. Obtain information about the client's past routines from family members or the client's primary caregivers. Inquire about the client's daily schedule and the safety measures implemented in the home.

3. Introduce yourself to the client, and explain your actions before providing care.

4. Face the client, and make eye contact before speaking. Once you have the client's attention, speak slowly and clearly using simple, short sentences. Use various communication aids, such as verbal or written cues, gestures, and pictures.

5. Note the client's nonverbal attempts to communicate.

6. Provide adequate lighting and stimulation as well as seasonal orientation in the environment.

7. Learn the client's usual hiding places.

8. Respond to the client's view of reality with empathy and support. Do not contradict delusional beliefs.

9. Closely monitor the client's response to medications.

Rationales

1. An initial assessment provides the nurse with a baseline against which to measure future behaviors.

2. A consistent routine can help decrease the client's anxiety. It also can help reinforce old habits and minimize memory deficits.

3. The client probably has lost the ability to interpret stimuli accurately. For example, the client may misinterpret your touching while bathing as sexual advances. Careful explanations can help prevent this kind of confusion.

4. Because the client's comprehension and concentration abilities are probably greatly impaired, attention-getting and attention-maintaining techniques are necessary to ensure comprehension.

5. The client with language deficits may use nonverbal means, such as facial expressions and hand gestures, to communicate with others.

6. Adequate and appropriate environmental stimuli can help overcome the confusion and disorientation that may result from the client's social and physical isolation.

7. The client may be unable to distinguish personal belongings from those of others and may inadvertently take something belonging to someone else. Knowing the client's hiding places enables the nurse to locate such items.

8. The client's ability to evaluate reality probably is severely impaired. Arguing will only decrease the client's trust in the nurse or increase agitation.

9. Because drug metabolism and absorption are altered in elderly persons, the demented client can easily become delirious after drug administration.

Nursing diagnosis: *Dressing or grooming self-care deficit related to cognitive impairment, weakness, memory impairment, and increased dependency needs*

NURSING PRIORITY: To foster the highest level of client independence while promoting safety

Interventions

1. Assess the client's ability to perform normal ADLs.

Rationales

1. Establishing a performance baseline for ADLs enables the nurse to more accurately measure changes in behavior and dependence.

2. Give direct, one-step directions. Address the client by name, and avoid the use of pronouns when referring to him. Repeat sentences, and discuss persons or objects that the client can readily observe.

2. Communicating clearly and precisely increases the probability that the client will understand. Avoiding abstract topics can help maintain the client's attention.

3. When necessary, assist the client in performing ADLs, such as brushing his teeth or combing his hair. Provide frequent cues, and encourage the client to complete the activities as independently as possible.

3. Though the client may retain the ability to perform routine activities, such as brushing teeth and combing hair, he may require some help.

4. Provide the client with limited choices (for example, in the morning, let the client choose from two shirts).

4. Being able to make choices can bolster self-esteem and increase the client's sense of control. Limiting the choices prevents the client from being overwhelmed, which can lead to agitation.

5. Anticipate the client's refusal of nursing care.

5. By refusing care, the client may be trying to achieve some sense of control. In addition, a suspicious client typically will refuse care.

Nursing diagnosis: *Social isolation related to cognitive impairment, decreased social awareness, impaired language, multiple losses, lack of support systems, and depressed mood*

NURSING PRIORITY: To help the client feel socially connected with others

Interventions

1. Interview the client and family to assess how introverted or extroverted the client was before the disorder's onset.

2. Provide the client with activities that stimulate multiple senses (for example, you might hand the client an orange and ask him to identify it).

3. In a relaxed manner, encourage the client to participate in group activities, such as a singing group; however, do not force participation.

4. Encourage the client and family to bring in personal articles, such as photographs, books, and clothing.

5. Regularly converse with the client, using short, simple sentences and nonverbal aids, such as smiling. Allow time for the client to respond.

6. Inform the client of current events, repeating information as needed. Avoid asking about facts, especially those related to recent events.

7. Assess the client's sense of hopefulness, and offer reassurance.

8. Listen to the client's reminiscences, and encourage or invite him to participate in a reminiscence group.

Rationales

1. Knowing the client's past socialization patterns can help the nurse set realistic expectations for social activities.

2. Such activities stimulate not only the client's recall ability but also the senses of touch, sight, and smell.

3. The client in the early stages of primary dementia of the Alzheimer's type may sense cognitive decline and feel ignored or left out of group activities.

4. Familiar objects may trigger the client's memory, facilitate conversation, and decrease feelings of isolation and alienation.

5. Conversation fosters a sense of connectedness. Patience on the nurse's part can prevent the client from feeling frustrated and increase interest in conversation.

6. Routine communication and repetition will not bore the client and can provide security. Because memory of recent events is typically affected first, the nurse should avoid asking the client to relay facts that he cannot remember.

7. A hopeful attitude contributes to the client's physical and mental well-being.

8. Sharing stories about the past can give the client a sense of connection with others, thereby decreasing feelings of isolation.

9. Encourage visits from the client's family and friends. Educate family members about the client's deficits.

9. Regular visits from family and friends can decrease the client's feelings of isolation and enhance self-esteem. Knowing about the disorder can help family and friends to cope with the client's illness more effectively and sensitively.

Nursing diagnosis: *Bowel incontinence and altered urinary elimination related to weak bladder or bowel muscle tone, confusion, disorientation, or lack of awareness of toileting needs*

NURSING PRIORITY: To help the client maintain adequate elimination patterns and avoid bowel or urinary complications

Interventions

1. Assess the client's usual elimination pattern and use of medications or enemas to maintain that pattern.

2. Check with the client about toileting needs every 2 hours during the day and every 4 hours or as needed at night.

3. Record the time, consistency, and amount of bowel movements.

4. Encourage the client to drink adequate amounts of fluid during the day, but limit fluid intake in the evening.

5. Encourage the client to eat a well-balanced diet that is rich in bulk and fiber. Also encourage him to exercise (walking and stretching) daily.

6. Administer prescribed stool softeners, and monitor the client's response.

7. Be accepting and empathetic when the client is incontinent.

8. Help the client to maintain proper skin care.

9. Be aware of the client's use of nonverbal cues, such as searching or restlessness, that might indicate a toileting need.

Rationales

1. By reinforcing the client's usual elimination pattern, the nurse can help the client remain aware of toileting needs and avoid confusion.

2. Establishing a regular pattern can help minimize incontinence.

3. The client may be unable to recall when he had a bowel movement or if he was constipated.

4. Adequate hydration prevents constipation and urinary tract infections.

5. Regular exercise and eating foods rich in bulk and fiber can help prevent constipation.

6. Because the client may have a history of laxative abuse, monitoring prescribed medications is essential. Psychotropic medications with anticholinergic effects can cause constipation.

7. By being empathetic, the nurse can minimize the client's embarrassment and preserve self-esteem.

8. Skin care can help preserve the client's skin integrity.

9. The client may be unable to recognize or articulate his toileting needs.

Nursing diagnosis: *Sleep pattern disturbance related to disorientation, brain dysfunction, or reversed sleep-awake cycle*

NURSING PRIORITY: To help the client achieve adequate sleep and rest

Interventions

1. Encourage the client to remain awake and active during the day, and provide short, scheduled rest periods.

2. Provide the client with a comfortable pillow, blankets, and loose-fitting bed clothes.

3. Assist the client to the toilet every 4 hours or more often if needed during the day. Limit the client's fluid intake in the evening.

4. Provide a night light, and keep the client's bathroom well lit.

Rationales

1. By increasing his activity level, the client will be tired in the evening and better able to sleep. Short rest periods during the day help to refresh the client, thereby preventing daytime fatigue.

2. The client may be unable to verbalize that he is cold or in need of other comforts. Extra pillows may facilitate breathing, and comfortable bedding can help induce sleep.

3. Attending to the client's elimination needs during the day and limiting the fluid intake in the evening can avert premature arousal.

4. Adequate night lighting helps keep the client oriented to the surroundings and provides security.

Nursing diagnosis: *Altered nutrition, less than body requirements, related to chewing difficulties, smell and taste changes, memory loss, decreased coordination, and depressed mood*

NURSING PRIORITY: To help the client maintain a nourishing diet

Interventions

1. Assess the client's food preferences, and collaborate with the dietitian in planning nutritious meals that include the client's favorite foods.

2. Prepare the client's food, but allow him to eat as independently as possible.

3. Tolerate the client's diminished table manners and unusual mixtures of food. If possible, avoid isolating the client when dining.

4. Assist the client with oral hygiene and denture care.

5. Weigh the client weekly.

Rationales

1. The client is more likely to eat foods that he enjoys and that are prepared to his liking.

2. Being self-sufficient to any degree can enhance client self-esteem.

3. As the client's dementia progresses, he will probably regress and forget learned social behavior.

4. Providing oral hygiene and denture care enables the client to chew more effectively and to improve dietary intake.

5. The nurse should monitor the client for weight fluctuations, which may indicate poor food or fluid intake.

Nursing diagnosis: *Ineffective family coping related to the client's personality changes, behavior, and diminished functioning level*

NURSING PRIORITY: To help the family adapt to the disorder's impact

Interventions

1. Determine the relationship and roles of family members before the onset of the client's illness.

2. Educate family members about dementia, including its effects on the client and family system.

3. Listen empathetically to the family's fears and concerns regarding the client's condition, and help them to solve problems.

4. Encourage family visits and involvement with the client.

5. Encourage family members to seek support for themselves. Suggest appropriate support groups or respite care.

6. Encourage the family's use of stress-management strategies, such as relaxation and respite care.

7. If the client is returning home, explain to the family what is involved in home care and provide referrals for community resources, such as home health nursing.

Rationales

1. Establishing a baseline concerning the family's relationships and roles enables the nurse to more accurately determine the disorder's impact on the family and to implement appropriate interventions.

2. Family members can become frustrated or impatient when the client ceases to recognize them or becomes belligerent. By teaching the family about the disorder, the nurse can help prevent such reactions.

3. As roles shift, family members may be overwhelmed by increased responsibilities, and their problem-solving abilities can be compromised.

4. Participating in care can make the family feel useful and can strengthen family bonds.

5. Sharing their fears and concerns with other families in similar circumstances can help the client's family feel less alone and devastated.

6. By managing stress and improving their sense of well-being, family members can make themselves more available to the client.

7. The family may overestimate its ability to care for the client. Resource referrals can enable the family to obtain assistance, such as a home health nurse.

Nursing diagnosis: *Impaired home maintenance management related to cognitive deficits and increased dependency*

NURSING PRIORITY: To help the client's family adapt to interpersonal and environmental changes, thereby facilitating care and maximizing the client's independence

Interventions

1. Assess the client's capabilities and the degree of supervision needed.

2. Educate the family members about the client's disorder. Advise them of techniques for coping with problem behaviors, such as wandering, hoarding, delusions, and agitation.

3. Recommend environmental modifications that accommodate the client's needs. One such modification might involve moving the client's bedroom to the first level of the house.

4. Work with the physician to simplify the client's medication regimen.

Rationales

1. Such assessment can help the nurse determine the client's needs and ensure both the client's and family's safety.

2. Proper teaching can help the family feel more capable of handling difficult behaviors and decrease their anxiety.

3. Such modifications can help to maintain the client's safety and facilitate the family's caregiving responsibilities.

4. A simplified medication regimen is less burdensome to the family. It also helps ensure client compliance.

5. Support the family's efforts at caring for the client, and encourage their involvement in respite care and Alzheimer's support groups.

5. A well-developed network of professional and community resources can help the family to better care for the client and manage stress.

Outcome criteria

As treatment progresses, the client, family, or both should be able to:
• demonstrate feelings of security
• demonstrate a decrease or absence of threatening behavior towards others
• demonstrate optimum communication skills and an interest in the immediate environment
• maintain adequate elimination patterns and skin integrity
• maintain adequate rest and activity levels
• maintain adequate nutritional intake and optimum body weight
• verbalize an understanding of the disorder and its effects
• demonstrate the ability to adapt to client and family role changes
• identify necessary environmental changes that accommodate the client's needs and decrease potential risks
• demonstrate appropriate coping and stress-management strategies and problem-solving abilities.
• demonstrate improved behavioral control
• report feeling less agitated
• demonstrate an increased ability to tolerate frustration
• demonstrate or verbalize more adaptive coping skills
• verbalize a knowledge of signs and symptoms of increasing agitation or anxiety.

Discharge criteria

Nursing documentation indicates that the client has responded positively to treatment and care.

Nursing documentation also indicates that the family:
• has verbalized an understanding of the client's diagnosis, treatment, and expected outcome
• is aware of the client's problematic behaviors and how to manage them
• has demonstrated an ability to interact with the client and to meet the client's needs
• has been referred to appropriate family and community resources
• has demonstrated the ability to identify follow-up needs
• has verbalized an understanding of the risks involved in client care and of how to maintain environmental safety

• understands when, why, and how to contact the appropriate health care professional in case of an emergency.

Selected references

Abraham, I., Fox, J., Harrington, D., et al. (1990). A psychogeriatric nursing assessment protocol for use in multidisciplinary practice. *Archives of Psychiatric Nursing,* 4(4), 242-259.

Blakeslee, J.A. (1988). Untie the elderly. *American Journal of Nursing* 6, 833-834.

Bloom, C. (1991). Success with wanderers. *Geriatric Nursing,* 20.

Butson, T. (1990). Mrs. R.: The need to understand meaning behind behavior. *Perspectives,* 14(3), 5-7.

Calfee, E.E. (1988). Are you restraining your patient's rights? *Nursing88,* 5, 148-149.

Campbell, L. (1987). Hopelessness: A concept analysis. *Journal of Psychosocial Nursing,* 25(2), 18-22, 34-35.

Carpenito, L. (1991). *Nursing diagnosis: Application to clinical practice* (4th ed.). Philadelphia: Lippincott.

Cohn, M.D., et al. (1990). Behavior management training for nurses aides: Is it effective? *Journal of Gerontological Nursing,* 16(11), 21-25.

Cummings, J.L., and Miller, B.L. (Eds.). (1990). *Alzheimer's disease: Treatment and long-term management.* New York: Dekker.

Dawson, P., and Reid, D.W. (1987). Behavioral dimensions of patients at risk for wandering. *Gerontologist,* 27, 104-107.

Doenges, M.E., Townsend, M.D., and Moorhouse, M.F. (1989). *Psychiatric care plans: Guidelines for client care.* Philadelphia: Davis.

Farran, C.J., and Popovich, J.M. (1990). Hope: A relevant concept for geriatric psychiatry. *Archives of Psychiatric Nursing,* 4(2), 124-130.

Fletcher, K.R. (1990). Restraints should be a last resort. *RN,* 1, 52-59.

Fopma-Loy, J. (1988). Wandering: Causes, consequences, and care. *Journal of Psychosocial Nursing,* 26(5), 8-18, 40+.

Fopma-Loy, J. (1989). Geropsychiatric nursing: Focus and setting. *Archives of Psychiatric Nursing,* 3(4), 183-190.

Frengley, J.D., and Mion, L.C. (1986). Incidence of physical restraints on acute general medical wards. *Journal of the American Geriatrics Society,* 8, 565-568.

Given, B.A., King, S.K., Collins, C., et al. (1988). Family caregivers of the elderly: Involvement and reactions to care. *Archives of Psychiatric Nursing*, 2(5), 281-288.

Kikuta, S.C. (1991). Clinically managing disruptive behavior on the ward. *Journal of Gerontological Nursing*, 17(8), 4-8.

Kirk, D. (1990). Dealing with psychological stress. *Emergency*, 22(11), 44-47.

Lee, V.K. (1991). Language changes and Alzheimer's disease: A literature review. *Journal of Gerontological Nursing*, 17(1), 16-20, 35-37.

Lofgren, R., et al. (1989). Medical restraints in the medical wards: Are protective devices safe? *American Journal of Public Health*, 6, 735-738.

Lynch-Sauer, J. (1990). When a family member has Alzheimer's disease: A phenomenological description of caregiving. *Journal of Gerontological Nursing*, 16(9), 8-11, 37-38.

Macpherson, D.S., et al. (1990). Deciding to restrain medical patients. *Journal of the American Geriatrics Society*, 5, 516-520.

Masters, R., and Marks, S.F. (1990). Use of restraints. *Rehabilitation Nursing*, 1, 22-25.

Mayers, K., and Griffin, M. (1990). The play project: Use of stimulus objects with demented patients. *Journal of Gerontological Nursing*, 16(1), 32-39.

Mitchell-Pedersen, L., et al. (1989). Avoiding restraints—Why it can mean good practice. *Nursing 90*, 9, 66-72.

Moore, T.A. (1986). Protection of the patient from self-injury: Uses of restraints and searches. *Topics in Hospital Law*, 3, 19-26.

Morrison, J., and King, D. (1987). Formulating a restraint use policy. *Journal of Nursing Administration*, 339-42.

Negley, E., and Manley, J.T. (1990). Environmental interventions in assaultive behavior. *Journal of Gerontological Nursing*, 16(3), 29-35.

Northrop, C.E. (1987). A question of restraint. *Nursing 87*, 2, 14.

Robbins, L.J., et al. (1987). Binding the elderly: A prospective study of the use of mechanical restraints in an acute care hospital. *Journal of American Geriatrics Society*, 4, 290-296.

Roder, J. (1991). Modifying the environment to decrease the use of restraints. *Journal of Gerontological Nursing*, 17(2), 9-13.

Rose, J. (1987). When the care plan says restrain. *Geriatric Nursing*, 1, 20-21.

Smith, M., Buckwalter, K., and Albanese, M. (1990). Geropsychiatric education programs: Providing skills and understanding. *Journal of Psychosocial Nursing*, 28(12), 8-12.

Spar, J.E., and LaRue, A. (1990). *Concise guide to geriatric psychiatry*. Washington, DC: APA Press.

Stevens, G.L., and Baldwin, B.A. (1988). Optimizing mental health in the nursing home setting. *Journal of Psychosocial Nursing*, 26(10), 27-31, 35-36.

Taft, L.B. (1989). Conceptual analysis of agitation in the confused elderly. *Archives of Psychiatric Nursing*, 3(2), 102-107.

Taft, L.B. (1990). Drug abuse? Use and misuse of psychotropic drugs in Alzheimer's care. *Journal of Gerontological Nursing*, 16(8), 4-10, 36-37.

Werner, P. et al. (1989). Physical restraints and agitation in nursing home residents. *Journal of American Geriatrics Society*, 37(12), 1122-1166.

Zarit, S.H., Zarit, J.M., and Rosenberg-Thompson, S. (1990). A special treatment unit for Alzheimer's disease: Medical, behavioral, and environmental features. *Clinical Gerontologist*, 9(3/4), 47-63.

Zgola, J. (1987). *Doing things: A guide to programming activities for persons with Alzheimer's disease and related disorders*. Baltimore: Johns Hopkins University Press.

Alcoholism

DSM III-R classifications
303.90 Alcohol dependence
305.00 Alcohol abuse

Psychiatric nursing diagnostic class
Substance abuse

Introduction

A progressive and, in many cases, fatal disorder, alcoholism is characterized by continuous or periodic impaired control over drinking, preoccupation with alcohol, use of alcohol despite adverse consequences, and distorted thought processes—most notably a continual denial of the condition. Such denial may be supported inadvertently by family and friends who refuse to confront the alcoholic client about the condition.

Alcohol abuse is characterized by alcohol use that results in physical, cognitive, emotional, or spiritual problems. *Alcohol dependence* is characterized by the same problems as well as by a tolerance for increasing amounts of alcohol and the occurrence of withdrawal symptoms. (For more information on identifying alcoholism, see *Performing an alcohol screening test,* page 170.)

ETIOLOGY AND PRECIPITATING FACTORS
Biological studies indicate a genetic predisposition to alcoholism. According to these studies, alcoholic persons are more likely than nonalcoholic persons to have alcoholic fathers, mothers, siblings, or other relatives. Furthermore, children of alcoholic biological parents reared by nonalcoholic foster parents develop a significantly higher incidence of alcoholism than do children of nonalcoholic biological parents raised by alcoholic foster parents.

The predominant biochemical theory suggests that individuals exhibit varying alcohol metabolism rates. This theory also suggests that acetaldehyde, produced by alcohol metabolism, may play a role in the development of alcoholism in those individuals with an impaired ability to remove acetaldehyde from their system. Research also suggests that low levels of monoamine oxidase (MAO), an enzyme involved in neurotransmitter metabolism, may be an antecedent to the development of alcoholism.

The disease model developed by Jellinek views alcoholism as a chronic, progressive illness with three well-defined phases. The first (prealcoholism) phase is characterized by use of alcohol to control stress and relieve tension. The second (early alcoholic) phase is characterized by blackouts, increased tolerance of quantities of alcohol, and a preoccupation with alcohol.

During the third (frank addiction) phase, the individual cannot stop drinking. During the last phase, the individual needs to drink constantly.

Family theorists maintain that the alcoholic's family usually is dysfunctional and that the alcoholic member and the disorder become the focus of all family interactions. According to this theory, family members adopt roles, such as scapegoats or clowns, allowing them to function, even if an impaired way.

According to one psychodynamic theory, an alcoholic is a person with low self-esteem, coping difficulties, poor social skills, low frustration tolerance, and poor impulse control. Other psychodynamic theories suggest that alcoholic individuals are self-destructive. For a more complete psychological profile of addicts and their addictions, see *Three phases of addiction,* page 171.

Assessment guidelines
NURSING HISTORY (Functional health pattern findings)
The client may report or exhibit one or more of the findings grouped here according to functional health patterns.

Health perception–health management pattern
- complaints of general pain and discomfort
- headaches
- distorted pain perception
- depression

Nutritional-metabolic pattern
- inadequate food intake
- diminished taste
- lack of interest in food
- abdominal pain
- poor muscle tone or skin turgor
- weight loss or gain
- pale mucous membranes

Elimination pattern
- constipation or diarrhea
- nausea and vomiting
- gastrointestinal bleeding

Activity-exercise pattern
- restlessness
- difficulty performing normal daily activities
- activity intolerance

PERFORMING AN ALCOHOL SCREENING TEST

Several assessment tools, such as the 1971 Michigan Alcoholism Screening Test (shown here) and the shorter version of the test developed in 1975, can help pinpoint the nature and severity of your client's alcohol abuse. To use this test, ask your client the following questions. For each positive response (except where indicated), score the number of points shown in the right column; then total the points. Generally, a score of five or more points indicates alcoholism; a score of four points suggests alcoholism; and a score of three or fewer points indicates that the client isn't an alcoholic.

Questions	Points
1. Do you feel you are a normal drinker? (By normal, we mean do you drink less than or as much as most other people?)*	2
2. Have you ever awakened the morning after drinking the night before and found that you could not remember a part of the evening?	2
3. Does your spouse, a parent, or another near relative ever worry or complain about your drinking?	1
4. Can you stop drinking without a struggle after one or two drinks?*	2
5. Do you ever feel guilty about your drinking?	1
6. Do friends or relatives think you are a normal drinker?*	2
7. Are you able to stop drinking when you want to?*	2
8. Have you ever attended a meeting of Alcoholics Anonymous (AA)?	5
9. Have you gotten into physical fights when drinking?	1
10. Has your drinking ever created problems between you and your spouse, a parent, or another near relative?	2
11. Has your wife or husband (or another family member) ever gone to anyone for help about your drinking?	2
12. Have you ever lost friends because of drinking?	2
13. Have you ever gotten into trouble at work or school because you were drinking?	2
14. Have you ever lost a job because of drinking?	2
15. Have you ever neglected your obligations, your family, or your work for 2 or more days in a row because you were drinking?	2
16. Do you drink before noon fairly often?	1
17. Have you ever been told you have liver trouble? Cirrhosis?	2
18. After heavy drinking have you ever had delirium tremens (DTs) or severe shaking, or heard voices or seen things that weren't really there?**	2
19. Have you ever gone to anyone for help about your drinking?	5
20. Have you ever been a patient in a psychiatric hospital or on a psychiatric ward of a general hospital where drinking was a part of the problem that resulted in hospitalization?	5
21. Have you ever been seen at a psychiatric or mental health clinic, or gone to any doctor, social worker, or counselor, for help with any emotional problem where drinking was part of the problem?	2
22. Have you ever been arrested for drunk driving, driving while intoxicated, or driving under the influence of alcoholic beverages? (If, yes, how many times? ___)†	2
23. Have you ever been arrested or taken into custody, even for a few hours, because of other drunk behavior? (If yes, how many times? _____)†	2

Key
* Alcoholic response is negative.
** Score five points for delirium tremens.
† Score two points for each arrest.

Adapted from Selzer, M.L. (1971). "The Michigan alcoholism screening test: The quest for a new diagnostic instrument," *American Journal of Psychiatry*, 127(12):1653-58. Used with permission.

Sleep-rest pattern
- difficulty falling asleep
- not feeling rested
- sleep pattern reversal
- early awakening
- frequent nighttime awakenings
- restlessness during sleep

Cognitive-perceptual pattern
- disorientation about people, places, or time
- confusion
- slow information processing
- slow and slurred speech
- anxiety

- poor short-term memory
- bizarre thinking
- exaggerated emotional responses

Self-perception–self-concept pattern
- feelings of inadequacy, guilt, or shame
- feelings of grandiosity
- decreased self-esteem
- derogatory statements about self
- self-destructive behaviors

Role-relationship pattern
- difficulty with intimacy
- withdrawal from social contact
- ineffective family communication

- dysfunctional family roles
- inability to express feelings
- concerns about how family, friends, and coworkers will respond to the disorder

Sexual-reproductive pattern
- actual or perceived limited sexual ability
- decreased libido
- lack of sexual satisfaction
- disturbances in sexual relationships

Coping–stress tolerance pattern
- withdrawal from relationships
- tension, fearfulness, or nervousness
- impaired ability to concentrate
- feelings of helplessness or hopelessness
- feeling that life is beyond personal control
- financial stresses
- need for attention, help, and reassurance

Value-belief pattern
- feelings of hopelessness about addiction and treatment
- desire to become more or less involved in spirituality or religion
- lack of future plans
- inability to believe in anything or anyone

PHYSICAL FINDINGS
The client may report or exhibit one or more of the following physical findings.

Cardiovascular
- arrhythmias
- hypertension or hypotension
- increased or irregular heart rate
- shortness of breath

Respiratory
- asymmetrical chest movements
- diminished or loud breath sounds
- elevated temperature
- hypoxia
- respiratory depression
- tachypnea, especially during alcohol withdrawal

Gastrointestinal
- ascites
- diarrhea
- hematemesis
- hepatic pain
- jaundice
- esophageal mucosa inflammation
- nausea and vomiting
- esophageal varices

THREE PHASES OF ADDICTION

Phase one
In the *progressive or early phase,* the person addicted to drugs or alcohol:
- denies addiction
- sneaks alcohol or drugs
- experiences blackouts
- uses alcohol or drugs to cope
- becomes angry easily
- lies to cover up habit
- avoids references to alcohol or drugs
- develops increased tolerance
- begins to lose control.

Phase two
In the *crucial phase,* the addict:
- justifies behavior
- feels angry and guilty
- develops paranoid traits
- behaves extravagantly
- changes pattern of alcohol or drug use
- encounters job and marital problems
- maintains a constant supply of alcohol or drugs
- develops physical and psychological problems
- swears off alcohol or drugs
- experiences indefinable fears
- loses friends.

Phase three
In the *chronic phase,* the addict:
- experiences tremors
- deteriorates physically and psychologically
- becomes divorced
- spends time in jail
- suffers serious financial setbacks
- loses job
- experiences breakdown of value system
- faces collapse of support system.

From *Psychiatric problems.* NurseReview. Springhouse, PA: Springhouse Corp., 1990.

Genitourinary
- sexual dysfunction
- frequent urination

Musculoskeletal
- ataxia
- evidence of healed or new fractures
- muscle aches, pains, or tension
- trembling, shaking, or twitching

Neurologic
- confabulation
- confusion
- impaired judgment
- labile affect
- memory deficits
- sleep disturbances (such as insomnia or difficulty falling or remaining asleep)
- seizures (most commonly grand mal)

EFFECTS OF ALCOHOL ABUSE

Chronic alcohol abuse can lead to many physical and psychological complications, including the following:

Cardiovascular complications
- alcoholic cardiomyopathy
- increased systolic and pulse pressure
- tissue damage, weakened heart muscle, and heart failure

Gastrointestinal complications
- abdominal distention, pain, belching, and hematemesis
- acute and chronic pancreatitis
- alcoholic hepatitis leading to cirrhosis
- cancer of the esophagus, liver, or pancreas
- esophageal varices, hemorrhoids, and ascites
- gastritis, colitis, and enteritis
- gastric or duodenal ulcers
- swollen, enlarged fatty liver

Genitourinary complications
- swelling of prostate gland, leading to prostatitis and interference with voiding or sexual function
- prostate cancer

Hematologic complications
- abnormal red blood cells, white blood cells, and platelets
- anemia and increased risk of infection
- bleeding tendencies, increased bruising, and decreased clotting time

Neurologic complications
- Wernicke-Korsakoff syndrome, Marchiafava-Bignami disease, cerebellar degeneration, and peripheral neuropathy

Respiratory complications
- cancer of the oropharynx
- impaired diffusion, chronic obstructive pulmonary disease, infection, and tuberculosis
- respiratory depression causing decreased respiratory rate and cough reflex and increased susceptibility to infection and trauma

Miscellaneous complications
- acute and chronic myopathies
- alcoholic amblyopia
- beriberi
- electrolyte abnormalities
- osteoporosis
- scars, burns, and repeated injuries

From *Psychiatric problems*. NurseReview. Springhouse, PA: Springhouse Corp., 1990.

Integumentary
- bruises
- hematomas
- jaundice
- surface blood vessel vasodilation
- petechiae

Psychological
- anger
- depression
- manipulative behavior
- restlessness
- hostility or irritability
- violence
- mood swings

Potential complications

Chronic alcohol use can cause various physiologic impairments, including peripheral neuropathy, Wernicke's encephalopathy, Korsakoff's syndrome, alcoholic cardiomyopathy, esophagitis, esophageal varices, gastritis, pancreatitis, diabetes secondary to pancreatitis, alcoholic hepatitis, cirrhosis of the liver, cancer secondary to cirrhosis, and blood dyscrasias. Infants born to alcoholic women are at high risk for fetal alcohol syndrome. For a more complete list of complications, see *Effects of alcohol abuse*.

Nursing diagnosis: *Sensory-perceptual alteration (visual, auditory, or tactile) related to alcohol consumption*

NURSING PRIORITY: To help the client achieve detoxification and a normal level of consciousness

Interventions

1. Assess the client's degree of alcohol intoxication, and determine the withdrawal stage (see *Assessing alcohol withdrawal*).

Rationales

1. Determining the degree of intoxication and the withdrawal stage provides the nurse with baseline data for instituting appropriate nursing interventions for established medical protocols. (For details about interventions, see Appendix G, Managing Acute Substance Abuse.)

ASSESSING ALCOHOL WITHDRAWAL

Alcohol withdrawal affects your client's motor control, mental status, and body functions. This list of signs and symptoms of alcohol withdrawal can help you determine whether your client is experiencing mild, moderate, or severe withdrawal.

Mild withdrawal
- Hand tremor
- Mild restlessness and anxiety
- Restless sleep or insomnia
- Anorexia
- Nausea
- Oriented to time and place
- No hallucinations
- Tachycardia
- Normal or slightly elevated systolic blood pressure
- Slight sweating
- No seizures

Moderate withdrawal
- Visible tremulousness
- Obvious restlessness and anxiety
- Marked insomnia; nightmares
- Marked anorexia
- Nausea and vomiting
- Variable confusion

- Vague, transient hallucinations
- Pulse rate of 100 to 120 beats/minute
- Elevated systolic blood pressure
- Obvious sweating
- Possible seizures

**Severe withdrawal
(alcohol withdrawal syndrome)**
- Uncontrollable shaking
- Extreme restlessness and agitation
- Intense fear and anxiety
- Wakefulness
- Rejection of food and fluid except alcohol
- Dry heaves and vomiting
- Marked confusion and disorientation
- Frightening visual and occasional auditory hallucinations
- Pulse rate of 120 to 140 beats/minute
- Elevated systolic and diastolic blood pressure
- Marked hyperhydrosis
- Seizures

From *Psychosocial crises.* Clinical Skillbuilders. Springhouse, PA: Springhouse Corp., 1992.

---

2. Observe the client's behavioral responses, especially noting any signs of disorientation, confusion, irritability, or sleeplessness.

2. Sleep deprivation may aggravate disorientation and confusion. Worsening behavioral symptoms may indicate impending alcohol withdrawal syndrome (delirium tremens) or possibly withdrawal from other drugs.

3. Observe and document any auditory, visual, or tactile hallucinations exhibited by the client.

3. Hallucinations may occur during alcohol detoxification. Visual hallucinations commonly involve seeing insects or animals; tactile hallucinations, feeling bugs crawling over the body; and auditory hallucinations, hearing voices.

4. Provide a quiet, safe environment for the client.

4. Decreasing environmental stimuli during the hyperactive stage of detoxification can help reduce the client's delirium. The nurse may need to institute safety precautions to protect the client from self-harm caused by a distorted sense of reality.

5. Frequently orient the client to people, places, and time.

5. Such orientation can help reduce the client's confusion and misinterpretation of external stimuli.

6. Teach the client about alcohol withdrawal symptoms.

6. Understanding the relationship between alcohol use and withdrawal symptoms may increase the client's compliance with treatment.

Nursing diagnosis: *Sleep pattern disturbance related to alcohol abuse and decreased rapid eye movement (REM) sleep cycle*

NURSING PRIORITY: To help the client recognize the relationship between alcohol use and sleep disturbance and to improve the client's sleep patterns

Interventions

1. Monitor the client's sleeping patterns, and determine the type of sleep disturbance.

Rationales

1. Knowing the precise sleep disturbance enables the nurse to plan appropriate sleep-inducing interventions.

2. Establish a daily activity and rest schedule for the client.

2. Activity during the day, with rest but not naps, and a regular structured bedtime routine can help the client return to normal sleep patterns.

3. Recommend appropriate dietary changes, such as the elimination of caffeine.

3. Rebound insomnia can occur during alcohol withdrawal, but extended abstinence usually resolves the problem. Coffee and other caffeine beverages can interfere with REM sleep.

4. Provide the client with a quiet, darkened room for sleeping.

4. A quiet environment reduces stimuli and induces relaxation; a darkened room can help induce sleep.

5. Teach the client to use muscle relaxation techniques at bedtime.

5. Reducing muscle tension can help alleviate anxiety and promote sleep.

Nursing diagnosis: *Altered family processes related to role disruptions caused by the client's alcoholism*

NURSING PRIORITY: To help the family recognize their own needs for information and support and to learn to use available resources

Interventions

1. Assess the interaction styles, communication patterns, and role behaviors within the family.

2. Assess the learning needs of family members.

3. Teach the family about the parts they may be playing in the client's alcoholism.

4. Encourage the family members to communicate openly and honestly with each other.

5. Inform the family about appropriate resources and programs, such as Al-Anon, Al-Ateen, and Adult Children of Alcoholics.

Rationales

1. Understanding how the family functions can help the nurse to develop appropriate family interventions.

2. Family members usually need to be educated about alcoholism. In addition to teaching the family about the physiological and psychological effects of alcoholism, the nurse should discuss alcoholism as a family disorder.

3. Family members may be unaware of the ways in which they contribute to the client's disorder. By informing them of their roles, the nurse can help family members adopt new, positive behaviors.

4. Communication is essential before changes can occur in the family. Learning to communicate openly can be a slow process requiring long-term family therapy.

5. Such groups provide support for maintaining family integrity and functioning.

Nursing diagnosis: *Altered self-image related to unmet expectations, coping difficulties, guilt, and shame about alcohol abuse*

NURSING PRIORITY: To help the client develop and maintain an enhanced self-concept

Interventions

1. Establish a trusting relationship with the client.

Rationales

1. Establishing a trusting relationship with the client fosters a secure environment in which the client can discuss feelings of denial, shame, guilt, and helplessness. Such open discussions enable the nurse to help the client to develop a positive self-image.

2. Assess the client's suicide risk.

2. Depression commonly accompanies alcohol withdrawal. By assessing the client's suicide risk, the nurse can take necessary measures to help prevent any self-harm to the client.

3. Continually encourage the client to express his feelings.

3. Ongoing expression of feelings can help the client to recognize what triggers certain feelings and ultimately to develop more constructive ways of handling them.

4. Encourage the client to accept responsibility for his alcoholism.

4. Assuming responsibility is an important step in developing a positive self-concept.

5. Help the client to explore and accept both positive and negative traits and behaviors.

5. A positive self-concept is based on a realistic appraisal and acceptance of one's strengths and weaknesses.

6. Reinforce the client's positive efforts to cope with feelings.

6. The nurse's reinforcement of positive behavior changes can help the client to recognize and value them.

7. Inform the client of support groups and programs, such as Alcoholics Anonymous.

7. Peer encouragement in group settings can enhance self-concept and support the client's efforts to remain sober.

Nursing diagnosis: *Anxiety related to alcohol withdrawal, real or perceived threats to physical safety, or poor self-concept*

NURSING PRIORITY: To help the client recognize anxiety and to use adaptive coping mechanisms to cope with stress

Interventions

1. Assess the client's anxiety level and coping skills.

Rationales

1. During alcohol withdrawal, the client probably will experience moderate to severe anxiety. The nurse must be prepared to handle the client's anxious behavior.

2. Convey a sense of acceptance to the client.

2. The client probably will detect, and be sensitive to, condescending or biased attitudes or behaviors. By avoiding such attitudes and behaviors, the nurse can decrease the client's anxiety and promote a trusting relationship.

3. Encourage the client to talk about his anxious feelings.

3. Many alcoholic clients fear being dependent or out of control. Being able to talk about this anxiety can help relieve it.

4. Help the client to learn adaptive coping strategies that reduce anxiety, such as using relaxation techniques and verbalizing concerns.

4. Learning new ways to cope with anxiety can encourage the client to accept personal responsibility for making and maintaining positive changes.

5. Administer prescribed medications.

5. Minor tranquilizers, such as benzodiazepines, may be used during acute alcohol withdrawal to help the client relax, reduce hyperactivity, and feel more in control.

6. Teach the client stress management techniques, including cognitive and relaxation techniques.

6. Stress management training involves not only muscle relaxation but also cognitive restructuring, problem solving, and real-life rehearsals. Successful stress management can help the client regain control and increase self-esteem.

Nursing diagnosis: *Potential for injury related to alcohol withdrawal, seizures, depression, or suicidal ideation*

NURSING PRIORITY: To prevent the client from self-injury and injury to others

Interventions	Rationales
1. Assess the client's alcohol withdrawal stage.	1. Early assessment enables the nurse to implement appropriate interventions that may halt symptom progression and prevent injury.
2. Monitor and document any seizures the client may experience.	2. Seizures in a client with no history of seizures usually stop spontaneously and require only symptomatic treatment. Grand mal seizures are most common. In some treatment facilities, anti-convulsant medication may be used.
3. Provide a safe environment for the client as needed.	3. Sensory-perceptual alterations, such as hallucinations, lack of coordination, confusion, and disorientation, can result in potentially dangerous behavior. A client who is anxious and frightened may also become agitated and combative, striking out at others.
4. Assess the client's suicide risk.	4. During the early stages of alcohol withdrawal, the client may become depressed and entertain thoughts of suicide.

Nursing diagnosis: *Altered nutrition, less than body requirements, related to the client's poor dietary intake while consuming alcohol, the effects of chronic alcohol intake on the client's digestive organs, and the interference of alcohol in absorption and metabolism of nutrients*

NURSING PRIORITY: To help the client change dietary patterns and improve nutrition

Interventions	Rationales
1. Evaluate the presence and quality of the client's bowel sounds, and note any signs of abdominal distention.	1. Irritated gastric mucosa may result in nausea and hyperactive bowel sounds. Early detection of gastric irritation can prevent unnecessary nausea and vomiting.
2. Assess the client for nausea, vomiting, and diarrhea.	2. These symptoms typically occur early during alcohol withdrawal and may interfere with achieving adequate nutrition.
3. Provide frequent, small, and easily digested meals and snacks.	3. Such meals and snacks can limit gastric distress and enhance the client's dietary intake. As the client's appetite and food tolerance increase, the nurse can adjust the diet to increase calories and nutrients needed for cellular repair.
4. Provide the client with a protein-rich diet, ensuring that at least half of the daily calories come from carbohydrates.	4. A diet high in protein and carbohydrates can help stabilize the client's blood glucose level, thereby reducing the risk of hypoglycemia while providing nutrition for energy needs and cellular regeneration.
5. Add vitamins and thiamine to the client's diet as needed.	5. Chronic alcoholics commonly experience vitamin— especially thiamine—deficiencies. Some treatment facilities use megavitamin therapy during alcoholism recovery.

Outcome criteria

As treatment progresses, the client, family, or both should be able to:
• verbalize an understanding that alcohol alters sensory-perceptual abilities
• use appropriate interventions to facilitate sleep, and report an improved sleep pattern
• report improved communication among family members
• demonstrate increased self-esteem and confidence
• recognize dependency needs and fulfill them by non-self-destructive means
• recognize anxiety and use adaptive coping mechanisms to decrease anxiety without resorting to alcohol
• recognize the need for support, seek assistance, and use appropriate resources
• verbalize an awareness that alcohol ingestion can reduce dietary intake and alter nutrition
• demonstrate behavioral and life-style changes that will help maintain appropriate nutrition.

Discharge criteria

Nursing documentation indicates that the client:
• has demonstrated an understanding of alcoholism, its signs and symptoms, and its effects on the family
• can use newly learned coping strategies and skills
• is aware of available community and family support services
• has arranged to participate in an ongoing recovery and therapy program.

Nursing documentation also indicates that the family:
• has verbalized an understanding of the diagnosis, treatment, and expected outcomes
• has demonstrated an ability to use newly acquired adaptive coping mechanisms to enhance the client's recovery
• has been referred to the appropriate community resources for continuing recovery and support
• plans to participate in an ongoing therapy program
• understands when, why, and how to contact the appropriate health care professional in case of an emergency.

Selected references

American Nurses' Association. (1988). Standards of addictions: Nursing practice with selected diagnosis and criteria. St. Louis: ANA (PMH-10 4M).

Barteck, J., Lindeman, M., Newton, M., Fitzgerald, A., and Hawks, J. (1988). Nurse identified problems in the management of alcoholic patients. *Journal of Studies on Alcohol,* 49, 62-70.

Brown, S. (1986). *Treating the alcoholic: A developmental model of recovery.* New York: Wiley.

Cermak, T.L. (1986). *Diagnosing and treating co-dependence.* MN: Johnson Institute.

Cloninger, C. (1987). Neurogenic adaptive mechanisms in alcoholism. *Science, 236,* 410-416.

Estes, N.J., & Heineman, E. (1986). *Alcoholism: Development, consequences & interventions* (3rd ed.). St. Louis: Mosby.

Haber, J., Hoskins, P., Leach, A., Sideleau, B., (1987). *Comprehensive psychiatric nursing.* New York: McGraw-Hill.

Jack, L. (1990). *The core curriculum of addictions nursing.* IL: NNSA.

Jack L. (ed) (1989). *Nursing care planning with the addicted client.* Vols. I & II. IL: NNSA.

Kinney, J. & Leaton, G. (1987). *Loosening the grip,* 3rd ed. St. Louis: Mosby.

Long, P. (1990). Changing nursing students' attitudes towards alcoholism. *Perspective on Addictions Nursing,* June: 3-5.

Stuart, G., and Sundeen, S. (1991). *Principles and practices of psychiatric nursing.* St. Louis: Mosby.

Sullivan, E.J., and Hale, R.E. (1987). Nurses' beliefs about the etiology and treatment of alcohol abuse. *Journal of Studies on Alcohol,* 48(5): 456-460.

Townsend, M. (1988). *Nursing diagnoses in psychiatric nursing.* Philadelphia: F.A. Davis.

U.S. Dept. of Health & Human Services. *Seventh Special Report to the U.S. Congress on Alcohol and Health,* Jan. 1987. Washington, DC: NIA

ADDICTION DISORDERS

Central Nervous System Depressant Dependence

DSM III-R classifications
Psychoactive substance-induced organic mental disorders
292.00 Uncomplicated sedative, hypnotic or anxiolytic withdrawal
292.00 Sedative, hypnotic, or anxiolytic withdrawal delirium
292.83 Sedative, hypnotic, or anxiolytic amnestic disorder
305.40 Sedative, hypnotic, or anxiolytic intoxication
305.50 Opioid intoxication
Psychoactive substance use disorders
304.00 Opioid dependence
304.10 Sedative, hypnotic, or anxiolytic dependence
305.40 Sedative, hypnotic, or anxiolytic abuse
305.50 Opioid abuse

Psychiatric nursing diagnostic class
Substance abuse

Introduction
Psychoactive substance abuse disorders resulting from use of central nervous system (CNS) depressants may manifest as either organic mental disorders or as behavioral changes associated with depressant use. CNS depressants—including benzodiazepines, barbiturates, opioids, opiates, skeletal muscle relaxants, and antihistamines—depress the overall functioning of the CNS, ultimately inducing drowsiness and sedation.

Hypnotics include benzodiazepines, such as diazepam (Valium), flurazepam (Dalmane), triazolam (Halcion), and temazepam (Restorial), as well as other nonbenzodiazepine substances, such as chloral hydrate (Noctec), methaqualone, meprobamate (Miltown), glutethimide (Doriden), and barbiturates. Used predominantly to treat anxiety, insomnia, and panic, these drugs can produce intoxication and withdrawal syndromes (see *Commonly abused CNS depressants*).

Opioids include natural opioids, such as heroin, as well as morphine and morphine-like synthetics. Representative opioids, such as codeine, hydromorphone (Dilaudid), merperidine (Demerol), and methadone (Dolophine), usually are prescribed for cough suppression, analgesia, or anesthesia (see *Understanding meperidine toxicity,* page 181). Several other compounds, such as pentazocine (Talwin) and buprenorphine (Buprenex), produce physiologic and behavioral effects similar to those of the pure opioids.

When developing CNS depressant dependence, an individual may experience alternating denial, guilt, and shame, accompanied by withdrawal and silence.

ETIOLOGY AND PRECIPITATING FACTORS
According to one psychodynamic theory, an addict is a person with low self-esteem, coping difficulties, poor social skills, low frustration tolerance, and poor impulse control. Other psychodynamic theories suggest that addicts are seeking self-destruction or that they have adjustment disabilities.

Family theorists view the addicted family as a dysfunctional system in which the addict and his drug use become the focus of all family interactions. According to this theory, family members adopt roles, such as scapegoats or clowns, which allow them to function, even in an impaired way.

Behavioral theories, which present addiction as a behavior rather than an illness, suggest that drug use is influenced by factors that reinforce the need for and use of drugs. Such factors include peer pressure, family conflicts, and drug-induced euphoria. One behavioral theory suggests that drug use is learned from others.

Assessment guidelines
NURSING HISTORY (Functional health pattern findings)
The client may report or exhibit one or more of the findings grouped here according to functional health patterns.

Health perception–health management pattern
• distorted pain perception
• headache
• general discomfort
• chronic pain or frequent emergency room visits for migraine headaches
• depression or anxiety
• numerous physical complaints
• frequent viral or bacterial infections
• inaccurate perception of health

Nutritional-metabolic pattern
• inadequate food intake
• lack of interest in food
• abdominal pain
• dental problems
• altered skin integrity (including abscesses) and poor skin turgor
• pale mucous membranes

COMMONLY ABUSED C.N.S. DEPRESSANTS

All central nervous system depressants have abuse potential, but some are abused more commonly than others. Diazepam is the most abused benzodiazepine. It may become addictive with prolonged use of high doses. Morphine sulfate is the most commonly abused opiod. Because it produces euphoria, morphine may become addictive. Secobarbital is the most abused barbiturate. Prolonged use of high doses may result in tolerance and psychological and physiological dependence.

Drug	Signs and symptoms of abuse	Signs and symptoms of withdrawal	Treatment of withdrawal
diazepam (Valium)	• Ataxia • Drowsiness • Slurred speech • Vertigo	• Anorexia • Anxiety • Ataxia • Diaphoresis • Diarrhea • Dysphoria • Hallucinations • Insomnia • Irritability • Memory impairment • Muscle cramps • Psychosis • Seizures • Tremors • Vomiting	• Administration of gradually decreasing doses of diazepam
morphine sulfate	• Behavioral changes • Constipation • Decreased sexual drive • Miosis • Urine retention	**First 24 hours** • Diaphoresis • Excessive yawning • Gooseflesh • Increased lacrimation • Mydriasis • Restlessness • Rhinorrhea **After first 24 hours; peak within 72 hours** • Anorexia • Acid-base imbalance • Dehydration • Hot and cold flashes • Hypertension • Increased body temperature • Increased urinary 17-ketosteroid excretion • Insomnia • Involuntary kicking • Leukocytosis • Muscle twitching and spasms • Nausea, vomiting, and diarrhea • Severe back, abdominal, and leg pain • Severe sneezing • Spontaneous ejaculation and orgasm • Tachycardia, tachypnea	• Administration of methadone (Dolophine) to control signs and symptoms (signs and symptoms of withdrawal should subside in 5 to 14 days) • Administration of sedatives to reduce anxiety and opiate craving • Use of antiemetics and I.V. fluids • Supportive counseling
secobarbital (Seconal)	• Distorted mood • Impaired judgment • Impaired motor skills • Residual sedation or "hangover"	• Anxiety • Cardiovascular collapse • Delirium, hallucinations • Insomnia • Muscle twitching • Nausea and vomiting • Postural hypotension • Seizures • Weakness • Weight loss	• Administration of stabilizing dose of phenobarbital, (Barbita) then gradually decreasing dosage over 2 to 3 weeks • Administration of I.V. fluids to support blood pressure • Supportive counseling

Adapted from *Springhouse drug reference*. Springhouse, PA: Springhouse Corp., 1988.

- weight loss
- poor muscle tone

Elimination pattern
- gastrointestinal cramps
- diarrhea, nausea, or vomiting

Activity-exercise pattern
- lethargy and fatigue
- restlessness
- inability to engage in physical activity
- intolerance to activity secondary to decreased strength and endurance
- decreased interest or participation in diversional activities
- inability to complete normal daily activities

Sleep-rest pattern
- difficulty falling and remaining asleep
- early morning awakenings and interrupted sleep
- reversed normal sleep cycle
- fatigue after sleep
- anxiety about inability to sleep
- use of additional prescribed sleep medications
- increased dreaming that interrupts sleep

Cognitive-perceptual pattern
- disorientation about people, places, and time
- confusion
- slowed information processing
- hallucinations
- short-term memory deficits
- belief that quitting the drug is possible anytime
- concentration difficulty
- difficulty following directions
- difficulty making decisions

Self-perception–self-concept pattern
- difficulty acknowledging or accepting bodily changes
- derogatory statements about self
- feelings of inadequacy, guilt, and shame
- anger over inability to control things or situations
- self-destructive behaviors
- feelings of hopelessness and powerlessness
- feelings of grandiosity

Role-relationship pattern
- difficulty with intimacy
- changes in usual role responsibility and functioning
- inability to express feelings
- isolation or subculture existence
- dysfunctional peer and family interactions
- dysfunctional roles, rules, and rituals within the family

Sexual-reproductive pattern
- actual or perceived sexual or reproductive limitations
- decreased libido
- difficulties achieving sexual satisfaction

- concern about acquiring sexually transmitted diseases
- disturbances in relationship with sexual partner

Coping–stress tolerance pattern
- inability to cope
- difficulty asking for help
- projecting blame and responsibility for the disorder on others
- refusal of health care attention
- social withdrawal and isolation
- presence of significant life stressors

Value-belief pattern
- hopelessness about addiction and treatment outcome
- anger with God or others for the disorder
- inner conflict about beliefs
- spiritual distress

PHYSICAL FINDINGS
The client may report or exhibit one or more of the following physical findings.

Cardiovascular
- anemia
- bradycardia
- cardiac arrest
- cyanosis
- diaphoresis
- arrhythmias
- elevated diastolic blood pressure
- hemorrhage
- hypotension
- petechiae
- shock
- tachycardia

Respiratory
- rapid or deep breathing
- respiratory paralysis
- slow or labored breathing
- tachypnea

Gastrointestinal
- abdominal pain
- anorexia
- bloody stools
- colic
- constipation
- nausea and vomiting

Genitourinary
- glycosuria
- urinary tract infection
- proteinuria
- sexually transmitted disease

UNDERSTANDING MEPERIDINE TOXICITY

Prolonged use of opioid agonists typically results in drug tolerance and physical dependency. Drug tolerance is influenced by the degree of central nervous system (CNS) depression resulting from opiate use and the length of time this depression continues. Although meperidine (Demerol) is classified as an opioid agonist and is similar to morphine, its pattern of tolerance and toxicity is distinctly different.

Tolerance to meperidine seems to develop more slowly than morphine tolerance. Prolonged administration of meperidine, because of its shorter duration of action, causes less CNS depression than morphine. Continued CNS depression occurs only when meperidine is given at less than 4-hour intervals.

Symptoms of meperidine toxicity, like those of morphine, include CNS depression, respiratory depression, cold and clammy skin, flaccid skeletal muscles, bradycardia, and hypotension. However, morphine causes miosis, whereas meperidine causes mydriasis. Furthermore, in patients or addicts with tolerance to the drug's depressant effects, large and frequently repeated doses produce tremors, muscle twitches, hyperactive reflexes, and seizures. These excitatory symptoms are from the accumulation of normeperidine, a metabolite of meperidine. Review the chart below, which lists the symptoms of meperidine toxicity.

Withdrawal symptoms after prolonged meperidine use usually occur within 3 to 4 hours after the last dose of meperidine and reach maximum intensity in 8 to 12 hours. These symptoms are normally considered milder than those of morphine withdrawal, but during the period of maximum intensity, muscle twitching, restlessness, and nervousness may be much worse. Normally, symptoms of meperidine withdrawal gradually subside and disappear within 4 to 5 days.

AFFECTED AREA	SYMPTOMS OF TOXICITY
Central nervous system	• Apnea • CNS depression (ranging from stupor to profound coma) • Delirium, disorientation, hallucinations† • Generalized motor seizures, tonic-clonic seizures† • Muscle tremors and twitches, hyperactive reflexes† • Respiratory depression (may progress to Cheyne-Stokes respiration)
Cardiovascular	• Bradycardia • Cardiac arrest • Circulatory collapse • Cyanosis • Hypotension • Tachycardia†
Eyes, ears, nose, and throat	• Mydriasis
Gastrointestinal	• Dry mouth†
Other	• Cold, clammy skin • Flaccid skeletal muscles • Hypothermia

†Symptoms of excitatory syndrome

From *Springhouse drug reference*. Springhouse, PA: Springhouse Corp., 1988

Integumentary
• abcesses
• alopecia
• bruises or hematoma
• bullae
• cyanosis
• dermatitis
• dryness
• flushed complexion
• hirsutism
• jaundice
• needle puncture marks
• paleness
• pruritis
• uriticaria
• abrasions

Musculoskeletal
• dysarthria
• old and healed fractures
• hypotonia
• muscle aches and pains
• muscle rigidity and tension

Neurologic
• acute delirium
• anesthesia
• ataxia
• blurred vision
• coma
• confusion
• depressed deep tendon reflexes
• dizziness
• auditory or visual hallucinations
• headaches
• hyperreflexia
• hyperthermia
• coordination loss
• miosis
• myoclonus
• "nodding off"
• horizontal or vertical nystagmus
• paresthesias
• pupil changes
• seizures
• sleepiness
• spasms

- stupor
- tetanic rigidity
- tinnitus
- tremors, twitching

Psychological
- agitation and anger
- anxiety
- depression or euphoria
- floating feelings
- hostility or irritability
- manipulative behaviors
- paradoxical excitement
- restlessness

- insomnia
- violence

Potential complications

If left untreated, CNS depressant abuse disorders can lead directly or indirectly to the following conditions: abcesses, osteomyelitis, AIDS, amenorrhea, bacterial endocarditis, bronchitis, cardiac arrest, cellulitis, coma, dehydration, hepatitis, hypoglycemia, frequent infections, malnutrition, overdose, pulmonary emboli, renal failure, respiratory arrest, seizures, sepsis, sexually transmitted disease, tetanus, vascular disorders, or withdrawal states. (For details on managing an acute episode of depressant abuse, see Appendix G.)

Nursing diagnosis: *Ineffective denial related to feelings of low self-esteem*

NURSING PRIORITY: To help the client accept responsibility for behavior and acknowledge the relationship between substance abuse and personal problems

Interventions

1. Convey an accepting attitude to the client.

2. Educate the client to correct misinterpretations about substance abuse and substance use to alleviate negative feelings.

3. Confront the client's use of defense mechanisms, including rationalization and blaming.

4. Explore with the client significant events and situations that led to substance use, as well as any consequential maladaptive behaviors resulting from drug use.

5. Confront the client with facts about and the reality of the disorder if the client begins fantasizing or romanticizing about a life-style revolving around substance abuse.

6. Schedule, encourage, and monitor the client's and family's participation in group and educational activities.

7. Provide the client with positive feedback whenever he recognizes connections between behaviors and substance abuse.

Rationales

1. An accepting attitude can promote feelings of dignity and self-worth.

2. Factual information, including the signs and symptoms of substance abuse or dependence, can help the client and family focus on their own behaviors and can decrease the ignorance of substance abuse that contributes to continued addiction.

3. These defense mechanisms can prolong the client's denial of his disorder. Exposing them is an important step toward recovery.

4. Helping the client to visualize the relationship between personal difficulties and substance abuse is an important first step in eliminating the client's denial of the disorder.

5. A realistic, yet supportive approach can facilitate the client's self-esteem and diminish the use of defense mechanisms.

6. The client may accept feedback more readily from peer groups than from the nurse or staff. A peer group setting also can decrease the client's feelings of uniqueness and isolation.

7. Positive reinforcement can increase the client's self-esteem and encourage healthy behaviors.

Nursing diagnosis: *Knowledge deficit related to information about the risks involving substance abuse*

NURSING PRIORITY: To teach the client about the effects of substance abuse on the body and to help incorporate this knowledge into the client's daily life and family relationships

Interventions

1. Assess the client's and family's knowledge of substance abuse, identifying any attitudes, misconceptions, and myths associated with the disorder.

2. Provide the client with factual information about substance abuse and dependence as well as addiction patterns. Include the following concepts: diseases associated with substance abuse and dependence, disease model of addiction, the philosophy of support and self-help groups, family interactions and dynamics associated with addiction, nutritional effects of addiction, assertiveness and communication skills, specific treatment strategies, the disorder's impact on both the client's and family's lifestyle, adaptive coping strategies, relapse prevention, and prescription addiction. Also include information about how substance use affects pregnancy and the relationship between I.V. drug abuse and sexually transmitted diseases, as they apply to the client.

3. Use various teaching methods, including discussion groups, lectures, role playing, family sculpting, group exercises, audiovisual aids, and handouts.

4. Elicit the client's and family's interpretation of information and concepts covered in the teaching plan.

Rationales

1. Assessing the client's and family's knowledge can help the nurse to design and implement an appropriate educational plan based on standards of addictions nursing practice (see *ANA standards of addictions nursing practice,* page 184).

2. Comprehensive client and family education is essential to recovery.

3. These various teaching techniques can help ensure and reinforce client and family learning.

4. Having the client and family verbalize their understanding of the disorder can help the nurse evaluate the effectiveness of the teaching plan and identify points that need clarification.

Nursing diagnosis: *Potential for infection related to compromised immunity, insufficient knowledge about disease, and participation in high-risk behaviors*

NURSING PRIORITY: To help the client identify existing high-risk behaviors and develop an alternative lifestyle

Interventions

1. Assess the client's existing risk factors, such as I.V. drug use, needle sharing, use of impure drugs, and malnutrition.

2. Develop and implement specific teaching plans related to the client's risk factors.

Rationales

1. Knowing the client's risk factors can help the nurse develop an appropriate care plan.

2. Increasing the client's knowledge of existing risk factors can promote behavioral change.

A.N.A. STANDARDS OF ADDICTIONS NURSING PRACTICE

In 1988, the American Nurses' Association, with consultation from nurses working in the addiction field, developed a set of standards to be used when caring for clients who are addicted to alcohol and other drugs. These standards provide a guide for the practice of addictions nursing.

Standard I. Theory
The nurse uses appropriate knowledge from nursing theory and related disciplines in the practice of addictions nursing.

Standard II. Data Collection
Data collection is continual and systematic and is communicated to the treatment team throughout each phase of the nursing process.

Standard III. Diagnosis
The nurse uses nursing diagnoses congruent with accepted nursing and interprofessional classification systems of addictions and associated physiologic and psychological disorders to express conclusions supported by data obtained through the nursing process.

Standard IV. Planning
The nurse establishes a plan of care for the client that is based upon nursing diagnoses, addresses specific goals, defines expected outcomes, and delineates nursing actions unique to each client's needs.

Standard V. Intervention
The nurse implements actions independently and/or in collaboration with peers, members of other disciplines, and clients in prevention, intervention, and rehabilitation phases of the care of clients with health problems related to problems of abuse and addiction.

Standard V-A. Intervention: Therapeutic Alliance
The nurse uses the "therapeutic self" to establish a relationship with clients and to structure nursing interventions to help clients develop awareness, coping skills, and behavior changes that promote health.

Standard V-B. Intervention: Education
The nurse educates clients and communities to help them prevent and/or correct actual or potential health problems related to patterns of abuse and addiction.

Standard V-C. Intervention: Self-Help Groups
The nurse uses knowledge and philosophy of self-help groups to assist clients in learning new ways to address stress, maintain self-control or sobriety, and integrate healthy coping behaviors into their life-style.

Standard V-D. Intervention: Pharmacological Therapies
The nurse applies knowledge of pharmacological principles in the nursing process.

Standard V-E. Intervention: Therapeutic Environment
The nurse provides structures and maintains a therapeutic environment in collaboration with the individual, family, and other professionals.

Standard V-F. Intervention: Counseling
The nurse uses therapeutic communication in interactions with the client to address issues related to patterns of abuse and addiction.

Standard VI. Evaluation
The nurse evaluates the responses of the client and revised nursing diagnoses, interventions, and the treatment plan accordingly.

Standard VII. Ethical Care
The nurse's decisions and activities on behalf of clients are in keeping with professional codes of ethics and in accord with legal statutes.

Standard VIII. Quality Assurance
The nurse participates in peer review and other staff evaluation and quality assurance processes to ensure that clients with abuse and addiction receive quality care.

Standard IX. Continuing Education
The nurse assumes responsibility for his or her continuing education and professional development and contributes to the professional growth of others who work with or are learning about persons with abuse and addiction problems.

Standard X. Interdisciplinary Collaboration
The nurse collaborates with the interdisciplinary treatment team and consults with other health care providers in assessing, planning, implementing, and evaluating programs and other activities related to addictions nursing.

Standard XI. Use of Community Health Systems
The nurse participates with other members of the community in assessing, planning, implementing, and evaluating community health services that attend to primary, secondary, and tertiary prevention of addictions.

Standard XII. Research
The nurse contributes to the nursing care of clients with addictions and the addictions area of practice through innovations in theory and practice and participation in research, and communicates these contributions.

From *Standards of Addictions Nursing Practice with Selected Diagnoses and Criteria* ©1988, American Nurses' Association, Kansas City. Reprinted with permission.

3. Monitor and review laboratory results with the client. Provide counseling before and after human immunodeficiency virus (HIV) screens are conducted.

3. Laboratory results help the nurse to identify possible causes of infection and to initiate early counseling and outpatient support referrals should the client test HIV-positive.

4. Closely monitor the client's vital signs.

4. An elevated temperature, heart rate, and respiratory rate may indicate infection, which can lead to sepsis.

Outcome criteria

As treatment progresses, the client, family, or both should be able to:
• identify substance abuse effects on bodily functions
• demonstrate a willingness to accept responsibility for behavior
• verbalize an understanding of the impact that the client's substance abuse's has on their personal lives
• verbalize an understanding of the addiction disease model
• acknowledge the need for ongoing support and treatment
• verbalize an awareness of resources for obtaining knowledge of and support for problems related to substance abuse.

Discharge criteria

Nursing documentation indicates that the client:
• understands about substance abuse and is aware of its impact on his life and the lives of family members
• has verbalized an understanding of the expected psychological, physiological, and spiritual responses during the first year of recovery
• demonstrates an ability to use newly acquired coping strategies to facilitate recovery
• is aware of available medical and community resources, including HIV counseling and follow-up treatments.
• has scheduled the necessary follow-up appointments.

Nursing documentation also indicates that the family:
• has verbalized an understanding of the diagnosis, treatment, and expected outcomes
• has been referred to the appropriate community resources for ongoing family support
• has verbalized an understanding of when, why and how to contact appropriate health care professionals in case of a relapse or other emergency.

Selected references

Bluhm, J. (1987). *When you face the chemically dependent patient: A practical guide for nurses.* Missouri: Ishiyaku EuroAmerica.

Boyer, P.A. (1989). A guide to therapy with families with a chemically dependent parent. *Psychotherapy,* 26(1), 88-95.

Cohen, S. (1988). The chemical brain: The neurochemistry of addictive disorders. Irvine, CA: Care Institute.

Compton, P. (1989). Drug abuse: A self-care deficit. *Journal of Psychosocial Nursing,* 27(3), 22-26.

Dodge, V.H. (1991). Relaxation training: A nursing intervention for substance abusers. *Archives of Psychiatric Nursing,* 5(2), 99-104.

Doenges, M.E., and Moorehouse, M.F. (1991). *Nursing diagnosis with interventions,* 3rd ed. Philadelphia: F.A. Davis.

Donovan, D., and Marlatt, G.A. (Eds.) (1988). *Assessment of addictive behaviors.* New York: Guilford Press.

Doweiko, H.E. (1990). *Concepts of chemical dependency.* Pacific Grove, CA: Brooks/Cole.

Ellis, P., and Carney, M. (1988). Benzodiazepine abuse and management of anxiety in the community. *International Journal of the Addictions,* 23(10), 1083-1090.

Froedricj, R.M., and Kus, R.J. (1991). Cognitive impairments in early sobriety: Nursing interventions. *Archives of Psychiatric Nursing,* 5(2), 105-112.

Giannini, A.J., and Slaby, A.E. (1989). *Drugs of abuse.* Oradell, NJ: Medical Economic Books.

Gold, M.S. (1988). Alcohol, drugs, and sexual dysfunction. *Alcoholism and Addiction,* 9(2), 13.

Gorski, T.T. (1989). *Understanding the twelve steps.* New York: Prentice Hall/Parkside Recovery Book.

Harper, J.M., and Hoopes, M.H. (1990). *Uncovering shame: An approach in integrating individuals and their family systems.* New York: W.W. Norton.

Inaba, D., and Cohen, W. (1989). *Uppers, downers and all arounders.* Ashland, OR: Ciremed.

Jack, L. (Ed.) (1989). *Nursing care planning with the addicted client,* volume 2. National Nurses Society on Addictions. Skokie, IL: Midwest Educational Association.

Jack, L. (Ed.) (1990). *The core curriculum of addictions nursing.* National Nurses Society on Addictions. Skokie, IL: Midwest Educational Association.

Kanwischer, R.W., and Hundley, J. (1990). Screening for substance abuse in hospitalized psychiatric patients. *Hospital and Community Psychiatry,* 41(7), 795-797.

Kennedy, J., and Faugier, J. (1989). *Drug and alcohol dependency nursing.* London: Heineman Professional Publishing.

Lerner, W.D., and Barr, M.A. (1990). *Handbook of hospital based substance abuse treatment.* New York: Permagon Press.

Leukefeld, C.G., and Tims, F.M. (1989). Relapse and recovery in drug abuse: Research and practice. *International Journal of the Addictions,* 24(3), 189-201.

Madow, L. (1988). *Guilt: How to recognize and cope with it.* NJ: Jason Aronson.

Miller, N.S., Cackis, C.A., and Gold, M.S. (1987). The relationship of tolerance and dependence to benzodiazepines in medical and nonmedical populations. *American Journal of Drug and Alcohol Abuse,* 17(1), 2737.

Miller, N.S., and Gold, M.S. (1990). Benzodiazepines: Tolerance, dependence and addiction. *Journal of Psychoactive Drugs,* 22(1), 23-33.

Murphy, G.E. (1988). Suicide and substance abuse. *Archives of General Psychiatry,* 45(6), 593-594.

Naegle, M. (1988). Substance abuse among women: Prevalence, patterns, and treatment issues. *Issues in Mental Health Nursing,* 9, 127-137.

Nakken, C. (1988). *The addictive personality: Roots, rituals, recovery.* Minneapolis: Hazelden.

Noyes, R., Garvey, M., Cook, B., and Perry, P. (1988). Benzodiazepine withdrawal: A review of the evidence. *Journal of Clinical Psychiatry,* 49(10), 382-389.

Orford, J. (1987). *Excessive appetites: A psychological view of addictions.* New York: John Wiley & Sons.

Platt, J.J. (1986). *Heroin addiction: Theory, research, and treatment.* Malabar, FL: Robert Krieger Publishing.

Rickels, K., Schweizer, E., Case, G., and Garcia-Espana, F. (1988). Benzodiazepine dependence, withdrawal, severity and clinical outcome: Effects of personality. *Psychopharmacology Bulletin,* 24(3), 415-420.

Townsend, M.C. (1991). *Nursing diagnoses in psychiatric nursing.* Philadelphia: F.A. Davis.

Treadway, D.C. (1989). *Before it's too late: Working with substance abuse in the family.* New York: W.W. Norton.

Treece, C., and Khantzian, E.J. (1986). Psychodynamic factors in the development of drug dependence. *Psychiatric Clinics of North America,* 9(3), 399-412.

Velicer, W.F., Diclemente, C.C., Rossi, J.S., and Prochaska, J.O. (1990). Replase situations and self-efficacy: An integrative model. *Addictive Behaviors,* 15, 271-283.

Wanigratne, S., Wallace, W., Pullin, J., Keany, F., and Farmer, R. (1990). *Relapse prevention for addictive behaviors.* Boston: Blackwell Scientific.

Williams, A., D'Aguila, R., and Williams, A. (1987). HIV infection in intravenous drug abusers. *Image: Journal of Nursing Scholarship,* 19(4), 179-183.

Zweben, J.E. (1987). Recovery-oriented psychotherapy: Facilitating the use of 12 step programs. *Journal of Psychoactive Drugs,* 19, 243-251.

Stimulant Dependence

DSM III-R classifications
304.40 Amphetamine or similarly acting sympathomimetic dependence
305.10 Nicotine dependence
305.60 Cocaine abuse
305.60 Cocaine intoxication
305.90 Caffeine intoxication

Psychiatric nursing diagnostic class
Substance abuse

Introduction
Stimulants include all forms of cocaine, amphetamines, caffeine, and nicotine. When these substances are ingested, inhaled, or injected, they commonly cause increased heart rate and blood pressure, appetite loss, and insomnia. Psychological symptoms commonly exhibited by the user include agitation, anxiety, mood swings, and paranoia. Pharmacodynamic, behavioral, and metabolic tolerance occur rapidly. Dependence results as the user adapts physiologically to the continued use of the drug (see *Cocaine effects,* page 188). Psychological dependence also may occur but remains a subjective phenomenon.

ETIOLOGY AND PRECIPITATING FACTORS
Stimulants cause biochemical alterations, specifically neurotransmitter release, which affect the central and peripheral nervous systems and the cardiovascular system. Research indicates that the biochemical effects on the brain reinforce drug use (for example, cocaine blocks norepinephrine and dopamine re-uptake at the synapse). This action leads to the euphoria associated with cocaine use.

According to one psychodynamic theory, an addict is a person with low self-esteem, coping difficulties, poor social skills, low frustration tolerance, and poor impulse control. Other psychodynamic theories suggest that addicts are self-destructive or have adjustment difficulties.

Family theorists view the addicted family as a dysfunctional system in which the addict and drug use become the focus of all family interactions. According to this theory, family members adopt roles, such as scapegoats or clowns, allowing them to function, even in an impaired way.

Behavioral theories present addiction as a behavior rather than as an illness and suggest that drug use is influenced by factors that reinforce drug taking. Such factors include peer pressure, family conflicts, and drug-induced euphoria. One behavioral theory suggests that drug use is learned from others.

Assesssment guidelines
NURSING HISTORY (Functional health pattern findings)
The client may report or exhibit one or more of the findings grouped here according to functional health patterns.

Health perception–health management pattern
• denial of medical or health care concerns
• grandiose perception of health
• preoccupation with physical complaints
• overconcern with health issues
• general anxiety regarding personal well-being
• inability to manage self-care
• feelings of hopelessness and powerlessness about health
• paranoia about health and fear of nonexistent illness
• hypervigilance over health care
• distorted body image
• integumentary alterations, including abcesses and needle marks from I.V. drug use

Nutritional-metabolic pattern
• chronic weight loss
• malnourishment symptoms, including muscle wasting and altered skin and hair condition
• denial of obvious nutritional needs
• poor dentition and bruxism
• increased or decreased appetite dependent on drug use
• irregular eating patterns

Elimination pattern
• heartburn, nausea, vomiting, or diarrhea
• frequent urination

Activity-excercise pattern
• mood swings
• hyperactivity
• chronic fatigue and apathy
• lack of excercise or leisure activity
• denial of normal activity disturbances
• repetitive activities and psychomotor agitation

Sleep-rest pattern
• insomnia
• violent nightmares
• disturbed sleep cycle
• hypersomnia when not using drugs
• need for sedative to aid sleep
• racing thoughts that interfere with resting
• sleep deprivation symptoms, including forgetfulness, emotional liability, and difficulty concentrating

COCAINE EFFECTS

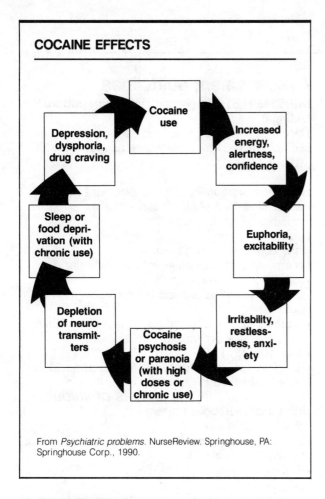

From *Psychiatric problems*. NurseReview. Springhouse, PA: Springhouse Corp., 1990.

• denial of sleep needs
• inability to stay awake

Cognitive-perceptual pattern
• ongoing inappropriate paranoia and suspicion
• racing thoughts, poor memory, fragmented thinking
• delusional thought patterns
• increased sensitivity
• increased alertness

Self-perception–self-concept pattern
• lack of control over drug use
• poor self-esteem
• feelings of grandiosity
• denial of drug dependence
• denial of feelings

Role-relationship pattern
• alienation from family and close friends
• shame or guilt concerning family or friends
• denial of intimacy needs

• problems with intimacy
• extreme financial or emotional dependence on family and friends
• abscence of a productive social role

Sexual-reproductive pattern
• hypersexuality
• irregular menstrual cycle
• promiscuity
• high-risk sexual practices, including multiple partners and unprotected sex
• concerns about unsafe sexual practices
• denial of unsafe sexual practices

Coping–stress tolerance pattern
• hand tremors and bruxism
• nervousness and impatience
• compulsive activity
• hyperalertness
• feelings of not being in control
• denial of obvious coping difficulties
• violent outbursts or emotional immaturity

Value-belief pattern
• breakdown of value system
• denial of spirituality
• heavy emphasis on drug use as a means of maintaining well-being
• powerlessness over drug use
• loss of trust in self and others

PHYSICAL FINDINGS
The client may report or exhibit one or more of the following physical findings.

Cardiovascular
• arrhythmias
• endocarditis
• cardiac depression
• increased body temperature
• increased blood pressure and heart rate
• palpitations
• sweating and chills

Respiratory
• bronchitis
• chest pain with deep inspiration
• chronic productive cough
• deviated nasal septum
• dry, hacking cough
• increased respiratory rate
• nasal mucosa irritation
• pulmonary congestion
• respiratory depression
• rhinitis
• shortness of breath on exertion

Gastrointestinal
- heartburn
- increased gastric acidity
- dry mouth
- nausea or vomiting

Genitourinary
- frequent urination

Musculoskeletal
- ataxia
- twitching
- motor agitation
- muscular rigidity
- muscle wasting
- tactile hallucinations

Neurologic
- dilated pupils
- headaches
- inability to concentrate
- intense agitation and irritability
- tinnitus

- seizures
- insomnia

Psychological
- aggression
- delirium
- depression
- emotional liability
- euphoria
- exhaustion
- mania
- paranoia
- violent outbursts
- visual and auditory hallucinations

Potential complications
Identifying medical complications is the first priority. The client free from medical or psychiatric problems will more readily benefit from treatment. Complications may include seizures, cardiovascular shock, cardiac arrhythmias, destruction of the nasal septum, intracranial hemorrhage, and cardiac arrest.

Nursing diagnosis: *Altered health maintenance related to the effects of stimulant dependence on the client's self-esteem*

NURSING PRIORITY: To help the client acknowledge the need for improvements in maintaining health and to implement healthy self-care

Interventions

1. Maintain a nonjudgmental and caring attitude toward the client and the client's condition.

2. Establish a trusting relationship with the client.

3. Encourage the client to participate in normal activities of daily living.

4. Educate the client about positive health habits.

5. Respond to the client's denial of stimulant dependence with genuine caring.

Rationales

1. Genuine concern and a nonjudgmental approach can enhance the client's self-esteem.

2. The client whose stimulant dependence may have caused paranoia and distrust can learn from the nurse's example how to trust again.

3. Participation in normal activities and personal care can enhance the client's self-worth and sense of control.

4. Learning positive health habits can enhance self-esteem.

5. Denial can be a persistant defense mechanism for the stimulant-dependent client. By making the client face the reality of his condition in a sensitive and caring manner, the nurse can help break down these defenses.

Nursing diagnosis: *Altered nutrition, less than body requirements, related to placing greater importance on drug use than on eating*

NURSING PRIORITY: To help the client establish an adequate, nutritious diet and increase the client's body weight

Interventions

1. Provide the client with well-balanced meals.

2. Provide the client with nutritional supplements if prescribed.

3. Educate the client about proper nutrition.

Rationales

1. The stimulant-dependent client may be experiencing nurtritional deficits from not eating during drug use, spending money on drugs rather than food, and eating junk food rather than well-balanced meals.

2. Nutritional supplements can help replenish vitamins and minerals that have been depleted by stimulant use.

3. Nutritional knowledge can help the client make appropriate dietary decisions.

Nursing diagnosis: *Potential altered body temperature related to stimulant use*

NURSING PRIORITY: To help the client maintain a normal body temperature

Interventions

1. Monitor the client's body temperature.

2. Administer antipyretics as necessary.

3. Monitor the client's fluid intake and output, and encourage the client to drink plenty of fluids.

Rationales

1. Because stimulant abuse can severely elevate body temperature, the nurse should monitor for such temperature changes and institute appropriate actions, such as applying ice packs or a hypothermia blanket, as prescribed. (For more information about interventions, see Appendix G, Managing Acute Substance Abuse.)

2. Antipyretics will help lower the client's body temperature to a safe level.

3. Adequate fluid intake is needed to replace fluids lost because of elevated body temperatures and to aid in lowering the client's body temperature. Sufficient fluid intake also helps prevent dehydration.

Nursing diagnosis: *Potential impaired skin integrity related to changes in health maintenance*

NURSING PRIORITY: To help the client maintain healthy skin integrity

Interventions

1. Assess the client's integumentary system, and explore any factors, such as I.V. drug use, that have led to skin breakdown.

2. Institute prescribed treatments and monitor the client's progress.

Rationales

1. I.V. drug use can lead to abcesses, skin breakdown, and infections. By assessing the client's integumentary system, the nurse can better plan appropriate interventions.

2. Proper treatment promotes healing. Monitoring helps prevent further complications.

Nursing diagnosis: *Decreased cardiac output related to stimulant use*

NURSING PRIORITY: To help the client maintain optimal cardiac function

Interventions

1. Assess and monitor the client's heart sounds, heart rate, and blood pressure.

2. Administer antihypertensives and antiarrythmics if prescribed.

3. Monitor the client's fluid intake and output.

Rationales

1. Stimulant abuse, especially cocaine abuse, increases the client's risk of cardiac arrest.

2. Cardiac output may be altered by stimulant use; various medications may effectively control and help prevent poor cardiac output.

3. An accurate measurement of fluid intake and output helps the nurse to monitor cardiac status.

Nursing diagnosis: *Dressing or grooming self-care deficit related to low self-esteem and ineffective coping mechanisms*

NURSING PRIORITY: To help reestablish the client's self-care and improve the client's self-perception

Interventions

1. Assess the client's self-care measures, reinforcing appropriately used measures and identifying those areas that need special attention.

2. Encourage independent self-care.

Rationales

1. Such assessment provides the client with a foundation upon which to develop additional appropriate self-care strategies.

2. Encouraging independent self-care can increase the client's self-esteem and decrease feelings of powerlessness.

Nursing diagnosis: *Sleep pattern disturbance related to stimulant use*

NURSING PRIORITY: To help the client establish and maintain a balanced wake-sleep cycle that enhances restfulness

Interventions

1. Provide the client with a comfortable sleeping environment.

2. Reassure the client that nightmares will diminish in time.

3. Encourage the client to take fewer naps during the day.

4. Encourage the client to engage in adequate exercise and other stimulating activities during the day.

5. Encourage the client to use nonpharmacologic sleep aids, such as drinking warm milk and practicing relaxation techniques, to promote sleep.

Rationales

1. Comfort and quiet will enhance the client's ability to obtain restful sleep.

2. Restless sleep and nightmares commonly occur with stimulant abuse and during withdrawal but tend to dissipate over time.

3. Avoiding daytime naps can help the client feel more fatigued at bedtime, facilitating a return to a normal sleep cycle.

4. Adequate exercise and activity can help the client return to a normal sleep cycle.

5. Warm milk and relaxation techniques both promote sleep. Because the chemically dependent client probably has used drugs to cope with most problems, he may benefit greatly from the nurse's encouragement in using nondrug solutions.

Nursing diagnosis: *Sensory-perceptual alteration (visual, auditory, and kinesthetic) related to sensory overload from stimulant use*

NURSING PRIORITY: To help the client establish a balanced sensorium and perception

Interventions

1. Promote a quiet, nonthreatening atmosphere by decreasing environmental stimuli.

2. Explain all nursing procedures to the client before beginning them.

3. Observe the client for seizures, and administer prescribed medications, such as Valium or Librium, as needed.

4. Institute and maintain safety precautions. For example, remove articles from the room that the client can use to harm the self and restrain the client, if necessary.

Rationales

1. Decreasing environmental stimuli promotes relaxation and helps prevent potential complications, such as seizures.

2. By sharing information, the nurse can help decrease the client's suspicion and paranoia.

3. The client withdrawing from stimulants may have seizures. Close monitoring by the nurse and administration of prescribed anticonvulsant medications can decrease the likelihood of seizures.

4. Because a client with a sensory disturbance is at risk for self-harm, the nurse should maintain a safe environment at all times.

Nursing diagnosis: *Fear related to an altered thought process*

NURSING PRIORITY: To establish a trusting and safe environment and help decrease the client's paranoia

Interventions

1. Speak calmly and confidently to the client, thoroughly explaining all procedures.

2. Repeatedly orientate the client to people, places, time, and situations.

Rationales

1. By creating an honest, trusting relationship with the client, the nurse can decrease anxiety and enhance trust.

2. The nurse should keep the client orientated during drug withdrawal when he may be experiencing perceptual distortions.

Nursing diagnosis: *Self-esteem disturbance related to perceived failure and dysfunctional family system*

NURSING PRIORITY: To promote the client's self-esteem

Interventions

1. Encourage the client's self-care, and provide appropriate positive feedback.

2. Encourage the client to explore his feelings and thoughts, focusing especially on areas of his life he would like to change.

3. Encourage the client to communicate with peers through group therapy and such support groups as Cocaine Anonymous (CA).

Rationales

1. By affirming positive behaviors, the nurse can increase the client's feelings of self-worth and hopefulness.

2. The client needs to become more self-aware about problem areas in his life, especially those related to drug use, before he can develop more positive behaviors.

3. In group therapy, the client can explore feelings and receive feedback and support from peers. Support groups, such as CA, encourage members to share their feelings and experiences in an effort to gain support from others who have similar experiences and problems.

Nursing diagnosis: *Impaired social interactions related to isolation associated with drug use*

NURSING PRIORITY: To promote the client's social interaction skills and self-esteem

Interventions	Rationales
1. Arrange for the client to participate in an ongoing therapy group.	1. Group therapy provides the client with support and feedback from peers as well as opportunities for practicing social interaction skills.
2. Discourage the client from remaining isolated from others by limiting the client's time spent alone.	2. Limiting the client's time alone helps promote interaction with others.
3. Encourage the client to participate in group role-playing sessions.	3. Group role playing enables the client to rehearse newly learned social skills.

Nursing diagnosis: *Potential for violence related to difficulty processing and interpreting thoughts and to sensory overload from stimulant use*

NURSING PRIORITY: To help the client maintain a safe environment and decrease violent outbursts

Interventions	Rationales
1. Remove all harmful objects from the client's room, and provide necessary safety precautions (such as soft restraints, one-to-one monitoring, and padding).	1. The nurse should monitor closely the client at risk for violence and take necesaary measures to prohibit the client's self-harm or harm of others.
2. Administer prescribed sedatives when necessary.	2. Sedatives usually are provided for their calming effects during the initial stages of stimulant detoxification.
3. Provide a quiet, nonthreatening environment for the client.	3. By providing a quiet environment, the nurse can decrease sensory stimuli associated with stimulant withdrawal.

Nursing diagnosis: *Spiritual distress related to feelings of powerlessness and hopelessness*

NURSING PRIORITY: To help the client regain a sense of hopefulness and establish an improved value system

Interventions	Rationales
1. Arrange for the client to participate in spiritual or religious services if the client desires them.	1. Such services enable the client to obtain support from a formal spiritual source, thereby fostering values and beliefs.
2. Teach the client to make affirmative statements and to use assertiveness skills.	2. Learning to give positive self-messages can help the client increase feelings of self-worth. Assertiveness training can help the client learn how to make needs and feelings known without resorting to aggression or passive behavior.

Nursing diagnosis: *Ineffective family coping related to poor communication*

NURSING PRIORITY: To help the client and family enhance their coping skills, thereby allowing for healthy communication

Interventions

1. Provide or arrange for therapy sessions for the client's family.

2. Educate the client's family regarding their dysfunction, and encourage them to attend self-help groups such as Cocaine Anonymous.

3. Encourage the client and his family to participate in role-playing sessions.

4. Refer the client and his family to outside support agencies as necessary.

Rationales

1. A family therapist can help sort out family dysfunction and communication problems. Through family therapy, the family can create a new system of healthy communication patterns and improved family functioning.

2. Self-help groups can provide support and assistance for the client's family.

3. Role playing enables the client and family to express their real needs and concerns within the safety of a therapeutic setting.

4. Support and assistance resources can become an important part of the family's follow-up therapy.

Nursing diagnosis: *Knowledge deficit related to denial of need for information*

NURSING PRIORITY: To educate the client and family about addictions and when to seek help

Interventions

1. Educate the client and family about addiction, including physical effects of drug use, treatment, and aftercare.

2. Instruct the client and family regarding signs of relapse, such as self-isolation, failure to follow aftercare plan, and stress.

Rationales

1. Such knowledge allows the client and family to make informed decisions.

2. Recognizing warning signs of relapse allows the client and family to seek assistance before relapse occurs.

Outcome criteria

As treatment progresses, the client, family, or both should be able to:
• recognize triggers that can lead to the client's relapse
• identify and use relapse prevention
• demonstrate an awareness of factors that can lead to infection and ways to control or prevent it
• practice appropriate sleep-enhancement methods
• report improved sleep patterns, normal sensorium, and decreased paranoia
• report increased social interaction
• report a decrease or absence of violent outbursts
• verbalize an understanding of family dysfunction related to drug abuse
• demonstrate increased family support
• demonstrate a willingness to participate in family therapy and aftercare plans.

Discharge criteria

Nursing documentation indicates that the client:
• has verbalized a knowledge of the addiction process and relapse triggers
• has demonstrated the ability to use relapse prevention
• has verbalized an understanding of the risk factors associated with stimulant use
• has demonstrated a willingness to participate in an appropriate self-help group, such as Cocaine Anonymous
• is aware of the need for follow-up appointments
• has demonstrated an ability to use skills learned in treatment to maintain a drug-free life-style.

Nursing documentation also indicates that the family:
• is willing to participate in ongoing therapy
• has been referred to appropriate community resources for ongoing recovery and family support.

Selected references

Banks, A., and Waller, T. (1988). *Drug misuse: A practical handbook for general practitioners.* Boston, MA: Blackwell Scientific.

Chychula, N.M., and Okore, C. (1990). The cocaine epidemic: A comprehensive review of use, abuse and dependence. *Nurse Practitioner,* 15(7), 3139.

Chychula, N.M., and Okore, C. (1990). The cocaine epidemic: Treatment options for cocaine dependence. *Nurse Practitioner,* 15(8), 33-40.

Doeneges, M.E., Townsend, M.C., and Moorhouse, M.F. (1989). *Psychiatric care plans, guidelines for client care.* Philadelphia: Saunders.

Frances, R.J., and Franklin, J.E. (1989). *Treatment of alcohol addictions.* Washington, DC: APA Press.

Gawin, F.H., and Ellinwood, E.H. (1988). Cocaine and other stimulants. *New England Journal of Medicine,* 318(18), 1173-1182.

Jack, L. (Ed.). (1990). *The core curriculum of addictions nursing.* Skokie, IL: Midwest Educational Association, Inc.

Khantzian, E.J. (1986). A contemporary psychodynamic approach to drug abuse treatment. *American Journal of Drug and Alcohol Abuse,* 12(3), 213-222.

King, P., and Coleman, J.H. (1987). Stimulants and narcotic drugs. *Pediatric Clinics of North America,* 34(2), 349-362.

McFarland, G.K., and Thomas, M.D. (1991). *Psychiatric mental health nursing.* Philadelphia: Lippincott.

National Clearing House for Alcohol and Drug Information. (1990). *"Ice" poses a new threat to public health.* R #MS403. Rockville, MD.

Pelletier, L.R. (1987). *Psychiatric nursing.* Springhouse, PA: Springhouse.

Perko, J.E., and Kreigh, H.Z. (1988). *Psychiatric and mental health nursing.* (3rd ed.). San Mateo, CA: Appleton & Lange.

Schuckit, M.A. (1989). *Drugs and alcohol abuse.* New York: Plenum Medical Books.

Silvis, G.L., and Perry, C.L. (1987). Understanding and deterring tobacco use among adolescents. *Pediatric Clinics of North America,* 34(2), 363-379.

Weiss, R.D., Mirin, S.M., Michael, J.L., and Sollogub, A.C. (1986). Psychopathology in chronic cocaine abusers. *American Journal of Drug and Alcohol Abuse,* 12(1,2), 17-29.

ADDICTION DISORDERS

Hallucinogen Dependence

DSM III-R classifications
Psychoactive substance–induced organic mental disorders
Cannabis
292.11 Cannabis delusional disorder
305.20 Cannabis intoxication
Hallucinogen
292.11 Hallucinogen delusional disorder
292.84 Hallucinogen mood disorder
292.89 Posthallucinogen perception disorder
305.30 Hallucinogen hallucinosis
Phencyclidine (PCP) or similarly acting arylcyclohexylamine
292.11 PCP or similarly acting arylcyclohexylamine delusional disorder
292.81 PCP or similarly acting arylcyclohexylamine delirium
292.84 PCP or similarly acting arylcyclohexylamine mood disorder
292.90 PCP or similarly acting arylcyclohexylamine organic mental disorder not otherwise specified
305.90 PCP or similarly acting arylcyclohexylamine intoxication

Psychoactive substance use disorders
Cannabis
304.30 Cannabis dependence
305.20 Cannabis abuse
Hallucinogen
304.50 Hallucinogen dependence
305.30 Hallucinogen abuse
PCP or similarly acting arylcyclohexylamine
304.50 PCP or similarly acting arylcyclohexylamine dependence
305.90 PCP or similarly acting arylcyclohexylamine abuse

Psychiatric nursing diagnostic class
Substance abuse

Introduction

Hallucinogens include naturally occurring plants, fungi, or roots, as well as synthetically produced substances. Naturally occurring hallucinogens include mescaline (peyote), psilocybin (mushrooms), harmine, harmaline, dimethyltryptamine (barks and seeds), and ibogaine (root). Synthetic hallucinogens include lysergic acid diethylamide (LSD), diethyltryptamine (DET), dipropyltryptamine (DPT), 2,5-dimethoxy-4-methylamphetamine (DOM, STP), 2,5-dimethoxy-4-

ethylamphetamine (DOET), and 3,4-methylenedioxymethamphetamine (MDMA, ADAM, ecstasy).

Other substances can produce hallucinations. Cannabis, or tetrahydrocannabinoids (marijuana), is a naturally occurring plant that may produce hallucinogenic experiences. Phencyclidine (PCP) and similarly acting arylcyclohexylamine (ketamine)—both anesthetic agents—can also cause hallucinations. PCP, which is inexpensive and easily synthesized, and other synthetic or designer drugs commonly contain toxic impurities that can cause various responses, including death.

Hallucinogen abuse and dependence is characterized by vivid and unusual changes in feelings, thoughts, and perceptions without delirium or severe generalized toxic physical effects. Such abuse and dependence can cause a wide range of psychological effects; individual experience is influenced by setting, personality, and expectations.

ETIOLOGY AND PRECIPITATING FACTORS
According to one psychodynamic theory, an addict is a person with low self-esteem, coping difficulties, poor social skills, low frustration tolerance, and poor impulse control. Other psychodynamic theories suggest that addicts are self-destructive or that they have adjustment inabilities.

Family theorists view the addicted family as a dysfunctional system in which the addict and drug use become the focus of all family interactions. According to this theory, family members adopt roles, such as scapegoats or clowns, allowing them to function, even in an impaired way.

Behavioral theories, which treat addiction as a behavior rather than an illness, suggest that drug use is influenced by factors that reinforce drug taking. Such factors include peer pressure, family conflict, and drug-induced euphoria. One behavioral theory suggests that drug use is learned from others.

Assessment guidelines
NURSING HISTORY (Functional health pattern findings)
The client may report or exhibit one or more of the findings grouped here according to functional health patterns.

Health perception–health management pattern
• denial of health problems even when faced with physical evidence
• use of mood-altering drugs or hallucinogens
• decreased goal-directed activity
• impaired social judgment

- poor school or work performance
- self-destructive behaviors or injury potential
- apathy
- compliance difficulties

Nutritional-metabolic pattern
- increased salivation
- erratic nutritional intake

Elimination pattern
- nausea or vomiting

Activity-exercise pattern
- unpredictable activity patterns
- verbal or physical assaults on others
- agitation

Rest-sleep pattern
- fatigue
- sleep deprivation
- nightmares
- daytime flashbacks

Cognitive-perceptual pattern
- body image changes
- visual and auditory distortions
- illusions
- feelings of depersonalization
- paranoia
- suspicion
- fear of losing control
- synesthesia (such as hearing colors or seeing sounds)
- increased sense of colors, sounds, smells, and tastes
- time or space alterations

Self-perception–self-concept pattern
- fearfulness
- guilt and shame
- denial of hallucinogen use

Role-relationship pattern
- social, interpersonal, and economic problems
- family history of substance abuse or dependence

Sexual-reproductive pattern
- sperm abnormalities
- sterility (in males)
- anovulatory cycles
- retarded sexual development (teenagers)
- sexually transmitted diseases

Coping–stress tolerance pattern
- anxiety or panic
- fatigue or stress resulting in increased flashbacks
- history of psychiatric problems
- substance abuse or dependence history
- family history of psychiatric or substance use disorders

Value-belief pattern
- religious or cultural belief systems that incorporate the drug use

PHYSICAL FINDINGS
The client may report or exhibit one or more of the following physical findings.

Cardiovascular
- coma or death from respiratory or cardiac failure (with PCP)
- diaphoresis
- hypertensive crisis (with PCP)
- increased blood pressure
- tachycardia or palpitations

Respiratory
- asthma-like symptoms (with THC)
- bronchitis (with THC)
- lung cancer (with THC)
- pneumonia (with THC)
- sinusitis (with THC)

Gastrointestinal
- increased salivation
- nausea or vomiting

Genitourinary
- decreased prostate and testes size
- impaired sperm production and increased chromosomal breakage rate (with THC)

Musculoskeletal
- muscle twitching

Neurologic
- ataxia
- confusion
- quickened deep tendon reflexes with intoxication
- delirium
- dilated pupils
- dizziness (with LSD)
- headache (with LSD)
- horizontal nystagmus (with PCP)
- lack of coordination
- muteness or catatonia
- numbness or tingling of the lower extremities (with LSD)
- piloerection
- respiratory or cardiovascular depression with higher doses
- restlessness
- seizures
- visual blurring

Psychological
- altered time or space perceptions
- anxiety or panic
- depersonalization

- distractibility
- euphoria or calm
- labile mood
- suggestibility

Potential complications

Halucinogen dependence can lead to various complications, including decreased vital capacity, chromosomal damage, hypothermia, cardiovascular collapse, panic reaction, and drug-induced psychosis.

Nursing diagnosis: *Sensory or perceptual alterations (visual, auditory, kinesthetic, gustatory, tactile, or olfactory) related to decreased cognitive function resulting from hallucinogen intake*

NURSING PRIORITY: To help the client respond appropriately to environment stimuli

Interventions

1. Monitor the client's intoxication symptoms hourly.

2. Monitor and document hourly the client's orientation to people, places, and time.

3. Document hourly the presence or absence of altered perceptions in the client.

4. Administer prescribed antianxiety or antipsychotic medications.

5. Approach the client calmly and use care when touching the client.

6. Encourage the client to keep his eyes open and to either sit-up or walk in a quiet environment.

Rationales

1. Because peak intoxication levels vary, determining the last dosage time can be difficult. Hourly monitoring can help the nurse implement appropriate interventions (see Appendix G, Managing Acute Substance Abuse, for more information about interventions).

2. Hallucinogens can cause misperceptions of time, place, and person. Accurate client orientation may indicate the alleviation of the drug's acute effects.

3. Altered perceptions are a major symptom of acute hallucinogen intoxication.

4. Benzodiazepines are indicated for extreme anxiety related to hallucinogen abuse. Haloperidol can diminish severe misperceptions.

5. Because the client may be experiencing visual and tactile alterations, the nurse should approach calmly and cautiously to avoid unnecessary agitation.

6. Because closed eyes can intensify altered perceptions, the nurse should keep the client focused on the current environment.

Nursing diagnosis: *Potential for injury related to impaired judgment and disorientation*

NURSING PRIORITY: To maintain the safety of the client and others

Interventions

1. Search the client and the client's belongings upon admission to the unit.

Rationales

1. The client might be carrying illicit drugs. If self-administered, these drugs can complicate assessment and withdrawal.

2. Provide a safe, quiet environment for the client.

2. Hallucinations can be frightening to the client and can foster self-aggression or aggression toward others. Decreasing the environmental stimuli can help prevent intensification of the hallucinations.

3. Use physical restraints on the client only after first trying psychological and chemical restraints.

3. An actively hallucinating client will not perceive restraints as a calming experience. Rather, such a client will be more likely to physically resist the restraints, possibly increasing the anxiety level.

4. If the client cannot comply with commands or requests, move the client to a calm environment.

4. Redirection and reorientation can help calm a hallucinating client, thereby promoting compliant behavior.

5. Encourage the client to verbalize fears and harmful impulses.

5. By encouraging the client to verbalize fears and harmful impulses, the nurse can begin to redirect and reorient the client.

Nursing diagnosis: *Altered thought processes related to hallucinogen abuse and evidenced by auditory or visual hallucinations, inattentiveness, problem-solving inabilities, impaired memory, or inability to retain information*

NURSING PRIORITY: To facilitate the client's ability to interpret reality appropriately

Interventions

1. Assess the client for hallucinations or altered thought processes hourly.

Rationales

1. Hourly assessment provides the nurse with critical information about peak intoxication levels and about the duration of the drug's effects. This knowledge also can help the nurse to implement safe, appropriate interventions during detoxification.

2. Encourage the client to drink plenty of fluids, especially water and fruit juices.

2. An increased fluid intake helps flush the body of drugs. Fruit juice provides the client with both calories and vitamins.

3. Reorient the client to people, places, and time.

3. Frequent reorientation can calm the client until the drug effects decrease and the client can regain and maintain baseline orientation.

4. Monitor the client's laboratory values for electrolyte imbalances, arterial blood gas alterations, and urine pH.

4. Laboratory values provide a data base for determining drug effects as well as the effects of nursing or medical interventions.

5. Provide a safe, calm environment for the client by decreasing external stimulation.

5. Hallucinations can be frightening to the client and can foster self-aggression or aggression toward others. Decreasing the environmental stimuli can help prevent intensification of the hallucinations.

6. Collaborate with multidisciplinary team members to ensure comprehensive client management.

6. Interdisciplinary approaches can provide the client with the highest care quality during acute intoxication and withdrawal.

Nursing diagnosis: *Sleep pattern disturbance related to hallucinogen abuse or intoxication as evidenced by verbal complaints of sleeping inability, nightmares, or interrupted sleep*

NURSING PRIORITY: To ensure that the client receives at least 4 hours of uninterrupted sleep per day

Interventions

1. Determine the client's usual sleeping pattern, and identify how exactly it has been altered.

2. Establish a daytime rest and activity schedule appropriate to the client's current detoxification status.

3. Educate the client and family about ways to promote normal sleep patterns, including decreasing caffeine intake, establishing consistent retiring and waking times, practicing relaxation techniques, decreasing environmental stimuli, drinking warm milk and eating snacks at bedtime, taking a warm bath before bedtime, and decreasing daytime napping.

4. Provide the client with a quiet environment.

Rationales

1. By identifying the client's usual sleeping pattern and the nature of the sleep disturbance, the nurse can more appropriately educate the client about hallucinogen abuse and dependence. Episodic disturbances may be directly related to the substance used and it may be six months to a year before the client is able to return to a normal sleep pattern.

2. Such a schedule can foster a normal sleep cycle that provides adequate rest.

3. The nurse should encourage the use of natural relaxation measures without chemical use to improve the client's sleep pattern. The client should avoid caffeine, a central nervous system stimulant.

4. A stimulating environment increases hypervigilance, thereby inhibiting the client from sleeping.

Nursing diagnosis: *Potential for injury related to poisoning by use of adulterated street drugs*

NURSING PRIORITY: To protect the client from the physical effects of adulterated drugs

Interventions

1. Teach the client about the specific drugs he is using and about the effects of adulterants.

2. Obtain a comprehensive toxicology screening of the client, and assess the client's risk for poisoning caused by adulterants.

Rationales

1. Such knowledge can increase the client's understanding of the drug and encourage appropriate behavioral changes.

2. Toxicology screens provide the nurse with information about possible adulterant substances in the client's system. This allows the nurse to seek appropriate medical assistance to prevent life-threatening complications.

Outcome criteria

As treatment progresses, the client, family, or both should be able to:
• display normal orientation to people, places, and time
• report a cessation of hallucinations
• report an absence of injury to himself or others
• verbalize an understanding of non-mood-altering substances and activities to promote rest
• demonstrate a willingness to seek assistance with abstaining from drugs.

Discharge criteria

Nursing documentation indicates that the client:
• has verbalized an intent to maintain abstinence
• is maintaining vital signs within normal limits
• understands what occurs in hallucinogen abuse and dependence
• has demonstrated a willingness to participate in on-going therapy
• has schdeuled the necessary follow-up appointments.

Nursing documentation also indicates that the family:
• understands the client's diagnosis, treatment, and expected outcomes
• has been referred to the appropriate community and family resources
• has demonstrated a willingness to participate in a self-help group.
• understands when, why, and how to contact the appropriate health care professional in case of an emergency.

Selected references

Americal Nurses' Association. (1988). *Standards of addictions nursing practice with selected diagnoses and criteria: Practice with selected diagnoses and criteria.* Kansas City, MO: ANA.

Bluhm, J. (1987). *When you face the chemically dependent patient: a practical guide for nurses.* St. Louis: Ishiyaku EuroAmerica.

Doenges, M.E., Townsend, M.C., and Moorehouse, M.F. (1989). *Psychiatric care plans: Guidelines for client care.* Philadelphia: Saunders.

Giannini, A.J., and Slaby, A.E., (Eds.) (1989). *Drugs of abuse.* Oradell, NJ: Medical Economics Co.

Grinspoon, L. (Ed.) (1990). Psychedelic drugs. *The Harvard Medical School Mental Health Letter,* 6(8), 1-4.

Leiker, T., (1990). *Nursing Detoxification Guidelines, Monograph.* Wichita, KS.

Lerner, W.D., and Barr, M.A. (1990). *Handbook of hospital-based substance abuse treatment.* New York: Pergamon Press.

McCormick, M. (1989). *Designer-drug abuse.* Franklin Watts.

Munoz, A.E., (1990). *Medical complications of drugs of abuse.* Tucson, AZ: Padre King Video Libreria.

NNSA., (1989). *Nursing care planning with the addicted client,* Volume I. Skokie, IL: Midwest Education Association.

NNSA., (1990). *Nursing care planning with the addicted client,* Volume II. Skokie, IL: Midwest Education Association.

NNSA., (1990). *The core curriculum of addictions nursing.* Skokie, IL: Midwest Education Association.

Schukit, M.A., and Slaby, A.E., (Eds.) (1989). *Drugs of abuse.* Oradell, NJ: Medical Economics Co.

Wilford, B., (1990). *Syllabus for the Review Course in Addiction Medicine.* Washington, DC: American Society of Addiction Medicine.

ADDICTION DISORDERS
Polysubstance Dependence

DSM III-R classification
304.90 Polysubstance dependence

Psychiatric nursing diagnostic class
Substance abuse

Introduction

Clinicians typically reserve *polysubstance dependence* for individuals who use at least three different psychoactive substances concurrently for more than 6 months. The substances used include any or all of the following: depressants (alcohol, sedatives, barbiturates, and benzodiazepines), stimulants (amphetamines, cocaine, and caffeine), opioids (morphine, codeine, and heroin), and hallucinogens (marijuana, LSD, and PCP). Many alcoholics also use marijuana or cocaine. Former heroin users on methadone maintenance have been found to use cocaine intravenously.

Individuals with polysubstance dependence expose themselves not only to the serious physical consequences of chronic alcoholism but also to diseases resulting from poor diet and poor personal hygiene. Furthermore, cocaine use can cause sudden death from cardiac arrhythmia, cerebrovascular accident, myocardial infarction, or respiratory arrest. Using contaminated needles for I.V. administration of amphetamines, cocaine, or heroin can expose users to various infections, including human immunodeficiency virus (HIV) and its related disorders.

Like other psychoactive substance use disorders, polysubstance dependence is characterized by intoxication; interference with work, family life, and social relationships; withdrawal symptoms; and physical diseases caused by the toxic effects of the drugs. Addicted individuals typically rely on the drugs to produce desired states and believe that they need the drugs to cope with life. They also need the drugs to avoid unpleasant withdrawal symptoms. As a result, they develop strong defense mechanisms to protect their habit and to avoid anxiety. Characteristic defense mechanisms include denial, rationalization, projection, and manipulation.

ETIOLOGY AND PRECIPITATING FACTORS

Research suggests that many polysubstance dependent individuals use alcohol and psychoactive substances to relieve anxiety, stress, or depression. Depressants may be combined with stimulants to alter moods and assist with sleep or relaxation. Narcotics may be used to produce a mellow euphoria that alleviates aggression and rage. Alcohol may be used to decrease or intensify the effects of other drugs, to modify withdrawal symptoms, or to substitute for an unavailable drug. Individuals vulnerable to this kind of polysubstance abuse typically have low self-esteem, poor coping skills, and an inability to control or master their environment.

Biological research suggests that a genetic vulnerability to addiction may play a part in polysubstance dependence. Neurologic changes, which follow prolonged drug exposure and which cause alterations in mood and drive, may further reinforce the addiction tendency.

Psychological research suggests that multiple drug and alcohol use is associated with an increased incidence of behavior problems, including depression, attention deficit disorder, and antisocial personality disorder.

Assessment guidelines
NURSING HISTORY (Functional health pattern findings)

The client may report or exhibit one or more of the findings grouped here according to functional health patterns.

Health perception–health management pattern
- denial of treatment need
- minimizing of addiction problems
- concern about alcohol or certain drug, while denying substance use
- underestimation of daily alcohol consumption
- overestimation of or bragging about functional abilities while under alcohol or drug influence
- exaggeration of drug use
- resistance to treatment
- hostility and defensiveness when questioned about drug use
- belief that drinking or drug use can be stopped at any time

Nutritional-metabolic pattern
- weight gain or loss
- lack of interest in nutritious foods and beverages
- tendency to buy drugs and alcohol rather than food
- overconsumption of junk food

Elimination pattern
- concern over gastrointestinal disturbances, including pain, diarrhea, nausea, constipation, vomiting, or bleeding
- frequent urination or urine retention

Activity-exercise pattern
• mobility problems related to automobile accidents, falls, or traumatic injuries
• hyperactivity or lethargy
• unexplained syncope and dizziness
• unsteady gait

Sleep-rest pattern
• insomnia or excessive sleep

Cognitive-perceptual pattern
• difficulty concentrating
• difficulty with decoding sensory input
• worry over inability to think clearly
• distorted perceptions
• grandiose thinking

Self-perception–self-concept pattern
• lack of eye contact
• isolation
• difficulty accepting positive reinforcement
• feelings of hopelessness and worthlessness
• excessive criticism of self and others
• anxiety about entering hospital for treatment
• little or no family support
• suicidal ideation or suicidal gestures
• blame of drug use on external sources
• description of self as dependent and controlled by psychoactive substances or as superior and in control of life-style

Role-relationship pattern
• concern about relationships with family and loved ones
• alienation from others
• job performance difficulties or frequent job changes

Sexual-reproductive pattern
• difficulties with intimacy
• reliance on chemicals to perform sexually
• sexual dysfunction
• concern about participation in high-risk sexual activity in conjunction with I.V. drug use

Coping–stress tolerance pattern
• denial of present anxiety
• feelings of being out of control
• fear of entering the hospital and of having to give up alcohol or other drugs
• reliance on chemicals to feel good
• inability to meet basic daily needs
• maladaptive defenses, such as denial, rationalization, and projection
• hostility when questioned
• low frustration tolerance

Value-belief pattern
• feeling powerless to achieve life goals
• lack of interest in anything
• guilt and shame
• diminished sense of spirituality

PHYSICAL FINDINGS
The client may report or exhibit one or more of the following physical findings.

Cardiovascular
• elevated or low blood pressure
• flushed face
• spider nevi or angioma
• orthostatic hypotension
• arrhythmias
• cold, clammy skin
• edema
• increased or decreased heart rate
• congestive heart failure
• dehydration and electrolyte imbalance

Respiratory
• respiratory depression or failure

Gastrointestinal
• emaciation
• hepatomegaly
• nausea and vomiting
• splenomegaly

Genitourinary
• gynecomastia
• small testes

Integumentary
• cigarette stains or burns on fingers
• many scars or tattoos
• poor personal hygiene
• unexplained bruises, abrasion, or cuts

Musculoskeletal
• muscle weakness

Neurologic
• agitated behavior
• dizziness
• lack of coordination
• nystagmus
• parotid gland enlargement
• seizures
• slurred speech
• staggered gait
• tremulousness

Psychological
• anxiety
• irritability
• sleep disturbances

Potential complications

Polysubstance dependence can lead to various complications, including acquired immunodeficiency syndrome, alcoholic hepatitis, anxiety, aspiration pneumonia, cardiac arrest, cardiomyopathy, cerebellar degeneration, cerebral hemorrhage, child abuse or neglect, cirrhosis, death from asphyxiation, dementia, fetal alcohol syndrome, hyperpyrexia, immunosuppression, legal problems, marital discord and family problems, nasal septum perforation, nose and throat cancer, acute or chronic pancreatitis, psychosis, pulmonary emboli, reduced testosterone and sperm count, respiratory depression and arrest, learning difficulties, sexual dysfunction, and Korsakoff's syndrome.

Nursing diagnosis: *Sensory and perceptual alterations related to multiple psychoactive substance withdrawal*

NURSING PRIORITY: To help the client achieve detoxification with minimum psychological and physiological effects

Interventions

1. Compile a history of the client's alcohol and drug use.

2. Determine the client's intoxication or withdrawal stage, assessing for orientation, hallucinations, speech pattern, and need for safety measures.

3. Monitor the client's response to medications given for withdrawal symptoms.

4. Provide the client with a safe, calm environment with minimal stimuli.

5. Monitor the client's vital signs at least four times daily for the first 72 hours after admission.

Rationales

1. By thoroughly assessing and documenting the client's drug and alcohol use, the nurse can better distinguish the withdrawal symptoms from other symptoms and behavior.

2. The nurse should complete a comprehensive assessment upon admission and continuously assess the client during the first 72 hours of treatment. This allows the nurse to determine if the client is experiencing complications caused by intoxication (signs of impending shock) or by the withdrawal of the drug((delerium tremens with alcohol or seizures with diazepam).

3. The nurse's observations help determine how much medication the client needs to relieve withdrawal symptoms and prevent severe physical or psychological complications.

4. Providing a safe environment helps the nurse prevent the client from harming himself or anyone else during withdrawal. A calm environment prevents unnecessary agitation.

5. Vital signs provide the most reliable information about the client's condition during acute detoxification.

Nursing diagnosis: *Ineffective individual coping related to maladaptive reliance on alcohol and other drugs*

NURSING PRIORITY: To help the client develop positive coping skills

Interventions

1. Establish a trusting relationship with client by being honest, keeping appointments, and being available.

2. Encourage the client to verbalize feelings, fears, and anxieties.

3. Provide the client with opportunities to rehearse problem-solving strategies within the treatment milieu.

Rationales

1. Establishing trust is the first step in convincing the client to develop more appropriate, positive behaviors.

2. Verbalizing feelings in a nonthreatening environment can help the client recognize and begin to resolve many uncomfortable feelings that may have led to polysubstance dependence.

3. Such rehearsals can improve the client's ability to use effective, healthy means to solve problems.

4. Teach the client positive long-term coping strategies that focus on assertiveness, sharing thoughts and feelings with others, and relaxing.

4. These strategies can help the client learn to cope with feelings and stress in a more constructive way.

5. Set limits on the client's manipulative and irresponsible behavior.

5. Limiting and enforcing the consequences of irresponsible behaviors can help the client learn to behave more appropriately.

6. Examine specific problems to help the client see that substance abuse is causing problems in his life.

6. Seeing the relationship between substance abuse and problems can help the client break down his defenses and develop positive coping methods.

7. Positively reinforce the client's efforts to solve problems constructively.

7. Reinforcement enhances self-esteem and encourages the client to adopt acceptable behaviors.

8. Encourage the client to become involved in support groups, such as Alcoholics Anonymous or Narcotics Anonymous.

8. The client will probably need long-term support for effective coping.

Nursing diagnosis: *Self-esteem disturbance related to perceived failures and lack of positive feedback*

NURSING PRIORITY: To help the client develop and maintain feelings of increased self-worth

Interventions

1. Communicate acceptance of the client and his condition.

2. Spend adequate time with the client.

3. Work with the client to identify and focus on personal strengths and accomplishments.

4. Encourage the client to participate in group and family therapy sessions.

5. Encourage the client to participate in treatment-related decisions and to accept responsibility for the condition.

6. Reinforce the client's belief in the ability to change.

7. Help the client to explore both positive and negative traits and behaviors.

Rationales

1. By conveying an accepting attitude, the nurse can enhance the client's feelings of self-worth.

2. Time spent with the client provides the nurse with opportunities to convey acceptance and to enhance the client's feelings of self-worth.

3. Doing so can help the client develop a more positive outlook.

4. Positive feedback and support from others can enhance the client's feelings of self-worth. Group and family therapies allow the client to develop open and honest communication.

5. Such participation promotes an attitude of self-care and encourages the client to adopt positive behaviors.

6. Reinforcing the client's belief in self-change can instill an attitude of hope and self-control over drug dependence.

7. The client may be using drugs to deny the existence of such traits and behaviors. Encouraging discussions and exploration of feelings will help to validate the client's feelings and enhance the client's self-worth.

Nursing diagnosis: *Powerlessness related to lack of control over psychoactive substance use*

NURSING PRIORITY: To help the client develop values and skills that will enable him to regain a sense of control and meaning in life

Interventions

1. Help the client to identify feelings of powerlessness, such as intense cravings and resentment about the substance dependency.

2. Encourage the client to make choices and establish goals.

3. Help the client to differentiate situations that can be changed from those that cannot.

4. Encourage the client to accept the spiritual dimension of 12-step treatments, such as Alcoholics Anonymous.

Rationales

1. The client probably has been coping with feelings through denial and drug use and must now begin to recognize and resolve feelings in more positive ways.

2. By actively participating in decision-making activities and establishing short- and long-term goals, the client can regain a sense of control over the condition and work toward a more productive life.

3. By identifying what is—and is not—within the client's control, the client can learn to direct his energies productively.

4. Twelve-step groups stress reliance on a higher power, which is said to provide relief from anxiety caused by feelings of powerlessness.

Outcome criteria

As treatment progresses, the client, family, or both should be able to:
• verbalize awareness of anxiety and low self-esteem
• identify ineffective coping behaviors and their negative consequences
• acknowledge that polysubstance abuse is a problem
• demonstrate improved problem-solving skills
• report the absence of psychoactive substance withdrawal symptoms
• exhibit no evidence of physical injury obtained during detoxification
• demonstrate an ability to cope with stress constructively
• verbalize positive personal traits
• demonstrate acceptance of responsibility for self-care.

Discharge criteria

Nursing documentation indicates that the client:
• has verbalized an understanding of how alcohol and other drugs affect the body
• has demonstrated an improved self-concept and an increased feeling of control
• can use positive coping skills to control cravings and anxiety
• has verbalized an understanding of situations that trigger alcohol and other drug use
• has verbalized an awareness of the relationship between high risk behaviors, such as I.V. drug use, and AIDS

• has demonstrated an awareness of safe sex practices that decrease the risk of spreading the HIV infection
• has verbalized an intent to participate in ongoing therapy through a 12-step group in the community
• is aware of available community support services
• has expressed a willingness to participate in an ongoing treatment program.

Nursing documentation also indicates that the family:
• has been referred to the appropriate community and family support resources.

Selected references

American Nurses' Association and National Nurses Society on Addictions (1988). *Standards of addictions nursing practice with selected diagnoses and criteria.* Kansas City, MO: ANA and NNSA.

Bluhm, J. (1987). *When you face the chemically dependent patient: A practical guide for nurses.* St. Louis: Ishiyaku EuroAmerica.

Finley, B. (1991). Patients with psychoactive substance use disorders. In McFarland, G., and Thomas, M. *Psychiatric/mental health nursing: Application of the nursing process.* Philadelphia: Lippincott.

Jack, L., (Ed.) (1989). *Nursing care planning with the addicted patient*, Vol. I. Skokie, IL: Midwest Education Association.

Jack, L., Ed. (1990). *Nursing care planning with the addicted patient*, Vol. II. Skokie, IL: Midwest Education Association.

Jack, L., Ed. (1990). *The core curriculum in addictions nursing*. Skokie, IL: Midwest Education Association.

Kaufman, E. (1990-91). Critical aspects of the psychodynamics of substance abuse and the evaluation of their application to a psychotherapeutic approach. *International Journal of the Addictions*, 25(2A):97-116.

Labouvie, E. (1990). Personality and alcohol and marijuana use: Patterns of convergence in young adulthood. *International Journal of the Addictions*, 25(3):237-252.

McAndrew, M. (1990). People who depend upon substances other than alcohol. In Varcarolis, E. *Foundations of psychiatric/mental health nursing*. Philadelphia: Saunders.

Miller, N., Gold, M., and Klahr, A. (1990). The diagnosis of alcohol and cannabis dependence (addiction) in cocaine dependence (addiction). *International Journal of the Addictions*, 25(7): 735-744.

Miller, N., Millman, R., and Keskinen, S. (1989). The diagnosis of alcohol, cocaine, and other drug dependence in an inpatient treatment population. *Journal of Substance Abuse Treatment*, 6:37-40.

Miller, N., and Mirin, S. (1989). Multiple drug use in alcoholics: Practical and theoretical implications. *Psychiatric Annals*, 19(5):250-255.

Scavnicky-Mylant, M., and Keltner, N. (1991). Chemical dependency. In Keltner, N., Schwecke, L., and Bostrom, C. *Psychiatric nursing: A psychotherapeutic management approach*. St. Louis: Mosby-Year Book.

Smith-DiJulio, K. (1990). People who depend upon alcohol. In Varcarolis, E. *Foundations of psychiatric/mental health nursing*. Philadelphia: Saunders.

Townsend, M. (1988). *Nursing diagnoses in psychiatric nursing: A pocket guide for care plan construction*. Philadelphia: F.A. Davis.

Wallace, J. (1986). The other problems of alcoholics. *Journal of Substance Abuse Treatment*, 3:163-171.

Anorexia Nervosa and Bulimia Nervosa

DSM III-R classifications
307.10 Anorexia nervosa
307.51 Bulimia nervosa

Psychiatric nursing diagnostic class
Self-destructive behavior

Introduction

Eating disorders are characterized by grossly imbalanced eating behaviors. Individuals with these disorders tend to alternate between anorexia nervosa and bulimia nervosa, or between bulimia nervosa and obesity.

Anorexia nervosa has at least two distinct presentations. Restricting anorexics are those who lose weight by an extremely decreased food intake in conjunction with intense physical exercise. Bulimarexics are those who alternate between periods of excessive and minimal food intake.

Bulimia nervosa is primarily characterized by episodes of binge eating accompanied by any or all of the following: feelings of being out of control, self-induced vomiting, laxative or diuretic use, strict dieting or fasting, or vigorous exercise. The purpose of these behaviors is to prevent weight gain.

Although not classified as a mental disorder, obesity exhibits some of the same characteristics as anorexia and bulimia. Similarities include dissatisfaction with body shape and size and preoccupation with eating.

ETIOLOGY AND PRECIPITATING FACTORS
Biogenetic theories focus on the role of the hypothalamus and its relationship to the pituitary, thyroid, adrenal, and hormone-secreting glands. A decreased hypothalamic norepinephrine activation produces behaviors similar to those of anorexia. A dysfunction in the lateral hypothalamus produces aphagia and lower body weight. Some of these abnormalities also resemble those noted in depressed or alcoholic individuals.

Other biological research has linked anorexia nervosa and bulimia nervosa to certain affective disorders. Some studies have shown that anorexic and bulimic individuals may have abnormal dexamethasone suppression test findings similar to those of individuals with depression or a family history of affective disorders. Individuals with bulimia may have a low serum serotonin level, which correlates with an increased carbohydrate need.

Biological studies also suggest that obesity may be associated with certain physical disorders. Localized hypothalamic tumors can precipitate excessive eating.

Altered hormone functioning, such as hypothyroidism, adrenal insufficiencies, and excessive insulin secretion can result in a significantly decreased basal metabolic rate, which can cause obesity.

Psychodynamic theory associates eating disorder behaviors with an arrested childhood development. According to this theory, the individual fails to reconcile the natural tendency toward autonomy. Rather than adjusting normally into adulthood, the individual expresses autonomy by actively controlling the body.

Other psychological characteristics common to all eating disorders include low self-esteem, a sense of powerlessness in life and over the environment, and an inability to identify and express clearly feelings and needs. Food may be used to suppress feelings, provide comfort, or achieve self-control.

According to family theorists, individuals with eating disorders typically come from families with rigid rules and roles, blurred or nonexistent boundaries, and overprotective parents. Typically, the family might have rules against talking, expressing feelings, and discussing sexuality. Perfectionism is usually a family expectation.

Finally, sociocultural influences and peer pressure can affect how individuals perceive themselves, which in turn can influence eating behavior. Many individuals perceive the images projected by manufacturing advertisers and the entertainment field—such as physical beauty and thinness—as desirable and equate the attainment of these images as a sign of personal achievement, self-control, and success. Setting such expectations may contribute, in part, to the development of eating disorders.

Assessment guidelines
NURSING HISTORY (Functional health pattern findings)
The client may report or exhibit one or more of the findings grouped here according to functional health patterns.

Health-perception–health management pattern
• inability to control feelings
• denial of health problems even when confronted with concrete evidence indicating physical problems
• hypervigilance about weight and body shape
• use of alcohol, caffeine, nicotine, or other drugs

Nutritional-metabolic pattern
• restricted daily food intake
• binge eating
• purging behaviors, including vomiting, intense exercise, and fasting

• use of diuretics, cathartics, and diet pills
• obsession with counting calories
• hiding and hoarding food
• frequent weight fluctuations
• being underweight (at least 15% of ideal body weight)
• increased incidence of dental problems, including caries
• hair loss
• dry or yellowish skin

Elimination pattern
• constipation or diarrhea
• use of cathartics and diuretics
• rebound water retention after purging
• bowel obstruction

Activity-exercise pattern
• compulsive exercise
• sedentary life-style
• normal daily activity disruptions

Sleep-rest pattern
• inability to sleep without interruption

Cognitive-perceptual pattern
• difficulty concentrating
• distorted body-image perception

Self-perception–self-concept pattern
• perception of eating as a problematic behavior
• preoccupation with food
• description of self as fat even when emaciated
• overconcern with and intense fear of gaining weight
• guilt and shame
• negative self-concept
• obsession with body image and appearance
• feelings of powerlessness

Role-relationship pattern
• overprotective family system
• high and unrealistic family expectations
• role reversal, characterized by feeling responsible for nurturing parents
• avoidance of intimate relationships

Sexual-reproductive pattern
• history of amenorrhea
• breast atrophy
• confusion or anxiety over sexual role
• promiscuity
• significantly delayed psychosexual development
• decreased libido

Coping–stress tolerance pattern
• use of food and eating behaviors as primary coping mechanisms
• inability to identify and name feelings
• anxiety

• depression
• difficulties with impulse control
• sexual abuse or incest
• low self-esteem
• substance use or abuse

Value-belief pattern
• inability to achieve goals
• belief that perfectionism is unattainable
• difficulty trusting others

PHYSICAL FINDINGS
The client may report or exhibit one or more of the following physical findings.

Cardiovascular
• anemia
• arrhythmias
• cyanosis of extremities
• dehydration
• peripheral edema
• emetic-induced cardiomyopathy
• orthostatic hypotension
• hypertension (with obesity)
• hypochloremia, hyponatremia, or hypokalemia
• rebound water retention after purging

Respiratory
• aspiration pneumonia
• pulmonary insufficiency (with obesity)

Gastrointestinal
• parotid galnd swelling
• bleeding gums
• bloating secondary to delayed gastric emptying
• cachexia
• constipation
• caries
• diarrhea
• emaciation
• esophagitis
• gastric rupture
• hematemesis
• mouth sores
• rectal bleeding
• rectal prolapse

Genitourinary
• amenorrhea
• vaginal mucosa atrophy
• dyspareunia
• irregular menses
• renal calculi

Musculoskeletal
• muscle weakness
• osteoporosis

Neurologic
- dizziness or faintness
- light-headedness
- reduced attention and concentration

Psychological
- apathy
- anxiety
- depression
- guilt
- irritability
- mood lability
- obsession with body-image and thinness
- shame
- sleep disturbances
- social withdrawal

Potential complications

Eating disorders can have numerous medical consequences and severe complications (for more information, see *When should an anorexic client be hospitalized?*). The most life-threatening complications include cardiac arrhythmias, coronary artery disease, dehydration, gastrointestinal bleeding, hypokalemia, hypothermia, metabolic acidosis, pancreatic dysfunction, pulmonary insufficiency, substance abuse or dependence, an undiagnosed affective disorder, or sudden death.

WHEN SHOULD AN ANOREXIC CLIENT BE HOSPITALIZED?

Hospitalization is necessary if the anorexic client:
- rapidly loses 15% or more of total body weight
- develops persistent bradycardia (50 beats/minute or less)
- becomes hypotensive (a systolic reading of 90 mm Hg or lower)
- becomes hypothermic (a core body temperature of 97° F [36° C] or lower)
- develops medical complications
- expresses suicidal thoughts
- persistently sabotages or disrupts outpatient treatment
- adamantly denies the need for help.

From *Psychosocial crises.* Clinical Skillbuilders. Springhouse, PA: Springhouse Corp., 1992.

Nursing diagnosis: *Altered nutrition, less than body requirements, related to refusal to eat, purging activities, or excessive physical exercise*

NURSING PRIORITY: To help the client reduce the incidence of food restriction and purging behaviors

Interventions

1. Collaborate with the client and multidisciplinary team to identify a target weight range (about 90% of the client's ideal body weight), and determine the calories necessary to provide adequate nutrition and achieve the targeted weight.

2. Establish a weight gain range and make a contract with the client for attaining this goal.

3. Explain to the client the benefits of compliance and the consequences of noncompliance with the established behavioral program.

Rationales

1. Including both the care team and the client in such decisions can enhance the client's sense of self-control and offers reassurance that staff members are not plotting to make the cllient overweight.

2. A weight range can help the client learn to accept small weight fluctuations as normal. A contract enhances the client's sense of self-control.

3. The client should understand that when body weight falls to 15% below ideal body weight (IBW) and body fat levels are 10% below ideal levels, weight restoration treatment becomes a priority. If the client fails to demonstrate appropriate meal patterns and weight restoration after several weeks, an inpatient hospital setting becomes necessary for the client's physical well-being and safety.

4. Establish and monitor a behavioral program appropriate to the client's condition. Parameters might include some or all of the following:
- weighing the client daily to three times per week
- using the same scale and maintaining a consistent weighing schedule
- having the client wear the same amount of clothing for each weighing
- inspecting the client's clothing for objects or weights that would artificially increase weight
- monitoring and limiting the client's fluid intake to not more than 500 ml at one time
- directly observing the client at mealtime for food hoarding and hiding
- establishing a defined time for finishing meals (approximately 30 minutes)
- arranging specific times for prescribed and monitored physical activity
- monitoring the client's vital signs and intake and output
- establishing a primary nurse or case manager system
- incorporating behavioral and social rewards for appropriate eating.

4. A complete, well-defined behavioral modification program typically is prescribed on inpatient psychiatric units to enhance the client's compliance with treatment. Privileges should be granted or restricted based on compliance and weight restoration.

5. Assure the client that a quick weight gain is not desirable and that a slow, regulated weight gain is the goal.

5. This can allay any client anxiety over rapid weight gain.

6. Begin exploring the client's fear of gaining weight as the nutritional status stabilizes and normal eating behaviors become established. Have the client take an eating attitudes test to help identify specific problem areas.

6. The client must begin identifying and acknowledging underlying emotional issues if maladaptive responses are to be changed.

7. Check the client's belongings for laxatives, diuretics, and diet medications upon admission and when the client returns from therapeutic passes and off-unit activities.

7. The client may seek out and conceal such substances if compulsive purging needs are not met or addressed in a therapeutic atmosphere.

8. Encourage the client to participate in group sessions and to ask for feedback about food intake and activity.

8. Group feedback provides the client with support during attempts to establish an appropriate balance between food intake and amount of physical activity; many anorexics also exercise compulsively.

9. For the client in an outpatient setting, establish specific behavioral criteria that would signal a need for inpatient care. Criteria might include a life-threatening weight loss or medical complication, suicidal ideation or attempts, uncontrolled purging, and concomitant chemical dependency.

9. Negotiating a contract with the client about potential inpatient care can facilitate a trusting relationship between the client and nurse and promote client safety.

Nursing diagnosis: *Altered nutrition, potential for less than body requirements, related to binging and purging*

NURSING PRIORITY: The client will exhibit no signs of binging and purging by discharge

Interventions

1. Sit with the client during meals.

Rationales

1. This provides support for the client and permits observation of intake.

2. Teach the client delay and distraction measures to use when faced with the urge to binge. Measures might include speaking with a staff member, calling a friend, attending a support group meeting, calling a sponsor, or using relaxation techniques.

2. Distraction measures can help the client learn to differentiate an emotional response from hunger. They also can help the client learn the relationship between mood changes and the eating disorder.

3. Once nutritional status has improved, explore the client's feelings associated with weight gain.

3. Emotional issues need to be resolved if the client is to refrain from maladaptive eating behavior.

4. Help the client identify high-risk times for binging and purging, such as when bored or feeling lonely.

4. This allows the nurse and the client to explore better ways to deal with those times, such as by calling a friend, taking a bath, or going for a walk instead of eating.

Nursing diagnosis: *Body-image disturbance related to the client's misperceived physical appearance*

NURSING PRIORITY: To help the client verbalize misperceptions of body image, including those of shape and size

Interventions

1. Ask the client to define an ideal body shape and size, then determine the client's perception of meeting that standard. Point out the client's positive physical attributes.

2. Provide the client with positive reinforcement and factual feedback, but do not argue or challenge the client's distorted perceptions. Encourage the client to seek community or group feedback.

3. Refer the client to art and movement therapies that will provide objective body-image information.

4. Acknowledge and discuss the client's cultural and family values, beliefs, and stereotypes, especially those related to thinness and attractiveness.

5. Limit the client's discussions and comments about actual weight gain.

Rationales

1. Identifying positive physical attributes can enhance the client's self-worth and self-esteem.

2. Positive reinforcement and factual feedback can enhance the client's self-esteem and provide opportunities for initiating and practicing independent functioning. Arguments or power struggles will only increase the client's underlying need to control.

3. External, objective feedback can help the client begin to recognize that his body-image perceptions are unrealistic and unhealthy.

4. Such information can help the client realize how family and cultural factors have fostered an unrealistic body image.

5. Any attention on actual weight gain may escalate the client's anxiety, thereby increasing phobic behaviors.

Nursing diagnosis: *Knowledge deficit about nutrition and eating disorders*

NURSING PRIORITY: To teach the client about nutrition and about eating disorders and their influence on physical and emotional well-being

Interventions

1. Collaborate with the dietitian to teach the client and family about nutrition, calories, food values, a balanced dietary plan, and foods that promote normal bowel function.

2. Arrange for the client to attend meal-planning classes, and encourage the client's participation in helping to plan a unit meal.

Rationales

1. Factual nutrition information can help the client challenge myths, fantasies, and misperceptions about food. Maintaining normal bowel function by diet may encourage the client to reduce laxative and cathartic use.

2. Participation in unit activities can enhance the client's sense of sharing and self-control and can decrease the client's sense of isolation.

Nursing diagnosis: *Potential for injury related to excessive exercise or potentially harmful behaviors*

NURSING PRIORITY: To help the client maintain personal safety

Interventions	Rationales
1. Explain to the client the physiologic impact of excessive exercise.	1. The client should learn that excessive exercise can cause significant shifts in hormonal and metabolic functioning. This can result in amenorrhea, ketosis, and vitamin deficiency.
2. Collaborate with the client and multidisciplinary team to establish an appropriate activity schedule. Observe and monitor the client during private time.	2. Collaborating in the care plan can enhance the client's sense of control; initially, however, the client may need protection from compulsive behaviors and possibly from escalating anxiety, guilt, and shame, which can precipitate a relapse into injurious compulsive exercising.
3. Help the client to develop specific diversionary activities that can be used when the client feels a need to exercise.	3. Diversionary activities can serve as concrete options to exercising. During a crisis, these activities can decrease the client's overwhelming anxiety and compulsive behaviors.

Nursing diagnosis: *Altered family processes related to a dysfunctional family system as evidenced by a pervasive sense of perfectionism, overprotectiveness, or chaos*

NURSING PRIORITY: To help the client and family identify roles, rules, and rituals that impede autonomous, differentiated functioning among family members and contribute to the client's eating disorder

Interventions	Rationales
1. Explore the degree of dependency and enmeshment within the client's family.	1. Dependency and enmeshment impede the normal separation process and the development of autonomy within the family.
2. Teach the client and family about family functions, roles, boundaries, and messages. Explore family patterns that reinforce the client's compulsive behavior.	2. Group educational sessions enable the client and family members to identify and validate feelings in a supportive, safe environment.
3. Teach the client to develop problem-solving skills, and rehearse ways in which to use them.	3. The client needs to develop skills and strategies that decrease the overinvolvement of family in the client's life. Such skills can increase the client's sense of self-control.
4. Encourage the client and family to participate in multiple family psychodrama or family sculpting sessions.	4. Family psychodrama and sculpting can help the client and family to clarify dysfunctional roles and messages in a safe, therapeutic environment.
5. Initiate family therapy, or refer the family to an appropriate therapist within the community.	5. The nurse can help the client and family identify alternative ways to meet their present and future needs.

Nursing diagnosis: *Ineffective denial related to a lack of knowledge about real or potential dangers associated with eating disorders*

NURSING PRIORITY: To challenge the client's denial and facilitate the client's participation in a treatment plan

Interventions

1. Ask the client's family and peers to encourage the client to seek treatment. Allow the client to express any anger or fears about being involved in treatment.

2. Collaborate with the client to identify problems and to establish mutually determined priorities.

Rationales

1. The client may require some pressure from others into starting treatment. Allowing the client to express anger and fear about treatment can foster a trusting nurse-client relationship.

2. Allowing the client to participate in the plan of care can enhance feelings of self-control and decrease anxiety.

Nursing diagnosis: *Impaired social interaction related to withdrawal from peer group, fear of rejection, and preoccupation with eating behaviors or rituals*

NURSING PRIORITY: To help the client develop positive strategies that facilitate socialization

Interventions

1. Individually or in a group, instruct and rehearse with the client interpersonal communication, socialization, and assertiveness skills. Use didactic and role-playing methods to reinforce learning.

2. Identify leisure activities that require minimal productivity from the the client, and teach the client relaxation techniques for use during leisure time.

3. Arrange for the client to attend a self-help or support group, such as Overeaters Anonymous or Anorexics and Bulimics Anonymous.

Rationales

1. Social withdrawal may result from feelings of inadequacy in social situations and interpersonal relationships. Learning strategies for dealing with these feelings can draw the client out of isolation.

2. The client should learn to enjoy leisure activities as a counterbalance to a probably too-rigid need to be productive and successful.

3. Participation in such groups can diminish the client's sense of social isolation and foster feelings of hope for recovery.

Outcome criteria

As treatment progresses, the client, family, or both should be able to:
• demonstrate knowledge about the causes and effects of the eating disorder
• demonstrate a willingness to participate in treatment
• obtain and maintain an appropriate healthy food intake
• report a decrease in or absence of binging or purging
• demonstrate an increased knowledge of nutrition
• verbalize a realistic body image
• demonstrate a decrease in or absence of self-destructive behaviors
• demonstrate the ability to establish appropriate boundaries and autonomy within the family
• demonstrate increased socialization skills.

Discharge criteria

Nursing documentation indicates that the client:
• has demonstrated an increased ability to recognize signs and symptoms of eating disorders
• can use newly learned skills for managing anxiety, guilt, shame, and triggers that induce compulsive eating
• can identify appropriate internal and external support resources
• can use alternate coping skills
• has verbalized a desire to participate in an ongoing treatment program.

Nursing documentation also indicates that the family:
• has verbalized a knowledge of the client's diagnosis, treatment and expected outcomes
• has been referred to the appropriate family and community resources
• has expressed a willingness to participate in an ongoing therapy program
• understands when, why, and how to contact the appropriate health care professional in case of an emergency.

Selected references

Agras, W.S. (1987). *Eating disorders: management of obesity, bulimia and anorexia nervosa.* New York: Pergamon Press.

APA (1987). Diagnostic and statistical manual of mental disorders. Washington, DC: APA Press.

Cattanach, L., and Rodin, J. (1988). Psychosocial components of stress process in bulimia. *International Journal of Eating Disorders,* 7, 7588.

Deering, C.G. (1987). Developing a therapeutic alliance with the anorexia nervosa client. *Journal of Psychosocial Nursing,* 25(3), 10-17.

Dippel, N.M., and Becknal, B. (1987). Bulimia. *Journal of Psychosocial Nursing,* 25(9), 12-17.

Ebbitt, J. (1987). *The eating illness workbook.* Parkside Press.

Garfinkel, P.E., and Garner, D.M. (1987). *The role of drug treatment for eating disorders.* New York: Brunner-Mazel.

Garner, D.M., and Garfinkel, P.E. (1988). *Diagnostic issues in anorexia nervosa and bulimia nervosa.* New York: Brunner-Mazel.

Garner, D.M., Rockert, W., Olmstead, M.P., Johnson, C., and Coscina, D.V. (1985). Psychoeducational principles in the treatment of bulimia and anorexia nervosa. In D.M. Garner and P.E. Garfinkel (Eds.) *Handbook of psychotherapy for anorexia nervosa and bulimia.* New York: Guilford Press.

Geary, M.C. (1988). A review of treatment models for eating disorders. *Holistic Nursing Practice,* 3(1), 39-45.

Grigg, D.N., and Friesen, J.D. (1989). Family patterns associated with anorexia nervosa. *Journal of Marital and Family Therapy,* 15(1), 2942.

Head, S.B., and Williamson, D.A. (1990). Association of family environment and personality disturbances in bulimia nervosa. *International Journal of Eating Disorders,* 9(6), 667-674.

Henderson, M., and Freeman, C.P.L. (1987). A self-rating scale for bulimia: The "BITE." *British Journal of Psychiatry,* 150, 18-24.

Hsu, L.K.G. (1990). *Eating disorders.* New York: Guilford Press.

Jack, L. (ed) (1989). *Nursing care planning with the addicted client,* Vol 1. Skokie, IL: National Nurses Society on Addictions.

Katz, J. (1990). Eating disorders: A primer for the substance abuse specialist. Clincal features. *Journal of Substance Abuse Treatment,* 7(2), 143-149.

Kreitter, S., and Chemerin, A. (1990). Body-image disturbance in obesity. *International Journal of Eating Disorders,* 9, 409-418.

Laube, J.J. (1990). Why group-therapy for bulimia. *International Journal of Group Psychotherapy,* 40, 169-187.

Marcus, R.N., and Kate, J.L. (1990). Inpatient care of the substance-abusing patient with a concomitant eating disorder. *Hospital and Community Psychiatry,* 41(1), 59-63.

McFarland, B., and Baker-Baumann, T. (1990). *Shame and body image: Culture and the compulsive eater.* Deerfield Beach, Fla.: Health Communications, Inc.

Mitchell, J.E., Pyle, R., Eckert, E.D., and Hatsukami, D. (1990). The influence of prior alcohol and drug abuse problems on bulimia nervosa treatment outcome. *Addictive Behaviors,* 15(2), 169-173.

Norring, C.E.A. (1990). The eating disorder inventory: Its relation to diagnostic dimensions and follow-up status. *International Journal of Eating Disorders,* 9(6), 685-694.

Norring, C., and Sohlberg, S. (1991). Ego functioning in eating disorders: Prediction of outcome after one and two years. *International Journal of Eating Disorders,* 10(1), 1-13.

Picard, F.L. (1989). *Family intervention: Ending the cycle of addiction and co-dependency.* Kingsport, TN: Beyond Words Publishing.

Pomeroy, C., and Mitchell, J. (1989). Medical complications and management of eating disorders. *Psychiatric Annals,* 19(9), 488-493.

Powers, P.S., et al (1987). Perceptual and cognitive abnormalities in bulimia. *American Journal of Psychiatry,* 144(11), 1456-60.

Riebel, L.K. (1989). Communication skills for eating-disordered clients. *Psychotherapy,* 26(1), 69-74.

Riebel, L.K. (1990). The dropout problem in outpatient psychotheraphy groups for bulimics and compulsive eaters. *Psychotherapy,* 27(3), 404-410.

Root, M., Fallon, P., and Friedrich, W. N. (1986). *Bulimia: A systems approach to treatment.* New York: Norton.

Root, M.P.P. (1991). Persistent, disordered eating as a gender specific, post-traumatic stress response to sexual assault. *Psychotherapy,* 28(1), 96-102.

Root, M.P.P. (1990). Recovery and relapse in former bulimics. *Psychotherapy,* 27(3), 397-403.

Schlundt, D.G., and Johnson, W. G. (1990). *Eating disorders: Assessment and treatment.* Boston: Allyn & Bacon.

Siegel, M., Brisman, J., and Weinshel, M. (1988). *Surviving an eating disorder.* San Francisco: Harper & Row.

Steiner, H. (1990). Defense styles in eating disorders. *International Journal of Eating Disorders,* 9(2), 141-151.

Stierlin, H., and Weber, G. (1989). *Unlocking the family door.* New York: Brunner-Mazel.

Thompson, R.A., and Sherman, R.T. (1989). Therapist errors in treating eating disorders: Relationship and process. *Psychotherapy,* 26(1), 62-68.

Townsend, M.D. (1991). *Nursing diagnoses in psychiatric nursing: A pocket guide for care plan construction*, 2nd ed. Philadelphia: F.A. Davis.

Vandereycken, W. (1987). The constructive family approach to eating disorders: Critical remarks on the use of family therapy in anorexia nervosa and bulimia. *International Journal of Eating Disorders*, 6, 455-465.

Vandereycken, W. (1990). The addiction model in eating disorders: Some critical remarks and a selected bibliography. *International Journal of Eating Disorders*, 9(1), 95-101.

Williams, D.A., Prather, R.C., McKenzie, S.J., and Blouin, D.C. (1990). Behavioral-assessment procedures can differentiate bulimia-nervosa, compulsive overeater, obese, and normal subjects. *Behavioral Assessment*, 12, 239-252.

Wright, K., Smith, M.S., and Mitchell, J. (1990). Organic diseases mimicking atypical eating disorders. *Clinical Pediatrics*, 29, 325-328.

Psychophysiologic Disorders

DSM III-R classifications
300.11 Conversion disorder
300.70 Hypochondriasis
300.70 Body dysmorphic disorder
300.81 Somatization disorder
307.80 Somatoform pain disorder

Psychiatric nursing diagnostic class
Psychophysiologic disorder

Introduction
Psychophysiologic disorders suggest physical causes without demonstrable organic findings or identified physiologic mechanisms. The symptoms of these disorders are probably linked to psychological conflicts or factors.

Conversion disorder is characterized by a lost or altered physical function without the presence of any physiological disorder.

Hypochondriasis involves a preoccupation with the fear of developing or having a serious disease or disorder. This unwarranted fear, which typically is accompanied by physical signs or sensations, usually persists even after a comprehensive evaluation has eliminated physical causes.

Body dysmorphic disorder is characterized by a preoccupation with an imagined physical appearance defect. The most common complaints involve facial flaws.

Somatization disorder is characterized by recurrent and multiple somatic complaints, which usually begin before age 30. Generally, no evidence of a physical disorder can be found.

The individual with *somatoform pain disorder* has a preoccupation with pain, which usually cannot be explained by physical findings.

ETIOLOGY AND PRECIPITATING FACTORS
Intrapersonal theories maintain that anxiety, anger, frustration, or disappointment can give rise to psychophysiologic disorders. Because the emotion's underlying cause remains unrecognized or unacknowledged, consequent emotional discomfort is manifested by physical symptoms or disorders.

Behavioral theory suggests that psychophysiologic symptoms result from learned behavior. According to this theory, children learn from parents or other family members to deal indirectly with stressors. For example, a child who is unprepared for a school test may develop physical symptoms and subsequently may be kept home. As a result, the child begins to identify the physical symptoms with avoidance of stressors.

Social, cultural, and interactional stressors also may precipitate psychophysiologic disorders. These stressors include stressful occupations, overcrowding, poverty, prejudice and persecution, and inadequate social relations.

Psychoneuroimmunology attempts to address the etiology of these disorders in a holistic rather than reductionist manner. Research focuses on the immunological and physiological responses to stress and how they increase the individual's susceptibility to illness.

Assessment guidelines
NURSING HISTORY (Functional health pattern findings)
The client may report or exhibit one or more of the findings grouped here according to functional health patterns.

Health perception–health management pattern
• extreme worry over general health
• obsessive interest in bodily processes, concerns, or diseases
• preoccupation with an imagined appearance defect
• physical symptoms involving one or various body systems
• severe and prolonged pain as primary symptom
• inability to use a specific body part or system
• intense fear of a serious disease
• numerous, comprehensive evaluations for physical symptoms
• overuse of health care system to ease physical symptoms
• annoyance with or failure to follow through psychiatrist or psychotherapist referrals

Nutritional-metabolic pattern
• weight gain or loss
• rigorous monitoring of reactions to dietary intake
• concern about hair, nails, skin, or glands
• hypervigilance about small wounds or bruises
• concern about infection
• extreme concern about dentition

Elimination pattern
• numerous gastrointestinal symptoms
• frequent urination
• concern over sweating or cold, clammy skin
• intense worry about bowel elimination patterns

Activity-exercise pattern
• decreased ability to engage in occupation due to physical symptoms
• decreased interest in leisure activity

• concern about becoming easily fatigued following activity
• concern about life changes due to restricted activity caused by physical symptoms

Sleep-rest pattern
• sleep disturbance
• fatigue after sleep
• sleep aid use, not always reported

Cognitive-perceptual pattern
• sudden inability to hear or see
• hearing loss
• concern about hearing one's own heart beat
• memory difficulties

Self-perception–self-concept pattern
• perception of self as not feeling good
• difficulty describing feelings
• denial of anger, anxiety, frustration, or fear
• perception of self as dependent
• concern over body image, self-esteem, or self-worth

Role-relationship pattern
• concern about physical symptom impact on family
• fear about inability to function at job
• needing loved one's presence during testing, examinations, procedures, or explanations of treatment options
• concern about being socially isolated or alienated
• family system that does not discuss or resolve problems

Sexual-reproductive pattern
• lack of satisfaction or interest in sexual relations
• menstruation problems
• sexual intercourse problems

Coping–stress tolerance pattern
• denial as a coping mechanism
• significant life-style changes that may contribute to physical symptoms
• difficulty identifying anyone to discuss and assist with feelings or problems
• excessive analgesic use with minimal pain relief

Value-belief pattern
• feeling powerless to achieve life goals

PHYSICAL FINDINGS
The client may report or exhibit one or more of the following physical findings.

Cardiovascular
• chest pain
• palpitations

Respiratory
• shortness of breath
• smothering sensation

Gastrointestinal
• abdominal pain
• bloating
• burning sensation in rectum
• diarrhea
• food intolerance
• nausea or vomiting

Genitourinary
• impotence
• painful intercourse
• painful, irregular, or excessive menstruation
• pseudocyesis
• urinary retention or difficulty urinating

Musculoskeletal
• aches or pains
• muscle spasms
• muscle weakness

Neurologic
• akinesia or dyskinesia
• amnesia
• anesthesia or paresthesia
• anosmia
• aphonia
• blindness
• blurred or double vision
• coordination disturbances
• deafness
• dizziness or fainting
• dysphagia
• loss of consciousness
• seizures
• back or joint pain
• urination pain
• pain in extremities

Psychological
• anhedonia
• anxiety
• denial of feelings
• dependency
• depression
• insomnia
• sleep disturbances

Potential complications
The most common complications of psychophysiologic disorders include extensive hospital admissions, repeated or unnecessary surgical procedures, drug dependence, marital conflict or divorce, and suicide attempts. Contractures or disuse atrophy from paralysis related to prolonged function loss may accompany *conversion disorder*. Numerous attempts to obtain medical validation for multiple symptoms may cause an individual with *hypochondriasis* to overlook a real physical problem.

Nursing diagnosis: *Body-image disturbance related to low self-esteem evidenced by preoccupation with real or imagined altered body structure or function*

NURSING PRIORITY: To help the client realize that the perceived body changes are exaggerated

Interventions

1. Assess the body change with which the client is preoccupied. If the client's normal appearance or functioning has changed, help the client to explore his feelings about the change.

2. Collaborate with the client to identify misperceptions regarding body image. Provide accurate feedback in a direct and nonthreatening manner.

3. Encourage the client to participate in body-image group activities and movement therapy activities.

4. Encourage and reinforce the client's independent, self-care activities, participating or assisting only when necessary.

5. Encourage the client to use cognitive restructuring strategies, such as saying "Okay, just because I made a mistake doesn't mean I'm stupid," instead of "That was a stupid thing to do."

Rationales

1. By exploring and expressing feelings about a real change, the client can begin to resolve those feelings. Doing so can also help the client identify which feelings are appropriate and which are exaggerated.

2. Collaborating with the client in a nonjudgmental, nonthreatening manner can help establish a trusting nurse-client relationship.

3. Group activities, including a judicious use of touch, can help the client feel accepted by others and diminish fears of being rejected because body structure or function changes.

4. Active participation in self-care activities can enhance the client's self-esteem and provide opportunities for confronting bodily functions realistically.

5. Cognitive restructuring strategies can enhance the client's self-esteem and help the client develop new thinking patterns and eliminate negative messages about the self.

Nursing diagnosis: *Chronic pain related to unmet dependency needs or repressed anxiety as demonstrated by verbal complaints with no pathophysiologic validation*

NURSING PRIORITY: To help the client recognize and understand the relationship between pain and psychological problems

Interventions

1. Review the client's past and present medical records, and monitor any laboratory studies and reports. Assist the multidisciplinary team in developing a thorough diagnosis.

2. Observe and record the duration, location, and intensity of the client's pain. Collaborate with the client to identify factors that precipitate and help alleviate the pain.

3. Acknowledge the client's pain perception as a real event.

4. Collaborate with the client, multidisciplinary team, and a chronic pain specialist (if one is available) to determine appropriate treatment, such as the client's participation in a chronic pain program. Provide the client with pain medication as prescribed.

5. Collaborate with the client to identify additional strategies that can produce comfort. Strategies might include back rubs, warm baths or showers, applications of heating pads or ice packs, splinting, and use of a TENS unit.

Rationales

1. A comprehensive assessment can help ascertain the presence or absence of an organic condition or problem.

2. A comprehensive pain assessment can enable the nurse to develop a more effective care plan.

3. Denying or challenging the client's pain perception will only heighten the client's need to convince the health care team of the pain, draining the client of energy.

4. Including a chronic pain specialist in the multidisciplinary team can facilitate skill-building among staff members while providing quality client care.

5. Such strategies may be physically comforting to the client.

6. Encourage the client to begin identifying and using alternate coping strategies to manage stress.

6. Using alternate coping strategies may diminish the client's reliance on physical pain as a maladaptive response to stress.

7. Teach the client pain-cycle disrupting strategies to use when stress symptoms begin. Include visual and auditory distractions, breathing exercises, guided imagery and visualization, therapeutic massage, relaxation techniques, and cold and heat application. Encourage family member participation.

7. Disrupting the pain cycle can help eliminate the client's need to use pain as a response to stress.

8. Encourage the client to verbalize feelings about pain, to connect pain to increased anxiety, and to identify specific anxiety-causing situations.

8. Encouraging the client to verbalize feelings in a supportive environment can facilitate expression, problem solving, and the resolution of disturbing issues.

9. Help the client's family to develop a positive reinforcement program. Encourage family members to participate in family sessions, and provide referrals for outpatient family therapy.

9. By reinforcing and encouraging client self-control, family members can decrease the amount of time they spend attending to the client's pain behaviors.

Nursing diagnosis: *Ineffective individual coping related to the client's inability to manage emotional conflict, extreme need for approval and acceptance, unmet dependency needs, or low self-esteem*

NURSING PRIORITY: To help the client acquire and use adaptive coping strategies that manage conflict while reducing reliance on physical symptoms

Interventions

1. Use a time-line chart to determine when the client's somatic symptoms first appeared and which social, financial, emotional, familial, and occupational events were transpiring. Also note any symptom flare-ups, treatments, and hospitalizations that occurred. With the client, determine what roles the need for attention and distraction from problems play in the disorder.

2. Help the client to identify and determine the causes of any anger or resentment the client might feel.

3. Teach and rehearse with the client methods for directly expressing feelings. Positively reinforce the client's use of adaptive coping strategies.

4. Collaborate with the multidisciplinary treatment team to develop a comprehensive, consistent approach to the client's somatic complaints.

5. Teach the client assertiveness skills and incorporate these skills in role-playing sessions.

6. Collaborate with the client to identify positive personal characteristics. Encourage the client to use personal affirmations based on these characteristics.

Rationales

1. Such a history can help the nurse to develop a more appropriate plan of care and may illuminate some connections between crises or conflicts and the emergence of the disorder's symptoms.

2. The time-line chart can help the client target the source of the anger or resentment. Identifying and exploring these feelings can help decrease the maladaptive use of physical symptoms to express emotions.

3. Role modeling and rehearsing alternate behaviors can increase the client's ability to use and modify new behaviors. Reinforcement encourages the client to continue desired behaviors.

4. A coordinated treatment team can dissuade the client from trying to persuade staff members to side with him against other staff members about his condition. A consistent approach of limit setting and feedback can enhance behavioral change.

5. Learning assertiveness skills can help the client communicate more openly and honestly and can decrease conflict avoidance.

6. Building the client's self-esteem can help decrease his excessive dependency needs.

7. Teach the client how to ask for attention, nurturing, and support.

7. Learning to communicate needs directly can help decrease the client's reliance upon physical complaints as a means of getting emotional needs met.

Nursing diagnosis: *Knowledge deficit related to denial, intense repressed anxiety level, preoccupation with self and pain, or lack of interest in learning*

NURSING PRIORITY: Help the client understand the psychological foundation of physical symptoms

Interventions

1. Assess the client's knowledge about psychological problems and their effects on physiologic functioning.

2. Assess the client's overt and covert anxiety level and his ability to participate in educational sessions.

3. Consult with occupational, physical, recreational, and movement therapists to establish appropriate treatment plans and to determine adaptive coping strategies.

Rationales

1. Identifying knowledge deficits and misperceptions can enable the nurse to develop an appropriate care plan to confront the client's denial system.

2. Intense anxiety can inhibit the client's ability to learn and retain information.

3. Comprehensive team consultations can provide individualized and specialized techniques for identifying and dealing with stressors. Techniques might include decision making and problem solving, art therapy, horticultural therapy, leisure time management, pet therapy, movement therapy, and psychodrama.

Nursing diagnosis: *Ineffective family coping, compromised, related to struggles for control and power*

NURSING PRIORITY: Help the client's family to develop and use positive coping strategies that can decrease the reliance on physical symptoms as a coping means

Interventions

1. Explore specific family member roles and ways in which the client's disorder has changed the family organization.

2. Identify underlying situations that inhibit the family's ability to provide the client with needed assistance, support, or nurturing. Encourage family members to verbalize feelings.

3. Discuss with the client and family how they get needs met within and outside the family. Explore with family members the issues of power and control within their system.

4. Provide the family with referrals for ongoing family therapy after discharge.

Rationales

1. Family perceptions may have prevented the client from being identified as the family member with a disorder. Understanding the family's perspective of their roles can help the nurse understand the family's dynamics.

2. Doing so can help the family to reestablish appropriate boundaries and to express feelings honestly.

3. By learning and using a more democratic family process, the client and family can decrease the use of illness as a manipulative tool.

4. Ongoing therapy can promote progress in behavioral changes within the family and provide an additional avenue for managing family stress.

Nursing diagnosis: *Self-care deficit related to activity intolerance, neuromuscular or musculoskeletal impairment, pain, discomfort, or perceptual or cognitive impairment*

NURSING PRIORITY: Help the client regain the ability to perform normal daily functions

Interventions

1. Assess client's impairment in relation to feeding, bathing and hygiene, dressing and grooming, and toileting. Document strengths and inabilities.

2. Modify the client's environment to enable him to perform normal daily functions at his ability level.

3. Allow the client enough time to perform daily functions and positively reinforce successful performance. Be available to help the client if symptoms interfere with his ability to function independently.

4. Consult occupational and physical therapists when appropriate.

5. Encourage the client to participate in group therapy to discuss feelings about his disability or impairment and the dependency need it produces.

Rationales

1. This information can enable the nurse to develop an adequate client care plan.

2. Environmental adjustments can increase the client's chances of successfully performing daily functions, thereby increasing his self-esteem and promoting self-care.

3. Positive reinforcement enhances client self-esteem and encourages repetition of desired behaviors.

4. Teaching by occupational and physical therapists can facilitate optimal client functioning.

5. As the client becomes able to explore his feelings about his impairment and dependency needs, he can begin to address unresolved conflicts.

Nursing diagnosis: *Sensory-perceptual alteration evidenced by lost or altered physical functioning suggesting a physical disorder but without evidence of organic pathology*

NURSING PRIORITY: Help the client and family recognize relationship between emotional conflict and altered physical functioning

Interventions

1. Encourage client and family participation in education sessions describing stress responses and psychophysiologic conditions.

2. Offer only limited attention to the client's preoccupation with his disability or impairment, and encourage independence within the client's physical limits.

3. Have the client keep a daily log of feelings, thoughts, and symptoms. Regularly review the log with the client.

4. Encourage the client to participate in scheduled therapeutic activities. Do not permit the client to avoid participation because of his disability or impairment, withdrawing attention when he pursues this as rationale.

Rationales

1. Education can help the client and family understand the relationship between emotional stress and physical symptoms.

2. Attention paid to the client's preoccupation with his disability can reinforce the continued use of the maladaptive response to fulfill dependency needs. Support and encouragement for achievements can foster repetition of desired behaviors.

3. A daily log can provide the client the opportunity to discover the links between conflicts and physical symptoms.

4. Participating in scheduled therapeutic activities can enhance the client's self-esteem and reinforce positive behaviors.

Nursing diagnosis: *Social isolation related to physical symptoms or disability*

NURSING PRIORITY: Provide the client with opportunities for increased socialization

Interventions	Rationales
1. Collaborate with the client and multidisciplinary team to determine appropriate diversionary and expressive therapies, including occupational, recreational, art, movement, music, and pet therapies.	1. Structuring the client's day with different activities can decrease preoccupation with physical symptoms.
2. Work with the client to identify concrete ways to increase social contacts within physical limitations.	2. Broadening the client's social contacts can increase his support sources.
3. Identify and discuss community resources, self-help groups, and volunteer groups that may benefit the client.	3. Engaging in group activities can begin to alleviate the client's social isolation.

Outcome criteria

As treatment progresses, the client, family, or both should be able to:
• demonstrate a realistic perception and self-acceptance of bodily appearance or function
• demonstrate the ability to complete daily activities without pain interference
• verbalize an understanding of the relationship between emotional conflicts and problems and physical symptoms
• demonstrate the ability to use specific strategies that manage stress responses and prevent physical symptom exacerbation
• demonstrate increased independence in self-care
• verbalize an awareness of support and on-going therapy needs.

Discharge criteria

Nursing documentation indicates that:
• the client has recognized and acknowledged psychological reasons for physical symptoms
• the client has demonstrated the ability to use newly learned skills to manage emotional conflict
• the client has demonstrated the ability to use appropriate internal and external support sources
• the client and family have verbalized an understanding of the diagnosis, treatment, and expected outcomes
• the client and family have verbalized a willingness to participate in ongoing therapy
• the client and family have verbalized an awareness of community support groups and programs, such as chronic pain management program and vocational retraining program, and their referrals
• the client and family have verbalized an understanding of when, why, how, and whom to contact in case of an emergency.

Selected references

Adler, R., Felten, D.L., Cohen, N. (eds) (1991). *Psychoneuroimmunology*. New York: Academic Press.

Adler, C.S., Adler, S.M., and Packard, R.R. (1987). *Psychiatric aspects of headache*. Baltimore: Williams & Wilkins.

Alexander, R. (1987). *Psychosomatic medicine: Its principles and applications*. New York: W.W. Norton.

A.P.A. (1987). *Diagnostic and statistical manual of mental disorders*. (DSM III-R). Washington, DC: APA Press.

Barry, P.D. (1989). *Psychosocial nursing assessment and intervention: care of the physically ill person*. 2nd edition. Philadelphia: Lippincott.

Barsky, A. J. (1988). *Worried sick: Our troubled quest for wellness*. Boston: Little Brown.

Barsky, A.J., Geringer, E., Wood, C.A. (1988). A cognitive-educational treatment for hypochondriasis. *General Hospital Psychiatry*, 10(5), 322-327.

Basolo-Kunzer, M., Diamond, S., Maliszewski, M. et al (1991). Chronic headache patients' marital and family adjustment. *Issues in Mental Health Nursing*, 12(2), 133-148.

Baur, R. (1988). *Hypochondria*. CA: University of California Press.

Birket-Smith, M., Knudsen, H.C., et al (1989). Life events and social support in prediction of stroke outcome. *Psychotherapy and Psychosomatics*, 52(1-3), 146-150.

Brown, F.W., Golding, J.M., and Smith, R. (1990). Psychiatric co-morbidity in primary care somatization disorder. *Psychosomatic Medicine*, 52(3), 445-451.

Camara, E.G., and Danao, T.C. (1989). The brain and the immune system: a psychosomatic network. *Psychosomatics*, 30(2), 140-146.

Cook, J. S., and Fontaine, K. L. (1991). *Essentials of mental health nursing*, (2nd ed.). New York: Addison-Wesley.

Corbin, L.J., et al. (1988). Somatoform disorders: How to reduce overutilization of health care services. *Journal of Psychosocial Nursing and Mental Health Services*, 26(9), 31-34.

Costa, P.T., and Vanden Bos, G.R. (1990). *Psychological aspects of serious illness: chronic conditions, fatal diseases, and clinical care*. Hyattsville, MD: American Psychological Association.

Daruna, J.H., and Morgan, J.E. (1990). Psychosocial effects on immune function: neuroendocrine pathways. *Psychosomatics*, 31(1), 4-12.

Dossey, B. et al (1988). *Holistic nursing: a handbook for practice*. Rockville, MD: Aspen Publisher.

Escobar, J. I. (1987). Cross cultural aspects of the somatization trait. *Hospital and Community Psychiatry*, 38(2), 174-180.

Fabrega, H., Mezzich, J., and Jacob, R. et al (1988). Somatoform disorder in a psychiatric setting. *Journal of Nervous and Mental Disorders*, 176(7), 431439.

Fava, G. A., Grandi, S., Saviotti, F.M., and Conti, S. (1990). Hypochondriasis with panic attacks. *Psychosomatics*, 31(3), 351- 353.

Fisch, R.Z. (1987). Masked depression: its interrelations with somatization, hypochondriasis, and conversion. *International Journal of Psychiatry in Medicine*, 17(47), 367-379.

Flach, F. (1988). *Resilience: Discovering a new strength at times of stress*. New York: Fawcett Columbine.

Flor, H., Kerns, R.D., and Turk, D.C. (1987). The role of the spouse reenforcement, perceived pain and activity levels of chronic pain patients. *Journal of Psychosomatic Research*, 31(2), 251-259.

Green, S.A. (1985). *Mind and body: The psychology of physical illness*. Washington, DC: American Psychiatric Press.

Harter, L. (1988). Multi-family meetings on the psychiatric unit. *Journal of Psychosocial Nursing*, 26(8), 18-22.

Hollard, J.C., and Rowland, J.H. (1989). *The handbook of psychooncology: Psychological care of the patient with cancer*. New York: Oxford University Press.

Jones, L.R., Mabe, P.A., and Riley, W.T. (1988). Illness coping strategies and hypochondriacal traits among medical inpatients. *International Journal of Psychiatry in Medicine*. 19(4), 327-329.

Katon, W., Lin, E., Vonkorff, M., and Russo, J. et al. (1991). Somatization: a spectrum of severity. *American Journal of Psychiatry*, 148(1), 34-40.

Kellner, R. (1986). *Somatization and hypochondriasis*. New York: Praeger Press.

Koblenzer, C.S. (1987). *Psychocutaneous disease: a practical guide to clinical evaluation and management*. New York: Grune & Stratton.

Lambert, V. A., et al. (1989). Social support, hardiness and psychological well being in women with arthritis. *Image*, 21(3), 128-131.

Levenson, J.L., and Bemis, C. (1991). The role of psychological factors in cancer onset and progression. *Psychosomatics*. 32(2), 124-132.

Lewis, M.C. (1988). Attribution and illness. *Journal of psychosocial nursing*, 26(4), 14-21.

Lipowski, Z.J. (1990). Somatization and depression. *Psychosomatics*, 31(1), 13-21.

Lloyd, G.G. (1986). Psychiatric syndromes with a somatic presentation. *Journal of Psychosomatic Research*, 30(2), 113-120.

Locke, S., Ader, R., Besedovsky, H., Hall, N., et al. (eds) (1984). *Foundations of psychoneuroimmunology*. Hawthorne, NY: Aldine.

Manu, P., Lane, T. J., and Mathews, D.A. (1989). Somatization disorder in patients with chronic fatigue. *Psychosomatics*, 30(4), 388-395.

McCaffery, M., and Beebe, A. (1989). *Pain: Clinical manual for nursing practice*. St Louis: Mosby.

Miranda, J., Perez-Stable, E., and Munoz, R.F., et al. (1991). Somatization, psychiatric disorder and stress in utilization of ambulatory medical services. *Health Psychology*, 10(1), 46-51.

Moore, I.M., Gliss, C.L., and Martinson, I. (1988). Psychosomatic symptoms in parents two years after the death of a child with cancer. *Nursing Research*, 37(2), 104-107.

Moorey, S., and Greer, S. (1989). *Psychological therapy for patients with cancer*. Washington, DC: APA Press.

Moran, M.G. (1991). Psychological factors affecting pulmonary and rheumatologic diseases. *Psychosomatics*, 32(1), 14-23.

Morrison, J. (1989). Histrionic personality disorder in women with somatization disorder. *Psychosomatics*, 30(4), 433-437.

Othmer, E., and DeSouza, C. (1985). A screening test for somatization disorder (hysteria). *American Journal of Psychiatry*, 142(10), 1146-49.

Paulley, J.W., and Pelser, H.E. (1989). *Psychological managements for psychosomatic disorders*. New York: Springer-Verlag.

Priest, R.G. (1985). *Psychological disorders in obstetrics and gynecology*. London: Butterworth Publishing Co.

Savron, G., Grandi, S., Michelacci, L., et al. (1989). Hypochondriacal symptoms in pregnancy. *Psychotherapy and psychosomatics*, 52(1-3), 106-109.

Scott, A.L. (1988). Human interaction and personal boundaries. *Journal of Psychosocial Nursing*, 26(8), 23-27.

Simmermacher, D. (1981). *Self-image modification: Building self-esteem*. Deerfield Beach, FL: Health Communications.

Sternbach, R. A. (1986). *The psychology of pain*. New York: Raven Press.

Stewart, D. E. (1990). The changing faces of somatization. *Psychosomatics*, 31(2), 153-158.

Stoudemire, A., and Hales, R. E. (1991). Psychological and behavioral factors affecting medical conditions and DSM-IV: an overview. *Psychosomatics*, 32(1), 5-13.

Taylor, G.D., Bagby, R.M., and Parker, J.D.A. (1991). The alexithymia construct: A potential paradigm for psychosomatic medicine. *Psychosomatics, 32*(2), 153-164.

Todarello, O., LaPesa, M. W., Zaka, S., et al. (1989). Alexithymia and breast cancer. *Psychotherapy and Psychosomatics, 51*(1), 51-55.

Townsend, M.C. (1991). *Nursing diagnoses in psychiatric nursing,* (2nd ed.). Philadelphia: F.A. Davis.

Vollhardt, L.T. (1991). Psychoneuroimmunology: A literature review. *American Journal of Orthopsychiatry, 61*(1), 35-47.

Whitney, J.D., Sanger, E., Thomas, M.D., and Wolf-Wilets, V. (1988). A validation study of the nursing diagnosis "somatization." *Archives of Psychiatric nursing, 2*(6), 345-349.

Wolman, B.B. (1988). *Psychosomatic disorders.* New York: Plenum Medical Book Co.

Zahourek, R.P. (1988). *Relaxation and imagery: tools for therapeutic communication and intervention.* Philadelphia: Saunders.

Sleep Disorders

DSM III-R classifications
Dyssomnias
307.40 Dyssomnia not otherwise specified
307.42 Primary insomnia
307.42 Insomnia related to another mental disorder (nonorganic)
780.50 Insomnia related to a known organic factor
Parasomnias
307.40 Parasomnia not otherwise specified
307.46 Sleep terror disorder
307.46 Sleepwalking disorder
307.47 Dream anxiety disorder (nightmare disorder)
Hypersomnia disorders
307.44 Hypersomnia related to another mental disorder (nonorganic)
780.50 Hypersomnia related to a known organic factor
780.54 Primary hypersomnia
Sleep-wake schedule disorder
307.45 Sleep-wake schedule disorder

Psychiatric nursing diagnostic class
Sleep disturbance

Introduction

Sleep disorders can develop when an individual's normal cycle of sleep and wakefulness becomes altered. They are divided into two major groups: the dyssomnias and the parasomnias. The *dyssomnias* are characterized primarily by a disturbance in the amount, quality, or timing of sleep. The *parasomnias* are characterized by the occurrence of an abnormal event during sleep. The hypersomnia disorders are characterized by excessive daytime sleepiness. *Primary hypersomnia* is a persistent condition unrelated to organic factors or mental disorders. A *sleep-wake schedule disorder* is a mismatch between an environmentally determined sleep-wake schedule and the individual's circadian rhythm, resulting in insomnia or hypersomnia.

ETIOLOGY AND PRECIPITATING FACTORS
Sleep can be disrupted by illnesses and their accompanying symptoms, including pain, discomfort, pruritus, nocturia, confusion, palpitations, shortness of breath and other respiratory problems, diarrhea, and night sweats. Research also indicates that individuals recovering from surgical procedures experience fragmented sleep patterns that can lead to sleep disorders. Generally, sleep disturbance complaints increase with the severity of the underlying medical condition. Additionally, numerous prescription, over-the-counter (OTC), and illicit drugs can alter normal sleep.

Chronic insomnia may result from a disruption of the individual's circadian rhythm, specifically a delayed sleep phase. Some researchers speculate that individuals with chronic insomnia may be predisposed to higher activity levels of the reticular activating system. Research also suggests that life stress events, especially those related to loss or illness, also contribute to chronic insomnia.

Sleep disorders associated with shift work probably are caused by a disturbance in circadian rhythm regulation secondary to shift changes or sleep loss. Some researchers hypothesize that the sleep loss associated with shift work and the methods used to combat it, including alcohol, caffeine, nicotine, and benzodiazepines, are major contributing factors to this disorder. Jet lag is another example of circadian rhythm desynchronization.

Periodic limb movement, or nocturnal myoclonus, and restless leg syndrome apparently are transmitted as an autosomal dominant trait. These disorders usually appear in adolescence and persist throughout life. Both syndromes have been associated with various medical disorders, including peripheral neuropathies, anemia, uremia, and chronic pulmonary disorders. In addition, restless leg syndrome has been linked to mineral and vitamin deficiencies, uremia, cancer, and arthritis.

The daytime sleepiness associated with narcolepsy seems to result from a pathological intrusion of rapid-eye-movement (REM) sleep, resulting in wakefulness. An associated disturbance in the catecholamine systems, which are believed to control REM and non-REM sleep, also may be a contributing factor (see *Sleep stages* for information on the physiologic changes that occur during sleep stages). Furthermore, most narcoleptic individuals have in common the major histocompatibility antigen HLA-DR2. The familial incidence of narcolepsy, in conjunction with the presence of HLA-DR2, suggest a genetic defect.

Assessment guidelines
NURSING HISTORY (Functional health pattern findings)
The client may report or exhibit one or more of the findings grouped here according to functional health patterns.

Health perception–health management pattern
- frequent colds, viruses
- general lack of well-being

SLEEP STAGES

This chart indicates the physiologic changes that occur during the stages of sleep.

Stage	Description	Physiologic changes
Awake-alert	Normal daytime wakefulness	Normal vital signs
Stage I non-rapid eye movement (NREM)	Drowsiness; decreased reactivity to external stimuli; thinking no longer reality based	Decreased body temperature, heart rate, blood pressure, and respiratory rate
Stage 2 NREM	Light sleep	Decreased body temperature, heart rate, and blood pressure; slow, regular respiration
Stages 3 and 4 NREM	Deep sleep	Decreased body temperature, heart rate, and blood pressure; few body movements; release of growth hormone; markedly slow and regular respiration
Rapid eye movement (REM)	Rapid movement of eyes; dream state	Reduced muscle tone; bursts of eye movements and muscle twitching; decreased autonomic heart rate and blood pressure control; thermoregulation respiration; vivid dreaming; penile erection; increased bloodflow to brain

Nutritional-metabolic pattern
• significant daily caffeine intake
• obesity
• weight gain or loss

Elimination pattern
• gastric pain or discomfort
• nocturnal bowel irritability or diarrhea
• nocturnal urination
• night sweats

Activity-exercise pattern
• fatigue or lack of energy
• decreased interest in recreation activities
• decreased exercise

Sleep-rest pattern
• difficulty initiating sleep
• early morning awakening
• inability to sleep at desired time
• inability to remain asleep
• daytime sleepiness
• nightmares or terrors
• reliance on sleep aids
• increased dreaming
• not feeling rested or refreshed after sleep

Cognitive-perceptual pattern
• decreased alertness
• memory deficits
• difficulty concentrating
• distorted perceptions

• experiencing pain
• incomplete pain relief

Self-perception–self-concept pattern
• perception of self as anxious or depressed
• perception of self as inadequate or overwhelmed

Role-relationship pattern
• distressful family situation
• stressful work environment
• isolation

Sexual-reproductive pattern
• decreased libido
• difficulty with intimacy

Coping–stress tolerance pattern
• mood lability
• irritability
• tearfulness
• feeling vulnerable
• diminished coping ability after period of sleep disturbance

Value-belief pattern
• feeling powerless to achieve life goals
• spiritual distress or conflict

PHYSICAL FINDINGS
The client may report or exhibit one or more of the following physical findings.

General appearance
- dark circles under eyes
- eyelid ptosis

Cardiovascular
- cardiac arrhythmias
- chest pain
- co-existing cardiovascular disorders
- increased or decreased blood pressure (sleep-stage dependent)
- increased or decreased heart rate (sleep-state dependent)

Respiratory
- apnea
- decreased respiratory rate
- snoring

Gastrointestinal
- abdominal discomfort
- nausea or diarrhea
- abdominal pain
- dry mouth or oral mucus membranes

Genitourinary
- nocturnal penile erection

Musculoskeletal
- posture changes
- increased fatigue
- muscle aches, pain, soreness, or tension
- restless legs

Neurologic
- confusion
- delirium
- frequent yawning
- mild hand tremors
- fleeting nystagmus
- restlessness
- thick speech with mispronunciation and incorrect word use

Psychological
- agitation
- concentration problems
- irritability
- lethargic mood lability

Potential complications

If left untreated, sleep disorders can lead to cognitive impairment, confusional state delirium, impaired occupational and social functioning, self-injury, sleep terror disorder, and perceptual or memory deficits.

Various psychiatric and medical conditions can produce symptoms associated with sleep disorders; if left untreated, these disorders can cause serious, even life-threatening problems. For a list of specific conditions, see *Psychiatric and medical disorders that cause sleep disturbances.*

Nursing diagnosis: *Sleep pattern disturbance related to medical illness, pain, psychological stress, or external factors, such as hospital routines, environmental noise, and changing work shifts*

NURSING PRIORITY: To facilitate a normal sleep pattern that enables the client to fall asleep within 30 minutes of retiring and to sleep at least 6 to 8 hours per day

Interventions

1. Assess the client's current sleep pattern, and take a complete sleep history (see *Sleep history assessment,* page 230).

2. Identify both internal and external factors that are inhibiting the client's sleep. Such factors may include pain, itching, depression, metabolic disorders, noise, heat, and light.

3. Ascertain the client's sleep-related routines and rituals. Encourage the client to use the sleep-promoting methods described in *Promoting sleep,* page 231.

Rationales

1. A comprehensive assessment can help the nurse more accurately identify the client's sleep disorder.

2. By identifying sleep-inhibiting factors, the nurse can develop an appropriate, effective plan of care for the client.

3. The client may have ineffective sleep patterns and consequently may need to learn specific planning strategies for managing sleep. Many of these strategies are natural sedative measures that can promote sleep.

PSYCHIATRIC AND MEDICAL DISORDERS THAT CAUSE SLEEP DISTURBANCES

Certain psychiatric and medical disorders can produce various sleep disturbances, particularly insomnia and excessive daytime sleepiness. This chart includes some of the most common disorders.

Sleep disturbance	Psychiatric disorders	Medical disorders
Insomnia	• Adjustment disorder • Generalized anxiety disorder • Obsessive-compulsive disorder • Panic disorder • Bipolar disorder • Cyclothymic disorder • Dysthymic disorder • Hypomania • Major depression • Masked depression • Post-traumatic stress disorder • Psychoactive substance abuse disorder • Schizophrenia • Somatoform disorders	• Congestive heart failure • Myocardial infarction • Human immunodeficiency virus (HIV)-related disorders, including acquired immunodeficiency syndrome (AIDS) and AIDS-related complex (ARC) • Epstein-Barr virus • Chronic headache, neoplasms, head trauma, postencephalitic subdural hematoma • Neurosyphilis • Parkinson's disease • Addison's disease • Cushing's syndrome • Diabetes • Overeating, esophageal reflux, hiatal hernia, chronic inflammatory bowel disease, peptic ulcer • Anorexia nervosa • Arthritis • Cystic fibrosis
Excessive daytime sleepiness	• Atypical depression • Seasonal affective disorders associated with physiologic changes	• HIV-related disorders (AIDS and ARC) • Asthma • Chronic obstructive pulmonary disease

4. Encourage the client to maintain a sleep diary or chart and to make a practice of using sleep strategies. Inform the client that improvements may not occur for 4 or 5 weeks.

5. Provide comfort measures, such as back rubs, comfortable night clothes, and prescribed pain medications.

6. Arrange the timing of nursing care to provide at least a 4-hour block of uninterrupted time before sleep.

7. Assess the amount and types of psychoactive drugs the client is taking. Administer medications at bedtime if doing so is not contraindicated.

8. Collaborate with multidisciplinary team members to discuss the client's sleep history and sleep log. Consider referring the client to a sleep disorder assessment center or a sleep-related breathing disorder center.

9. If appropriate and needed, refer the client to a chronotherapy unit.

10. Teach the client and family about common sleep disturbances and methods of assessing and treating them.

4. The client should know that the sleep disorder will not be corrected quickly. Offering encouragement and support can help the client stay with a specific program.

5. Increasing the client's comfort can facilitate sleep.

6. Providing uninterrupted time by clustering care, treatments, medications, and other nursing procedures can decrease the number of awakenings and facilitate a normal sleep pattern.

7. Some psychoactive drugs interfere with normal sleep. A bedtime dosing schedule can facilitate sleep, especially if the drug has a sedative effect.

8. The client may require a comprehensive evaluation that is best accomplished in a sleep disorder assessment center. A sleep-related breathing disorders center can be helpful if the client has sleep apnea syndrome or a related disorder.

9. Participating in chronobiological therapy may help reset the body's sleep clock, especially if the client has delayed sleep onset insomnia.

10. Such instruction can enhance the client's and family's level of awareness and decrease the use of ineffective home sleep remedies, such as drinking a glass of wine or taking benzodiazepines before bed.

SLEEP HISTORY ASSESSMENT

An accurate sleep history is of utmost importance in evaluating a client's sleep disorder. The sleep history provides an assessment of the complaint in relation to environmental, familial, and medical factors, helping the nurse to determine the origin of the sleep disturbance. Typically, a thorough sleep history explores the client's daytime or awake behaviors, sleep patterns, sleep hygiene, and medical, psychological, and pharmacologic history. The form below includes appropriate questions to ask when assessing a client's sleep pattern.

1. a. When did these symptoms begin?
_____

   b. Which pattern best describes the frequency of the symptoms?
Occur persistently	Yes ☐	No ☐
Wax and wane	Yes ☐	No ☐
Occur seasonally	Yes ☐	No ☐

2. a. Are these symptoms associated with any of the following factors?
Medical problems	Yes ☐	No ☐
Job pressure	Yes ☐	No ☐
Stress	Yes ☐	No ☐

   b. If yes, how long have the factors persisted?
   _____

   c. Do these factors relate to the intensity of symptoms?
   Yes ☐   No ☐

3. a. Does anything seem to alleviate these symptoms?
   Yes ☐   No ☐

   b. If yes, what makes them better?
   _____

   c. What makes them worse?
   _____

   d. What happens on a vacation (for example, do they improve, worsen, or persist)?
   _____

4. How has this sleep disturbance made an impact on your life?
_____

5. What is your typical daily schedule?
_____

6. Describe your usual sleep hygiene (sleep routines and rituals).
_____

7. a. Do any other family members complain of sleep difficulties?
   Yes ☐   No ☐
   If yes, who?
   _____

   b. Are the complaints similar to yours?
   Yes ☐   No ☐
   c. If dissimilar, characterize the complaints.
   _____
   _____

8. a. Which sleep remedies or treatments have you tried so far?
   _____

   b. How effective have these treatments been?
   _____

9. a. Which drugs have you used in the past?
Prescribed	Yes ☐	No ☐
Over the counter	Yes ☐	No ☐
Illicit	Yes ☐	No ☐

   b. Which drugs are you currently using?
Prescribed	Yes ☐	No ☐
Over the counter	Yes ☐	No ☐
Illicit	Yes ☐	No ☐

   c. Do you smoke? Yes ☐   No ☐
   Frequency: _____

   d. Do you ingest caffeine-containing foods or beverages (such as coffee, tea, chocolate, or soda)?
   Yes ☐   No ☐
   Frequency: _____

10. a. Do you drink alcohol? Yes ☐   No ☐

    b. If yes, how often? _____

    c. In what quantity? _____

11. a. Do you ever have any unusual sleeptime experiences?
    Yes ☐   No ☐

    b. If yes, describe them.
    _____

12. What is your usual sleep time? _____

13. What is your usual awakening time? _____

14. How long do you usually take to fall asleep? _____

15. a. Do you awaken during sleep time?
    Yes ☐   No ☐
    b. If yes, why?
    _____

    c. Are you able to go back to sleep?
    Yes ☐   No ☐

16. Do you have a history of any of the following?
Bruxism (teeth grinding)	Yes ☐	No ☐
Kicking during sleep	Yes ☐	No ☐
Restless leg syndrome	Yes ☐	No ☐
Sleep talking	Yes ☐	No ☐
Sleep walking	Yes ☐	No ☐
Snoring	Yes ☐	No ☐

17. Do you feel rested and refreshed after sleeping?
    Yes ☐   No ☐

18. What is the condition of your bed linens after sleeping?

19. a. Do you experience daytime sleepiness?
    Yes ☐   No ☐
    b. Do you experience daytime fatigue?
    Yes ☐   No ☐

20. a. Can you provide any additional information that may be related to your sleep disturbance?
    _____

    b. If yes, describe.

PROMOTING SLEEP

If your client has difficulty falling asleep, suggest the following sleep-promoting techniques.

- Establish a regular time for going to bed.
- Schedule "worry time" separate from in-bed hours.
- Use relaxation techniques.
- Maintain a balance between rest, activity, and exercise.
- Engage in various social activities during the day.
- Restrict alcohol, coffee, tea, and caffeinated soft-drink intake, especially after 7:00 p.m.
- Restrict or discontinue nicotine intake.
- Exercise regularly in the late afternoon or early evening.
- Establish and maintain a quiet sleeping environment.
- Use dark shades or eye covers if needed.

- Adjust the room temperature to a comfortable level.
- Establish a regular time for rising in the morning.
- Avoid oversleeping.
- Determine how sleeping with a bed partner (spouse, loved one, or pet) affects sleep.
- Reduce external stimuli, such as a television or radio, in the bedroom.
- Schedule "wind down" time before bed; such activities as selecting clothes for the next day, reading a book, or taking a warm bath or shower promote relaxation.
- Go to bed when tired.
- Avoid daytime napping.
- Maintain a normal daily schedule even if fatigued.

---

11. Monitor the effects of the client's medication regimen, including the effects of ritalin (prescribed for narcolepsy) and pain medications.

11. Monitoring is necessary to determine the possible effects of medications on the client's sleep.

Outcome criteria

As treatment progresses, the client, family, or both should be able to:
- verbalize an understanding of sleep disorders
- identify specific sleep-inducing measures
- adjust life-style and daily schedule to accommodate chronobiological rhythms
- report an improved sleep pattern
- report feeling rested
- report less excessive daytime sleepiness
- verbalize an awareness of the possible need for a complete, comprehensive sleep disorder workup after discharge.

Discharge criteria

Nursing documentation indicates that the client:
- has displayed the ability to recognize the symptoms of an altered sleep pattern
- has displayed the ability to use newly learned strategies that facilitate a normal sleep pattern
- understands that further assessment and treatment may be necessary
- is aware of available social and family resources
- has scheduled any necessary follow-up treatments.

Nursing documentation also indicates that the family:
- understands the diagnosis, treatment, and expected outcomes
- has been referred to the appropriate community resources

- has demonstrated a willingness to schedule follow-up appointments and participate in ongoing psychotherapy if needed.

Selected references

Borbely, A. (1986). *Secrets of sleep*. New York: Basic Books.

Catesby-Ware, J. Blumoff, R., and Pittard, J.T. (1988). Peripheral vasoconstriction in patients with sleep related periodic leg movements. *Sleep*, 11(2), 182-187.

Closs, J. (1988). Assessment of sleep in hospital patients: A review of methods. *Journal of Advanced Nursing*, 13, 50-510.

Dicicco, B., Cooper, J., and Waldhorn, R. (1987). Sleep disorders in medical illness. *Psychiatric Medicine*, 4, 113-147.

Hauri, P.J., Friedman, M., and Ravaris, C.L. (1989). Sleep in patients with spontaneous panic attacks. *Sleep*, 12(4), 323-337.

Hobson, J.A. (1988). *The dreaming brain*. New York: Basic Books.

Horne, J.A. (1988). Sleep loss and "divergent" thinking ability. *Sleep*, 11(6), 528-536.

Knab, B., Engle, R. (1988). Perception of waking and sleeping: Possible implications for evaluation of insomnia. *Sleep*, 11, 265-272.

Kryger, M., Roth, T., and Dement, W. (1989). *Principles and practice of sleep medicine*. Philadelphia: Saunders.

Libert, J.P., Bach, V., Johnson, L.C., et al. (1991). Relative and combined effects of heat and noise exposure on sleep in humans. *Sleep*, 14(1), 24-31.

Meguro, K., Ueda, M., Yamaguchi, T., Sekita, Y., et al (1990). Disturbance in daily sleep-wake patterns in patients with cognitive impairment and decreased daily activity. *Journal of the American Geriatrics Society*, 38(11), 1176-1180.

Melles, R.B., Katz, B. (1988). Night terrors and sudden unexplained nocturnal death. *Medical Hypotheses*, 26, 149-154.

Regestein, Q.R. (1987). Sleep disorders in the medically ill. In A. Stoudemire and B.S. Fogel (Eds.), *Principles of medical psychiatry*. New York: Grune & Stratton.

Reite, M., Higgs, L., and Reed, N. (1989). Polysomnographic findings in chronic psychophysiological insomnia. *Sleep Research*, 18, 293.

Reite, M.C., Nagel, K.E., and Rudley, J.R. (1990). *The evaluation and management of sleep disorders*. Washington, D.C.: American Psychiatric Press.

Reynolds, C.F., and Kupfer, D.J. (1987). Neuropsychiatric aspects of sleep disorders. In (Eds) R.E. Hales and S.C. Yudofsky, *Textbook of neuropsychiatry*. Washington, D.C.: American Psychiatric Association Press.

Richards-Culpepper, K., and Bairnsfather, L. (1988). A description of night sleep patterns in the critical care unit. *Heart & Lung*, 17(1), 35-42.

Ruler, A., and Lack, L. (1988). Gender differences in sleep. *Sleep Research*, 17, 244.

Schenk, C.H., Bundie, S.R., Patterson, A.C., et al. (1987). Rapid eye movement sleep behavior disorder: A treatable parasomnia. *JAMA*, 257, 1786-1789.

Soldatos, C.R., Kales, J.D., et al. (1987). Classification of sleep disorders. *Psychiatric Annals*, 17, 454-458.

Spielman, A.J., Saskin, P., and Thorpy, M.J. (1987). Treatment of chronic insomnia by restriction of time in bed. *Sleep*, 10, 45-56.

Tan, T.L., Kales, J.D., Kales, A., et al. (1987). Inpatient multidimensional management of treatment resistent insomnia. *Psychosomatics*, 28, 266272.

Webb, W.B. (1988). An objective behavioral model of sleep. *Sleep*, 11(5), 488-496.

Williams, R.L., Karacan, I., and Moore, C.A. (1988). *Sleep disorders: Diagnosis and treatment* (2nd ed). New York: Wiley.

Gender Identity Disorder

DSM III-R classifications
302.50 Transsexualism
302.60 Gender identity disorder of childhood
302.85 Gender identity disorder of adolescence or adulthood, nontranssexual type
302.85 Gender identity disorder not otherwise specified

Psychiatric nursing diagnostic class
Sexual response variations

Introduction

Gender identity disorders occur when gender identity — a person's sense of being male or female — does not correspond to his or her sexual anatomy. Individuals with gender identity disorders usually experience persistent and intense distress about being their biological sex and wish to be the other sex. They even may insist that they are the other sex. Such individuals may be averse to wearing the stereotypical clothing of their sex, choosing rather to dress, or crossdress, in the clothes of the other sex. Some gender identity disorders are only mildly disturbing to the individual, whereas others may produce severe anxiety and personal dysfunction. Furthermore, behaviors that deviate from sexual norms imposed by society and culture are commonly harshly judged. Such judgments are a potential source of guilt and shame for the nonconforming individual.

In addition to the characteristics of other gender identity disorders, *transsexualism* includes a preoccupation for at least 2 years with eliminating primary and secondary sex characteristics and acquiring those of the other sex.

ETIOLOGY AND PRECIPITATING FACTORS
Biological research concerning the development of sexual responses focuses on genetic identity. An individual's somatotype includes chromosomes, hormones, internal and external genitalia, and gonads. If chromosomal patterns are not varied or altered, biological factors will produce a single, fully developed gender, either male or female.

Psychoanalytic theory maintains that congruent gender identity results from the successful resolution of libidinal conflicts, including the Oedipus and Electra complexes, during psychosexual development. According to this theory, the individual who successfully resolves these conflicts identifies with the same-sex parent as a role model. Unsuccessful resolution results in confusion.

Behavioral theory proposes that sexual responses are learned. Family, friends, social and cultural norms, the media, and life events all combine to create gender identity.

Assessment guidelines
NURSING HISTORY (Functional health pattern findings)
The client may report or exhibit one or more of the findings grouped here according to functional health patterns.

Health perception–health management pattern
• anxiety or depression

Self-perception–self-concept pattern
• belief that gender is incongruent with anatomy
• concern or confusion about personal identity
• discomfort with gender identity and expected sex-role behaviors
• cross-dressing
• severe anxiety over homosexual feelings

Role-relationship pattern
• disturbed interpersonal relationships
• discomfort with assigned sex roles
• dissatisfaction or confusion about sexual preference
• inability to establish satisfying sexual relationship
• dressing or life-style reflective of gender identity rather than anatomical sex

Sexual-reproductive pattern
• lack of interest in sex
• unsatisfactory sexual experiences
• sexual dysfunction or disorder
• desire to be the opposite sex
• discomfort over preferred means of sexual expression

Coping–stress-tolerance pattern
• extreme anxiety about sex or sexuality
• use of sexual behavior to cope with anxiety

Value-belief pattern
• belief that sexual activity is wrong

PHYSICAL FINDINGS
A complete physical examination and comprehensive sexual history are necessary for an accurate diagnosis of the client's condition. Psychological findings may include depression and anxiety (see *Sexual history*, pages 234 and 235).

(Text continues on page 236.)

SEXUAL HISTORY

The goal of the sexual history is to determine a client's level of sexual health and sexual functioning. Obtaining a sexual history, in addition to gathering data for assessment, may also be therapeutic by promoting the client's sexuality and sexual function as legitimate aspects of health and well being.

Sexual history formats include the brief sexual history, the comprehensive sexual history, and the sexual problem history. The brief sexual history can be part of a total health history or nursing assessment. The comprehensive sexual history supplements the brief sexual history and can be used in the context of sexual counseling. If a brief or comprehensive sexual history indicates that the client may have a sexual dysfunction disorder, a health care professional trained in sexual counseling or therapy should conduct a sexual problem history.

Brief Sexual History

1. Has anything (such as illness, pregnancy, or surgery) interfered with your roles and relationships as a spouse or parent?   Yes ☐   No ☐

2. Has anything (such as illness, surgery, hospitalization, injury, or medical treatment) changed the way you feel about yourself as a man or woman?   Yes ☐   No ☐

3. Has anything (such as surgery, medication, illness, or medical treatment) changed your ability to function sexually?   Yes ☐   No ☐

4. Are you currently sexually active?   Yes ☐   No ☐
   a. If no, does this make you uncomfortable?   Yes ☐   No ☐

b. If yes, are you satisfied with your sexual activity in terms of:
   1. Frequency?   Yes ☐   No ☐
   2. Arousal?   Yes ☐   No ☐
   3. Ability to attain erection?   Yes ☐   No ☐
   4. Orgasm?   Yes ☐   No ☐
   5. Comfort during intercourse?   Yes ☐   No ☐
   (If the client answers no to any of the five items, conduct a comprehensive sexual history.)

5. Do you have any questions or concerns that you would like to discuss at this time?   Yes ☐   No ☐
   If yes, please describe: _____
   _____
   _____
   _____

Comprehensive Sexual History *(Use information obtained from the Brief Sexual History.)*

General information
1. a. When you were growing up, from whom did you learn about sex?
   _____
   _____

   b. What did you learn?
   _____
   _____
   _____

   c. When was your first sexual encounter?
   _____
   _____

   d. Was your first sexual encounter:
   What you expected?   Yes ☐   No ☐
   Satisfying?   Yes ☐   No ☐
   Mutually desired?   Yes ☐   No ☐
   Safe?   Yes ☐   No ☐
   If you answered no to any of these items, please explain:
   _____
   _____

2. If you are currently sexually active, are you taking birth control measures?   Yes ☐   No ☐

3. Do you experience any physical or emotional discomfort during sexual activity?   Yes ☐   No ☐

4. Have you ever had or been exposed to a sexually transmitted disease?   Yes ☐   No ☐

Desire for sexual activity
5. Has your desire for sexual activity:
   Increased? _____
   Decreased? _____
   Fluctuated? _____

6. Do you have concerns about your sexual performance?   Yes ☐   No ☐

7. Please describe any specific feelings (positive or negative) about your body image and how it affects your desire for sexual activity:
   _____
   _____

Sexual interaction with partner
8. Describe your usual "preliminaries" to love making in terms of initiation and degree of communication:
   _____
   _____

SEXUAL HISTORY *(continued)*

9. Describe usual characteristics of "love play" in terms of:
   a. Behaviors that enhance the overall encounter:

   _____

   _____

   b. Behaviors that detract from the overall encounter:

   _____

   _____

   c. Sexual norms within the relationship:

   _____

   _____

   d. Extracoital alternatives:

   _____

   _____

10. Do you think your partner is satisfied with your sexual relationship? Yes ☐ No ☐

11. Have you or are you engaged in an extramarital relationship? Yes ☐ No ☐
    If yes, describe the frequency and duration of these relationships:

    _____

    _____

12. Have you engaged in any high-risk sexual activities, such as:

    Multiple sexual partners? Yes ☐ No ☐
    Unprotected sexual intercourse? Yes ☐ No ☐
    Sexual intercourse when under the influence of alcohol or drugs? Yes ☐ No ☐
    Sexual intercourse with an unknown partner? Yes ☐ No ☐

Male-specific questions

1. Please describe:
   Quality of erections:

   _____

   _____

   Situations that interfere with erection:

   _____

   _____

   Satisfaction with penis size:

   _____

   _____

2. a. Please describe:
   Frequency of orgasm or climax: _____
   How you achieve orgasm or climax:
vaginal penetration	Yes ☐	No ☐
by hand	Yes ☐	No ☐
orally	Yes ☐	No ☐
anally	Yes ☐	No ☐

   b. Has there been any change in the quality of orgasm? Yes ☐ No ☐

   c. Do you experience any discomfort or pain with orgasm? Yes ☐ No ☐

   d. Are your concerned with your partner achieving an orgasm? Yes ☐ No ☐

   e. Does this concern interfere with your experience? Yes ☐ No ☐

3. Do you use the same position during intercourse? Yes ☐ No ☐

Female-specific questions

1. a. Do you have enough time for vaginal lubrication before intercourse? Yes ☐ No ☐

   b. Please describe how long it takes you to become adequately lubricated:

   Has this time increased or decreased? _____

2. Do you ever experience pain during intercourse Yes ☐ No ☐
   If yes, please describe:

   _____

   _____

3. a. Do you usually achieve orgasm? Yes ☐ No ☐

   b. How do you achieve orgasm?
Masturbation	Yes ☐	No ☐
Orally	Yes ☐	No ☐
Manipulation by partner	Yes ☐	No ☐

   c. How often do you achieve orgasm? _____

   d. Please describe situations that interfere with orgasm:

   _____

   _____

Potential complications

Unresolved gender identify conflicts can lead to anxiety, depression, alcoholism, or drug abuse.

Nursing diagnosis: *Personal identity disturbance related to conflict between anatomical sex and gender identity*

NURSING PRIORITY: To help the client develop self-affirming social and psychological supports that can enhance a positive self-image

Interventions

1. Assess the client's knowledge and beliefs about sexuality.

2. Provide the client with accurate information about sexuality in an open, nonjudgmental manner.

3. Assess the degree to which the client's occupational, social, and interpersonal functionings have been affected by the condition.

4. Assess the effectiveness of social and psychological supports available to the client.

5. Assess the client's history of drug and alcohol use.

6. Whenever possible and with client approval, include the client's family in education sessions.

7. Inform the client of available community counseling and treatment resources.

Rationales

1. Such assessment can reveal conflicts concerning the client's sexual experiences and expectations.

2. By educating the client about sexuality, the nurse can correct misinformation and help the client see himself or herself in a wider, more realistic context of sexual behaviors.

3. Gender confusion and transsexual behaviors can cause extreme social isolation and limit occupational choices, sometimes to prostitution.

4. Because the client may be isolated or estranged from the family, social and emotional supports are often limited, manipulative, or exploitative. As a result, the client may have been forced to choose social environments that reinforce maladaptive behaviors.

5. The client's social environments and relationships, as well as anxiety about the disorder, may contribute to drug and alcohol use as the client tries to deal with anxiety and depression.

6. Because of ignorance of or misunderstandings about gender identity disorders, family members may have rejected the client. By educating everyone involved, the nurse can help rebuild disturbed family relationships.

7. Knowing available options and resources, such as hormonal or sex therapies, sexual reassignment, and support groups, can enhance the client's sense of self-control.

Nursing diagnosis: *Anxiety related to conflict between desires and expected sex role behavior*

NURSING PRIORITY: To decrease the client's anxiety and promote self-acceptance

Interventions

1. Convey to the client unconditional caring and positive regard.

Rationales

1. Acceptance can enhance self-esteem and help the client overcome fears of rejection.

2. Assess the degree to which the client is agitated and threatened by sexual impulses.

3. Assess the client's history for possible sexual abuse with a same-sex adult.

4. Provide a safe, nonthreatening, and nonjudgmental environment in which the client can discuss sexual feelings and impulses.

5. Educate the client about human sexuality and sexual responses.

6. Encourage the client to verbalize personal values, beliefs, and attitudes about sexuality and sexual preference.

7. Inform the client of available follow-up care or treatment alternatives.

2. The client's sexual impulses can produce agitated and aggressive gender behavior (macho or ultra-feminine) as a way of enhancing self-image and self-esteem. Recognizing these inappropriate responses is an important step toward developing positive behaviors.

3. Conflict and ambivalence over homosexual activity can generate considerable anxiety. Identifying such feelings can help the nurse develop a more appropriate plan of care.

4. A nonjudgmental environment can help the client express frightening and overwhelming feelings or thoughts.

5. Sex education can help alleviate the client's guilt over having experienced pleasure from homosexual or other sexual behaviors.

6. Talking about sexuality can help the client identify causes of anxiety and conflict.

7. Therapy that focuses on sexuality can help the client resolve, adapt to, and be comfortable with chosen sexual preferences.

Outcome criteria

As treatment progresses, the client, family, or both should be able to:
• demonstrate evidence of improved self-esteem
• demonstrate decreased anxiety
• identify available options and resources, such as support groups
• verbalize an increased knowledge of human sexuality.

Discharge criteria

Nursing documentation indicates that the client:
• has demonstrated increased self-acceptance
• has verbalized an increased knowledge of human sexuality and sexual responses
• has reported decreased anxiety when dealing with sexuality
• has verbalized a knowledge of available support and treatment resources.

Nursing documentation also indicates that the family:
• has demonstrated a knowledge and understanding of the client's condition
• has been referred to available community and family resources.

Selected references

Bancroft, John (1989). *Human sexuality and its problems*, (2nd ed). New York: Churchill Livingstone.

Cassell, C, and Wilson, P. (1989). *Sexuality education: A resource book*. New York: Garland Publishing.

Crooks, R., and Baur, K. (1987). *Our sexuality*, (3rd ed.). Reading, Mass.: Benjamin/Cummings.

Fogel, C., and Lauvar, D. (1990). *Sexual health promotion*. Philadelphia: Saunders.

Geist, R. (1988). Sexually related trauma. *Emergency Medicine Clinics of North America*, 6(3), 439-466.

Hogon, R.M. (1985). *Human sexuality: A nursing perspective*. Norwalk, CT: Appleton-Lange.

Hott, J.R. (1990). Speaking of sex. *American Journal of Nursing*, 90(1), 116.

Kaplan, H.S. (1987). *Sexual aversion, sexual phobias, and panic disorder*. New York: Brunner/Mazel.

Kaplan, H.S. (1988). Anxiety and sexual dysfunction. *Journal of Clinical Psychiatry*, 49 (Supplement) 21-25.

Katzin, l. (1990). Chronic illness and sexuality. *American Journal of Nursing*, 90(1), 54-59.

Lambert, C.E., Jr., and Lambert, V.A. (1987). Psychosocial impacts created by chronic illness. *Nursing Clinics of North America*, 22(3), 527-533.

Leiblum, S.R., and Rosen, R.C. (1989). *Principles and practice of sex therapy*, (2nd ed). New York: Guilford Press.

McCabe, S. (1988). Male-to-female transsexualism: A case for holistic nursing. *Archives of Psychiatric Nursing*, 2(1), 48-53.

Manley, G. (1990). Treatment and recovery for sexual addicts. *Nurse Practitioner,* 15(6), 37-41.

Nass, G., and Fisher, M. (1988). *Sexuality today.* Boston: Jones & Bartlett.

Nelson, R.P. (1987). Male sexual dysfunction: Evaluation and treatment. *Southern Medicare Journal,* 80(1), 69-74.

Poorman, S.G. (1988). *Human sexuality and the nursing process.* Norwalk, CT: Appleton & Lange.

Sanderson, M., and Maddock, J. (1989). Guidelines for the assessment and treatment of sexual dysfunction. *Obstetrics & Gynecology,* 73(1), 130135.

Schaffer, S., and Zimmerman, M. (1990). The sexual addict: A challenge for the primary care provider. *Nurse Practitioner,* 15(6) 25-26.

Schover, L. (1988). *Sexuality and chronic illness: A comprehensive approval.* New York: Guilford Press.

Seagraves, R. (1989). The effects of psychotropic drugs on human erection and ejaculation. *Archives of General Psychiatry,* 46(3), 275-284.

Shearer, S.L., and Herbert, C.A. (1987). Long-term effects of unresolved sexual trauma. *American Family Physician,* 36(4), 1313-1314.

Skeen, P., Walters, L., and Robinson, B. (1988). How parents of gays react to their children's homosexuality and to the threat of AIDS. *Journal of Psychosocial Nursing,* 26(12), 6-10.

Sladyk, K. (1990) Teaching safe sex practices to psychiatric patients. *American Journal of Occupational Therapy,* 44(3), 284-286.

Sexual Disorders

DSM III-R classifications
Paraphilias
302.20 Pedophilia
302.30 Transvestic fetishism
302.40 Exhibitionism
302.81 Fetishism
302.82 Voyeurism
302.83 Sexual masochism
302.84 Sexual sadism
302.89 Frotteurism
Sexual desire dysfunctions
302.71 Hypoactive sexual desire disorder
302.79 Sexual aversion disorder
Sexual arousal dysfunctions
302.72 Female sexual arousal disorder
302.72 Male erectile disorder
Orgasm dysfunctions
302.73 Inhibited female orgasm
302.74 Inhibited male orgasm
302.75 Premature ejaculation
Sexual pain dysfunction
302.76 Dyspareunia
306.51 Vaginismus
Miscellaneous sexual disorder
302.90 Sexual disorder not otherwise specified

Psychiatric nursing diagnostic class
Sexual response variations

Introduction

Sexual disorders are categorized primarily as paraphilias and sexual dysfunctions. The *paraphilias* involve different means of arousal. The means of arousal may be an object not normally considered sexually stimulating (fetish), an act involving humiliation or control (sadism or masochism), an act involving another's lack of awareness or consent (frotteurism, exhibitionism, voyeurism), or contact with children (pedophilia). (For a more complete list of paraphilias, see *Paraphilias.*) *Sexual dysfunctions* are characterized by a disturbed or disrupted ability to experience the complete sexual response cycle, the phases of which are desire, arousal, orgasm, and resolution.

ETIOLOGY AND PRECIPITATING FACTORS
Paraphilias generally are thought to involve learned behaviors. For example, an individual's sexual response somehow becomes associated with an object or experience that then becomes essential to sexual arousal and satisfaction. Evidence exists that paraphilias can be found in families in an intergenerational pattern; however their presence also is believed to be the result of

---

PARAPHILIAS

The paraphilias classified in *DSM III-R* as psychosexual disorders are marked by unusual or bizarre sexual behaviors that are necessary for sexual arousal and orgasm. Diagnosis should also consider the frequency of the behavior and its interference with function. Some paraphilias that violate social mores or norms are considered sex offenses or sex crimes. Everyone has sexual fantasies, and sexual behavior between two consenting adults that's not physically or psychologically harmful should not be considered a paraphilia.

TYPE OF PARAPHILIA	SOURCE OF SEXUAL AROUSAL
Fetishism	Use of clothing, such as leather or shoes
Transvestism	Recurrent and persistent cross-dressing by a heterosexual male
Frotteurism	Body contact with strangers in public places, such as buses or elevators
Voyeurism	Watching others engaged in sexual activity or undressing
Exhibitionism	Exposure of genitals in public
Sexual sadism	Inflicting physical/mental pain on sexual partner
Sexual masochism	Receiving physical/mental pain from sexual partner
Pedophilia	Sexual activity with children; may be homosexual or heterosexual or incestuous
Necrophilia	Sexual activity with a corpse
Zoophilia	Sexual activity with animals
Gerontophilia	Sexual activity that is not age-appropriate with an elderly person

From *Professional guide to diseases.* (4th ed.). Springhouse, PA: Springhouse Corp., 1992.

---

social learning or of disturbed or dysfunctional family systems.

Physiologic causes of sexual dysfunction include physical or mental illness, physical changes from surgery, trauma, aging, drug abuse, medication side effects, and gender identity disorders. These dysfunctions most commonly develop in early adulthood, after the individual has become sexually active. Dyspareunia and male erectile disorder usually occur in later life.

Assessment guidelines
NURSING HISTORY (Functional health pattern findings)
The client may report or exhibit one or more of the findings grouped here according to functional health patterns.

Health perception–health management pattern
- history of physical or emotional illness
- insistence that dysfunction is related to physical change

Self-perception–self-concept pattern
- poor self-image and self-esteem
- discomfort with sex role
- feelings of inadequacy or undesirability
- fear of sexual performance failure

Role-relationship pattern
- disturbed personal relationships
- fear of rejection
- inability to establish sexual relationships
- fear of intimacy

Sexual-reproductive pattern
- lack of interest in sex
- guilt or shame about sex
- distress about sexual expression
- fear of unwanted pregnancy
- fear of sexually transmitted diseases
- history of unsatisfying or difficult sexual experiences
- history of sexual assault or violence
- compulsive sexual activity
- high-risk sexual practices, including unprotected sex

Coping–stress tolerance pattern
- extreme anxiety about sex or sexuality
- use of sexual behavior to cope with anxiety

Value-belief pattern
- belief that sexual activity is wrong

PHYSICAL FINDINGS
The client may report or exhibit one or more of the following physical findings.

Cardiovascular
- angina
- congestive heart failure
- arrhythmias
- hypertension
- myocardial infarction
- palpitations

Respiratory
- chronic obstructive pulmonary disease
- cystic fibrosis
- lung cancer

Gastrointestinal
- abdominal pain
- colitis, especially with colostomy

Genitourinary
- benign prostatic hypertrophy
- bladder cancer
- cystitis
- end-stage renal disease
- erectile dysfunction
- penile, prostate, or testicular cancer
- Peyronie's disease
- priapism
- prostatism
- urinary incontinence

Gynecologic
- benign uterine tumors
- cervical cancer
- dysmenorrhea
- endometrial cancer
- endometriosis
- hysterectomy
- menopause
- ovarian tumors
- pelvic exenteration
- vaginal infections
- vaginal or vulvar tumors
- vulvectomy

Musculoskeletal
- ankylosing spondylitis
- fatigue
- lupus erythematosus
- muscular dystrophies
- pain
- rheumatoid arthritis or osteoarthritis
- stiffness or weakness

Neurologic
- central nervous system tumors
- closed head injury
- neuroendocrine disorders

Psychological
- conversion disorder
- eating disorders
- history of incest or sexual assault
- mood disorders
- psychoactive substance abuse disorders
- schizophrenia
- rape trauma syndrome
- somatization disorder

Potential complications

A complete physical examination is essential to determine potential organic causes for the dysfunction. Such conditions as diabetes, cardiovascular disease, neurologic problems, endocrine disorders, genitourinary and gynecologic disorders, and sexually transmitted diseases can disturb sexual functioning.

Nursing diagnosis: *Altered sexuality patterns related to inability to achieve sexual satisfaction in socially acceptable ways*

NURSING PRIORITY: To help the client develop alternative methods of achieving sexual satisfaction

Interventions

1. Obtain a complete medical, social, and sexual history from the client.

2. Assess the client's anxiety or discomfort about the disorder.

3. Remain nonjudgmental, and avoid seeming curious about or repulsed by the client's behavior.

4. Assess the client's knowledge of sexuality and sexual response patterns. Provide information and correct misinformation.

5. Inform the client of treatment options, including different kinds of sex therapies, and offer referrals.

6. When possible, provide education and support for the client's family or loved ones.

Rationales

1. A complete history can help the nurse identify causes of or precipitating factors for the client's disorder or dysfunction.

2. Anxiety can indicate that the client wants to change or learn about the disorder.

3. Both curiosity and repulsion can diminish the client's self-esteem. A nonjudgmental approach can both enhance client self-esteem and establish trust between the client and nurse.

4. Many people's knowledge about sexuality consists of myth and misinformation. Correct and accurate information can enable the client to understand and make informed choices.

5. Learning about the disorder as well as treatment options can help alleviate the client's anxiety.

6. Family members and loved ones also are affected by sexual disorders. Their participation in treatment can enhance the client's compliance.

Outcome criteria

As treatment progresses, the client, family, or both should be able to:
• verbalize an understanding of sexual disorders
• acknowledge the need for ongoing treatment
• demonstrate the ability to use adaptive coping methods
• identify the effects of disruptive behavior
• demonstrate improved self-esteem.

Discharge criteria

Nursing documentation indicates that the client:
• has demonstrated an understanding of the condition and of human sexual responses
• has demonstrated the ability to identify alternative methods of achieving sexual satisfaction
• has demonstrated an improved self-esteem

• has verbalized an awareness of the need for further treatment.

Selected references

Bancroft, J. (1989). *Human sexuality and its problems* (2nd ed.). New York: Churchill Livingston.

Kaplan, H.S. (1988). Anxiety and sexual dysfunction. *Journal of Clinical Psychiatry,* 49 (Supplement), 21-25.

Sanderson, M., and Maddock, J. (1989). Guidelines for assessment and treatment of sexual dysfunction. *Obstetrics & Gynecology,* 73(1), 130-135.

Wilson, H. and Kneisl, C. (1992)., *Psychiatric nursing* (4th ed.), Menlo Park, CA: Addison-Wesley.

Interpersonal Violence: Rape-Trauma Syndrome

Psychiatric nursing diagnostic class
Violence

Nursing diagnoses
Rape-trauma syndrome
Rape-trauma syndrome: compound reaction
Rape-trauma syndrome: silent reaction
Violence, potential for: directed at others
Post-trauma response

Introduction

Interpersonal violence occurs at an alarming rate in American society — some health care professionals describe it as an epidemic. Nurses in every practice setting face the challenge of caring for both the victims and perpetrators of violent behavior. Developing an understanding of the causes and effects of violent and abusive behavior enables the nurse to intervene in a therapeutic manner and provide comprehensive care.

Violent behavior is not limited to isolated populations. It crosses all social, ethnic, economic, and cultural boundaries and is ingrained in the way children are socialized. A failure to respond to violent behavior may condone it and perpetuate the cycle of violence. When treating and caring for the victims of violence, maintain objectivity and a systems perspective. Remember that the psychological and emotional consequences of violence may be more severe and long lasting than the physical injuries. Developing an understanding of victimization can help the nurse care for those caught in the cycle of violence. The first step comes in being able to identify victims of violence (see *Identifying and assessing victims of interpersonal violence*).

When dealing with the perpetrator of violence, assess for a history of violent behavior, including the type of violence and the situational and interactional factors associated with it. Aggressive behavior as a means of coping is not limited to persons with a diagnosed psychiatric disorder. Both the psychoanalytic and psychodynamic perspectives describe aggression as an innate striving, which when challenged in an adaptive manner helps people achieve goals and master the tasks of growth and development necessary for survival. In a maladaptive form, however, aggression may manifest itself as abusive and violent behavior, including child abuse (physical and sexual), spouse abuse, elder abuse, rape, and sexual assault.

The following plan of care addresses interpersonal violence within the context of rape.

ETIOLOGY AND PRECIPITATING FACTORS

Nurses in all practice settings must become more proficient at identifying and treating victims of sexual assault. Although many people assume that rape follows a surprise attack by a stranger in an isolated setting (blitz or fear rape), statistics indicate that victims typically are raped by someone they know (confidence or acquaintance rape). More attention is now paid to date rape, but marital rape is not widely discussed.

Violence involves force, including verbal and physical force, threats, and intimidation, which the victim is either unable to resist or complies with out of fear. The force involved in sexual violence can be described on a continuum ranging from free consent to violent rape (see *Sexual behavior: The force continuum*, page 244). The distinction is made to highlight the need for sensitive intervention with these victims.

While the long-term consequences of either blitz or confidence rape include post-traumatic stress disorder, the immediate response to confidence rape can be more emotionally devastating. Victims of blitz rape may question personal judgment about where they were or what they did to make themselves vulnerable to attack, and may even blame themselves for the rape. Victims of confidence rape are forced to question trust in others and examine personal responsibility for provoking the assault. The sense of betrayal and devastation is compounded by the fact that most assailants in confidence rape do not believe they have committed a crime, leaving the victim to question and doubt interpretations of the event.

While most victims of sexual assault are female, males also are sexually assaulted. Contrary to common beliefs, sexual assaults on males do not only occur in the absence of a suitable or preferred partner (such as in prison situations). As with females, assaults on males are acts of violence. Information about these assaults is minimal because of the shame and embarrassment of being victimized and because of the stigma of homosexuality.

What is known is that male victims respond to rape in much the same way as women. The prevailing myth that the rape victim somehow "wanted it" also applies to men, which then implies homosexuality or unfulfilled homosexual desires. If the victim is homosexual, he may fear the response of others. As with females, the male victim may feel that he may have done something to provoke or deserve the assault or that others will feel this way. Such fears and perceptions may be a significant factor in the low numbers of male rapes reported. Treatment of the male victim should

IDENTIFYING AND ASSESSING VICTIMS OF INTERPERSONAL VIOLENCE

The chart below describes nursing interventions and rationales appropriate when assessing possible victims of interpersonal violence.

Interventions	Rationales
• When assessing the client, determine whether the injury is consistent with the report of how it occurred.	• Most victims of abuse will not volunteer that someone harmed them, but instead will blame the action on an accident or their own clumsiness.
• Include questions about abuse, such as "This kind of injury can be caused by someone else. Has someone hurt you?"	• When asked directly, most victims will answer honestly. Victims of abuse are usually relieved when someone brings up the subject so that they can talk about it.
• Provide privacy and safety for the client when performing the assessment.	• The perpetrator of violence will usually insist that the victim not be left alone with the nurse. This should raise a red flag. Without privacy, fear of repercussions and further abuse will prevent the victim from telling the truth.
• Be alert for behavioral signs and symptoms common in victims of abuse, such as hypervigilance, anxiety, low self-esteem, apprehension or fear about answering questions, evasiveness, and difficulty making decisions.	• Victims of abuse may appear nervous or apprehensive in the presence of perceived authority. They also tend to place others' needs ahead of their own.
• Determine from hospital records or the client interview if the client has a history of previous injury.	• Although many victims of abuse may seek treatment from several different health care facilities, making tracking difficult, they will eventually revisit the same facility. A history of injuries attributed to accidents or clumsiness can signal abuse.
• Be alert for clients who repeatedly report vague, unfounded somatic complaints.	• Some victims develop gastrointestinal or neurologic symptoms. For these people, a physical complaint is more acceptable than admitting to abuse. This is not attention seeking behavior—it is a call for help.
• If a child shows any sign of physical, sexual, or emotional abuse or neglect, report it to the appropriate agency, such as the state's department of youth services.	• Health care workers are required to report all instances of confirmed or suspected child abuse. As mandated reporters, health care workers cannot be sued if their suspicions are unfounded.
• If the victim is an adult, share your suspicions and offer resources for help, such as shelters, hotlines, and support groups.	• Telling the client about suspicions and offering options can help the client acknowledge the problem.
• Do not insist that the client accept help immediately. Let the client think about the available options.	• The dynamics of abusive relationships can be so complex that the client may have difficulty sorting out the next aciton. Leaving an abusive relationship may be more frightening than staying. Accept this and support the client in making the decision that best meets personal needs.
• Maintain a supportive, nonjudgmental approach even if the client resists accepting help or making changes.	• A victim who chooses to return to an abusive situation can be extremely frustrating. Responding with anger will only alienate the victim and reinforce feelings of low self-esteem and victimization.
• Assess the client for signs and symptoms of post-traumatic stress disorder and dissociative disorders.	• Victims of abuse are at risk for these disorders. Adult survivors of untreated or unresolved childhood abuse are prone to behavior that reenacts the trauma or facilitates repeated victimization. Such behavior represents serious psychological problems requiring treatment beyond that for the current abusive situation.
• Understand that treating an abused client is a long-term process. Do not expect to treat or resolve the issue in a short-term encounter. Remember that engaging in dialogue and offering referral is invaluable to the victim of abuse.	• Nurses who feel they must resolve all problems they identify are setting themselves up for failure and a sense of futility. To keep their perspective, nurses must realize that starting the healing process is a great step.
• Be aware of the impact of absorbing the trauma of others. Seek adequate support and opportunities for personal ventilation and discussion.	• By virtue of their closeness to the trauma of others, nurses are susceptible to a phenomenon known as vicarious trauma. By being aware of their susceptibility and taking preventive measures, nurses can help maintain their mental health.

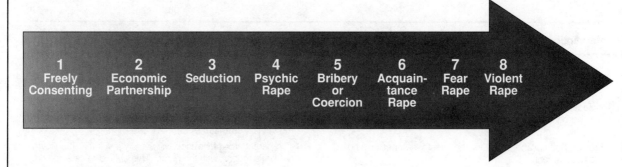

SEXUAL BEHAVIOR: THE FORCE CONTINUUM

| 1 Freely Consenting | 2 Economic Partnership | 3 Seduction | 4 Psychic Rape | 5 Bribery or Coercion | 6 Acquaintance Rape | 7 Fear Rape | 8 Violent Rape |

1. *Freely consenting.* Partners with equal power mutually choosing sexual activity. Equal power means each partner has equal status, knowledge, and ability to consent. This includes one partner agreeing to engage in sexual activity, even if not interested, as an expression of love and caring for the other person.

2. *Economic partnership.* One person agrees to sexual activity as part of an economic agreement. The type of sexual behaviors permitted are mutually determined as part of the economic agreement.

3. *Seduction.* One party attempts to persuade the other to engage in sexual activities.

4. *Psychic rape.* Assault to another person's dignity and self-respect, such as verbal abuse, street harassment, or the portrayal of violence or pornography in the media.

5. *Bribery or coercion.* The use of emotional or psychological force to persuade another to take part in sexual activities. This includes situations of unequal power between the individuals, especially when one person is in a position of authority.

6. *Acquaintance rape.* Sexual assault occurring when one party abuses the trust of a relationship and forces another into sexual activities.

7. *Fear rape.* When one party engages in sexual activities out of fear of potential violence.

8. *Violent rape.* When violence is threatened or occurs. This includes forced sexual activity between spouses, acquaintances, or strangers.

From Stuart, G.W., and Sundeen, S.J. (1992). *Principles and Practice of Psychiatric Nursing* (4th ed.). St. Louis: Mosby-Year Book. Used with permission.

proceed as for a female victim. Again, sensitivity, empathy, and respect are essential components of quality care.

Assessment guidelines
NURSING HISTORY (Functional health pattern findings)
The client may report or exhibit one or more of the findings grouped here according to functional health patterns. (Assessment findings may be similar to those found in anxiety disorder, especially generalized anxiety disorder, post-traumatic stress disorder, or dissociative disorders. Signs and symptoms may vary depending on the amount of time between the event and health care interventions.)

Health perception–health management pattern
• may deny severity of rape's impact
• may express disbelief
• may report symptoms of anxiety or panic
• may report or show signs of substance abuse

Activity-exercise pattern
• may report or show evidence of restlessness or trembling

Sleep-rest pattern
• may report difficulty falling asleep or staying asleep
• may report nightmares

Cognitive-perceptual pattern
• may report or demonstrate difficulty concentrating
• may report or demonstrate impaired recall of the rape
• may report or demonstrate a sense of depersonalization
• may appear hypervigilant

Self-perception–self-concept pattern
• may report or exhibit feelings of shame, humiliation, helplessness, guilt, or diminished self-esteem
• may express concerns about body image or self-concept
• may express feelings of responsibility for the rape

Role-relationship pattern
• may express concern about changes in relationships
• may express concern about other's responses to the rape
• may express fears about future intimacy with others

Sexual-reproductive pattern
• may express concerns about future sexual activity
• may express concerns about sexually transmitted diseases

Coping–stress tolerance pattern
• may exhibit physical tension
• may experience labile mood
• may report intrusive memories of the rape
• may exhibit or report psychological numbing

Value-belief pattern
• may report or exhibit feelings of powerlessness
• may use such defense mechanisms as denial, intellectualization, or rationalization

PHYSICAL FINDINGS
A comprehensive physical examination is conducted to assess the client for evidence of physical trauma. Findings from the physical exam must be carefully and completely documented because they will be an important part of the evidence used in any legal proceedings. Physical evidence is collected during the exam, and may include taking photographs of injuries, swabbing orifices for semen and sperm, and assessing for sexually transmitted diseases. Other evidence may be collected, such as fingernail scrapings, blood and saliva samples, clothing, and pubic hair. Awareness of institutional and municipal requirements for the proper collection and preservation of evidence is extremely important.

Specific physical findings may include cuts, bruises, fractures, and dislocations. Such injuries can appear anywhere on the body. Pay close attention to the head and neck for evidence of choking or attempted strangulation, and assess for loss of consciousness, which may indicate potentially serious head trauma.

Potential complications
Complications of rape may include disfigurement, physical injury, post-traumatic stress disorder, substance abuse, death from physical injuries, and suicide. (Refer to "Post-traumatic Stress Disorder," page 65, and "Dissociative Disorders," page 134, for more information.)

Nursing diagnosis: *Rape-trauma syndrome related to blitz rape*

NURSING PRIORITY: To help the client achieve optional adjustment to the rape and return to precrisis functioning

Interventions	Rationales
1. Assess for physical trauma.	1. Sexual assault may cause physical injury that is not readily apparent.
2. Establish a safe, trusting, empathetic, nonjudgmental environment in which the client can discuss the rape.	2. Because of a sense of violation, shame, and guilt, the client may have difficulty recounting the event. The clinician's objectivity and empathy are essential in helping the client regain self-esteem, self-confidence, and a sense of trust.
3. Explain the legal obligation to report the crime to the proper authorities and describe the client's rights.	3. Most rape victims are unable to make decisions immediately after the event and may not report the crime. By acknowledging this obligation, the nurse can alleviate the client's ambivalence about reporting the rape. The client also needs to know about personal rights and appropriate legal recourse.
4. Provide privacy for the client during the interview and physical examination.	4. Lack of privacy during the client's description of the rape can increase the sense of shame, guilt, and vulnerability.
5. Encourage the client to verbalize feelings and talk about the rape.	5. Verbalization provides an opportunity to dispel myths about rape and to help the client develop an accurate perception of the event.

6. Identify adaptive and maladaptive coping skills.

7. Do not challenge the client's coping style. Instead, provide education about rape as an act of violence and explain how people usually respond to this form of assault.

8. Help the client identify and mobilize resources and support systems.

9. Educate the family and loved ones about rape and the client's expected responses.

10. Refer the client to mental health personnel or an appropriate agency for rape counseling. With the client's permission, contact the facility's rape victim advocate.

11. If the victim is a child:
• Consult with a therapist with expertise in childhood sexual assault.
• Assess the child's level of knowledge about anatomy and sex.

• Identify the child's vocabulary for body parts and genitals, then use these words to ensure clear communication.
• Be consistent, honest, and reliable.

• Use visual aids when needed, such as anatomically correct dolls, pictures, or puppets, to help the child describe what happened.

• Explain all procedures. Allow the child to look at the examination room and touch equipment before the physical exam.

• Provide emotional support for and enlist the help of the child's caretaker during the examination.

• Educate the caretaker about the sexual assault and abuse of children. Dispel myths that hold the child responsible or that suggest the child fabricated the event.

6. Rape victims may express considerable self-doubt and recrimination, which can hinder recovery. Denial, repression, rationalization, and intellectualization may all be evident.

7. Most people do not think of rape as an act of violence. Education can help the client understand victimization and respond to it. Challenging the coping style will only undermine the client's damaged ego and may increase self-doubt and feelings of responsibility for the event.

8. Rape's emotional consequences may make victims reluctant to tell others, including the police and loved ones, about the event. Support will enhance the client's sense of safety and control.

9. Preparing the family and loved ones for the client's emotional responses helps ensure their ability to offer understanding and support.

10. Recovery from rape takes time. Emotional support, counseling, and therapy can help ensure optional client adjustment. Considering how long a rape case can take to come to trial and the emotional trauma that process creates, access to long-term support is essential.

11. Not all victims of sexual assault are adults.
• Children have special needs when dealing with the psychological aftermath of sexual assault.
• When dealing with children, some special issues arise. Most children lack the knowledge of anatomy, sexuality, and vocabulary usually involved in the assessment and care of victims of sexual assault. Gaining knowledge about the child's level of understanding can help the nurse gather accurate information, avoid misunderstandings, and prevent misinterpretation of information.
• Clinical terms may confuse or frighten the child, making data collection difficult.
• Fear, mistrust, and anger toward strangers and adults are common responses for child victims of assault. Feelings toward the abuser may be generalized to all adults.
• A child's lack of knowledge and understanding about sex and sexuality can complicate the telling of what happened. Visual aids can make the child's explanations clearer.
• For children, the physical examination can be more traumatic emotionally than the sexual assault. Developing as much trust and rapport as possible lessens the negative consequences and difficulties inherent in such an exam.
• The primary caretaker may feel guilt, shame, and anger or may express disbelief. Avoid alienating this person; support and praise the caretaker for bringing the child for examination and treatment.
• Children rarely make up stories about sexual assault. Sexual assault and abuse is the responsibility of the perpetrator, not the victim.

Outcome criteria

As treatment progresses, the client, family, or both should be able to:
• state that the traumatizing event produces less anxiety
• demonstrate age-appropriate ability to manage emotional reactions
• demonstrate appropriate life-style changes and actively pursue support from other family members
• express a sense of control over the present situation
• identify effective coping methods for eliminating negative self-perception
• verbalize an increased sense of self-esteem and hope.

Discharge criteria

Nursing documentation indicates that the client:
• has demonstrated an increased ability to recognize the impact of the rape and to use age-appropriate strategies that diminish that impact
• can effectively use age-appropriate strategies that diminish feelings of powerlessness
• has demonstrated a willingness to participate in the plan of care and decision making
• can use alternative coping skills
• is aware of available support resources.

Selected references

Brady, E.C. et al. (1991). Date rape: Expectations, avoidance strategies, and attitudes toward victims. *Journal of Social Psychology*, 131(3), 427-29.

Briere, J., and Runtz, M. (1989). The trauma symptom checklist (TSE-33): Early data on a new scale. *Journal of Interpersonal Violence*, 4(2), 151-62

Burgess, A. (1985). Rape-trauma syndrome: A nursing diagnosis. *Occupational Health Nurse*, 33(8), 405-06, 419-22.

Burgess, A.W., Hartman, C.R., and Grant, C. (1991). Drawing a connection from victim to victimizer. *Journal of Psychosocial Nursing*, 29(12), 9-14.

Campbell, J., and Humphreys, J. (1984). *Nursing care of the victims of family violence*. Reston, VA: Reston Publications.

Campbell, J.C., and Sheridan, D.J. (1989) Emergency nursing interventions with battered women. *Journal of Emergency Nursing*, 15(1), 12-17.

Cereen, A.H. (1988). Child maltreatment and its victims: A comparison of physical and sexual abuse. *Psychiatric Clinics of North America*, 11(4), 591-610.

Curry, L. et al. (1988). Breaking the cycle of family abuse. *American Journal of Nursing*, 18(9), 1188-90.

Dickstein, L. (1988). Spouse abuse and other domestic violence. *Psychiatric Clinics of North America*, 11(4), 611-28.

Donnelly, C. (1991). Ending the torment. *Nursing Times*, 87(11), 3638.

Faller, K.C. (1988). The myth of the collusive mother. *Journal of Interpersonal Violence*, 3, 190-96.

Finklehor, D., and Pillemer, K. (1988). The pre-violence of elder abuse: A random sample survey. *Gerontological Society of America*, 28(1), 5157.

Finkelhor, D., and Yllo, K. (1988). Rape in marriage. In M. Straus (Ed.) *Abuse and victimization across the life span*, Baltimore: Johns Hopkins University Press.

Gage, R.B. (1991). Examining the dynamics of spouse abuse: An alternative view. *Nurse Practitioner*, 16(4), 11-16.

Gise, L.H., and Paddison, P. (1988). Rape, sexual abuse, and its victims. *Psychiatric Clinics of North America*, 11(4), 629-48.

Goodwin, J. (1989). *Sexual abuse: Incest victims and their families*. Chicago: Yearbook Medical.

Grell, K. (1991). ENA sexual assault nurse examiners resource list. *Journal of Emergency Nursing*, 17(4), 31-35.

Hamilton, J.A. (1989). Emotional consequences of victimization and discrimination in "special population" of women. *Psychiatric Clinics of North America*, 12(1), 35-51.

Herman, J.L. (1988). Father-daughter incest. In F. Ochberg (Ed.) *Post-traumatic therapy and victims of violence*, New York: Brunner/Mazel.

Hyde, J. (1990) Treating the victim of rape. *Nursing Standard*, 4(17), 32-34.

Keltner, M., and Wright, L. (1987). *Psychiatric nursing: A psychotherapeutic management approach*. Philadelphia: Mosby.

Kramer, S., and Akhtar, S. (Eds.). (1991). *The trauma of transgression: Psychotherapy of incest victims*. Northvale, NJ: Jacob Aronson.

Lazzaro, M., and McFarlane, J. (1991). Establishing a screening program for abused women. *Journal of Nursing Administration*, 21(10), 24-29.

Leahy, M., and Wright L. (1987). *Families and psychosocial problems*. Springhouse, PA: Springhouse.

Levine, E.M., and Kanin, E.J. (1987). Sexual violence among dates and acquaintances: Trends and their implementation for marriage and family. *Journal of Family Violence*, 2(1), 55-65.

Lim, D. (1991). Nursing matters: Caring for a victim of rape. *Nursing Standard*, 6(1), 28.

Mackey, T.F. et al, (1991), Comparative effects of sexual functioning of child sexual abuse survivors and others. *Issues in Mental Health Nursing*, 12(1), 89-112.

McCann, I.L., and Pearlman, L. (1990). *Psychological trauma and the adult survivor*. New York: Brunner/Mazel.

McFarlane J., et al. (1991). Assessing for abuse: Self-report versus nurse interview. *Public Health Nursing*, 8(4), 245-50.

Mezey, G., and King, M. (1989). The effects of sexual assault on men: A survey of 22 victims. *Psychological Medicine*, 19(1), 205-09.

Minden, P. (1989). The victim care service: A program for victims of sexual assault. *Archives of Psychiatric Nursing*, 3(1), 41-46.

Mochling, K.S. (1988). Battered women and abusive partners: Treatment issues and strategies. *Journal of Psychosocial Nursing*, 26(9), 8-11.

Molleca, R.F., and Son, L. (1989) Cultured dimensions in the evaluation and treatment of sexual trauma, and overview. *Psychiatric Clinics of North America*, 12(2), 363-79.

Moss, V.A. (1991). Battered women and the myth of masochism. *Journal of Psychosocial Nursing*, 29(2), 18-23.

Moss, V.A., and Taylor W.K. (1991). Domestic violence: Identification, assessment, intervention. *AORN Journal*, 53(5), 1158-64.

Murphy, S.M., et al. (1988). Current psychological functioning of child sexual assault survivors. *Journal of Interpersonal Violence*, 3, 5579.

Nathanson, D.L. (1989). Understanding what is hidden: Shame in sexual abuse. *Psychiatric Clinics of North America*, 12(2), 381-88.

Newberger, E. and Bourne, R. (1985). *Unhappy families: Clinical research perspectives on family violence*. Littleton, MA: PSG Publishing.

Ochberg, F. (1988). *Post-traumatic therapy and victims of violence*. New York: Brunner/Mazel.

Peterson, D.L. and Pfost, K.S. (1989). Influence of rock videos on attitudes of violence against women. *Psychological Reports*, 64(1), 319-22.

Renshow, D.C. (1989). Treatment of sexual exploitation: Rape and incest. *Psychiatric Clinics of North America*, 12(2), 257-77.

Sampselle, C.M. (1991). The role of the nurse in preventing violence against women. *Journal of Obstetric, Gynecologic and Neonatal Nursing*, 20(6), 481-87.

Seirgess, A., Hartman, C.R., and Kelley, S. (1990). Assessing child abuse: The TRIADS checklist. *Journal of Psychosocial Nursing*, 28(4), 7-14.

Silverman, D.C., et al. (1988). Blitz rape and confidence rape: A topology applied to 1,000 consecutive cases. *American Journal of Psychiatry*, 145(11), 1438-41.

Sink, F. (1988). Sexual abuse in the lives of children. In M. Straus (Ed.) *Abuse and victimization across the life span*, Baltimore: Johns Hopkins University Press.

Sonnenberg, S.M. (1988). Victims of violence and post-traumatic stress disorder. *Psychiatric Clinics of North America*, 11(4), 581-90.

Straus, M. (Ed.). (1988). *Abuse and victimization across the life span*. Baltimore: Johns Hopkins University Press.

Struckman-Johnson, C, (1988). Forced sex on dates: It happens to men too. *The Journal of Sex Research*, 24, 234-41.

Tildon, V.P. (1989). Response of the health care delivery system to battered women. *Issues in Mental Health Nursing*, 10(3-4), 309-20.

Trevelyan, J. (1991). Marital rape. *Nursing Times*, 87(13), 40-41.

van der Kolk, B.A. (1988). Trauma in men: Effects on family life. In M. Straus (Ed.), *Abuse and victimization across the life span*, Baltimore: Johns Hopkins University Press.

van der Kolk, B.A. (1989). The compulsion to repeat the trauma: Reenactment, re-victimization, and masochism. *Psychiatric Clinics of North America*, 12(2), 389-411.

Walter, K. (1992). That was then: Elderly survivors of incest. *Journal of Psychosocial Nursing*, 30(1), 14-16.

Wilson, W. (1988). Rape as entertainment. *Psychological Reports*, 63(2), 607-10.

Wissow, L.S. (1990). *Child advocacy for the clinician: An approach to child abuse and neglect*. Baltimore: Williams & Wilkins.

DISORDERS ASSOCIATED WITH VIOLENCE

Vicarious Traumatization

Psychiatric nursing diagnostic class
Anxiety

Introduction

Health care professionals who work with trauma victims are susceptible to a parallel emotional process and behavioral response resulting from the secondary exposure to a traumatic event. This phenomenon is called *vicarious traumatization*. Although extensive research and clinical work has been done on the psychological impact of trauma on its victims, their families, and the community, less is known about trauma's effect on emergency and crisis workers and therapists. Research does show that health care professionals who work with trauma victims may experience profound psychological effects that can be disruptive and painful, persisting for months or even years. With long-term exposure to secondary trauma, therapists have shown signs of memory alterations and disruptions.

The concepts of burnout and countertransference are related to vicarious traumatization. Burnout symptoms may include cynicism, boredom, depression, loss of compassion, disillusionment, and discouragement. Such symptoms may result when the health care professional can no longer acknowledge, assimilate, or work through continual exposure to traumatic material—a process similar to the numbing-avoidant pattern trauma survivors sometimes employ. Through countertransference, the activation of the therapist's unresolved or unconscious concerns and conflicts within a psychotherapeutic relationship, the therapist may incorporate painful feelings, images, and thoughts from a trauma victim.

ETIOLOGY AND PRECIPITATING FACTORS

Health care professionals who have been exposed to the detailed and painful experiences of trauma victims are at risk for vicarious traumatization. Such exposure creates a sense of vulnerability and fragility; it also can awaken old memories and unresolved pain related to trauma in the health care professional's life.

Assessment guidelines

NURSING HISTORY (Functional health pattern findings)

The health care professional may report or exhibit one or more of the findings grouped here according to functional health patterns.

Health perception–health management pattern
• possible extreme concern about "going crazy"
• inattentiveness to medical and dental problems

Nutritional-metabolic pattern
• possible concern over eating behaviors, such as using food to suppress feelings
• weight fluctuations

Elimination pattern
• GI system disturbances, such as pain, flatulence, diarrhea, nausea, constipation, vomiting, and intestinal bleeding
• frequent urination
• increased sweating, cold and clammy skin, or both

Activity-exercise pattern
• agitation and restlessness
• fluctuations in energy and activity levels
• decreasing interest and participation in leisure and social activities

Sleep-rest pattern
• possible fatigue after sleep
• dreams or nightmares about traumatic events happening to others
• inability to fall or stay asleep or problems with early morning awakening
• possible use or dependence on aids (such as drugs or alcohol) to facilitate sleep

Cognitive-perceptual pattern
• memory impairment
• difficulty concentrating
• acute or chronic pain
• difficulty learning

Self-perception–self-concept pattern
• self-described anxiety or sense of inadequacy
• feeling detached or estranged from others

Role-relationship pattern
• inability to maintain relationships with family or significant others
• disillusionment with job
• inability to sustain job performance
• "compassion fatigue" or inability to care about others
• feeling alone and uninvolved with environment

Sexual-reproductive pattern
• decreased sexual desire
• difficulties in sexual performance or satisfaction

Coping–stress tolerance pattern
- high levels of anxiety
- feelings of tenseness most of the time
- flashbacks or recurrences of own traumatic events
- significant stress or number of stressful events during the last year
- feelings of "going crazy" or being unable to cope
- feelings of high vulnerability and fragility

Value-belief pattern
- increasing cynicism
- spiritual distress
- inability to achieve life goals

PHYSICAL FINDINGS
The health care professional may report or exhibit one or more of the following physical findings.

Cardiovascular
- excessive perspiration
- fatigue
- increased heart rate
- increased blood pressure

Gastrointestinal
- abdominal distress or pain
- diarrhea
- nausea
- ulcers

Genitourinary
- frequent urination

Musculoskeletal
- muscle aches
- muscle tension
- restlessness
- trembling

Neurologic
- headaches
- hyperalertness
- hypervigilance
- memory impairment
- sleep disturbance
- startle reaction
- tremors or tics

Psychological
- anger
- high anxiety
- constricted affect
- diminished interest
- feelings of detachment or estrangement
- illusions
- intrusive thoughts of events that happened to others
- nightmares
- numbing of responsiveness to environment
- process-behavioral addiction (such as compulsive gambling, spending, or working)
- recurrent dreams of traumatic events
- recurrent thoughts of own traumatic events
- significant irritability
- social withdrawal
- substance abuse or dependence
- sudden acting out or feeling as though traumatic event is recurring
- survivor guilt

Respiratory
- hyperventilation
- increased respiratory rate

Potential complications
Unacknowledged or untreated vicarious traumatization can lead to post-trauma response or post-traumatic stress disorder. It also may result in negative coping strategies, such as substance abuse or dependence, aggressive or violent behavior, and an inability to function in the workplace.

Nursing diagnosis: *Post-trauma response related to the subjective experience of single or multiple traumatic events through repeated exposure to trauma victims (vicarious traumatization)*

NURSING PRIORITIES: To assess the effect of secondary trauma on the health care professional, evaluate the degree of perceived threat, and minimize their impact

Interventions	Rationales
1. Assess for physical symptoms of vicarious traumatization, such as headaches, fatigue, palpitations, nausea, and abdominal distress.	1. These symptoms must be identified and differentiated from symptoms of other problems so that appropriate treatment can be initiated.
2. Identify any psychological and behavioral responses, such as emotional lability, crying, mood swings, and feelings of inadequacy or incompleteness.	2. Emotional responses to vicarious traumatization can vary. However, they must be acknowledged and managed in an adaptive manner to prevent ineffective coping behaviors.
3. Determine the degree of disorganization in thinking and coping.	3. The degree of disorganization determines the necessary level of intervention.

Nursing diagnosis: *Powerlessness related to inadequate problem-solving and coping skills and overwhelming anxiety*

NURSING PRIORITY: To help the health care professional regain a sense of control over feelings and behaviors

Interventions	Rationales
1. Determine the health care professional's previous coping abilities and level of mastery.	1. Reminding the health care professional of previous success enhances self-confidence, acknowledges options, and promotes self-control.
2. Explore cultural or religious beliefs that support helpless behavior.	2. Exploring these beliefs lets the health care professional acknowledge their ability to instill shame and guilt.
3. Collaborate with the health care professional to establish an effective plan of care that includes realistic and achievable goals.	3. Active involvement in treatment can enhance the health care professional's sense of control and mastery over a stressful situation.
4. Help the health care professional identify feelings of powerlessness and the factors that contribute to such feelings.	4. Awareness of these feelings and their causes can promote positive coping.
5. Instruct the health care professional about strategies to combat stress and escalating anxiety, such as using deep breathing exercises, suspending thought, using refocusing techniques, and seeking counsel from a trusted colleague or friend. Provide opportunities for practice and feedback.	5. Strategies for managing stress and anxiety provide alternative coping skills and increases the ability to manage feelings.
6. Encourage the health care professional to participate in individual and group clinical supervision.	6. Individual clinical supervision provides the health care professional an ongoing opportunity to deal with secondary trauma within a safe relationship. Group clinical supervision allows the health care professional to learn and share with peers who have also experienced secondary trauma and its consequences.

Nursing diagnosis: *Sleep pattern disturbance related to recurrent nightmares or dreams of personal death, and fear of their recurrence*

NURSING PRIORITY: To promote sleep by reducing the incidence of intrusive thoughts and dreams

Interventions

1. Determine the health care professional's normal and current sleep patterns. Ask the client to describe any changes.

2. Assess usual sleep routines, including use of sleep aids.

3. Instruct the health care professional in effective sleep hygiene measures, such as retiring and rising at the same times, avoiding naps and time spent awake in bed (such as reading in bed), eliminating caffeine and alcohol intake before bedtime, and, if unable to fall asleep within 15 minutes, performing a quiet activity outside the bedroom.

4. Help the health care professional arrange a restful sleep environment that is neither too warm nor too bright. Suggest using a night-light or having a light switch next to the bed.

5. Suggest that the health care professional develop an individualized relaxation program. Refer the client to an appropriate program, such as self-hypnosis, visualization and imagery, or progressive muscle relaxation; encourage practice.

Rationales

1. Subjective and objective information provides baseline assessment of the sleep disturbance and focuses interventions.

2. Sedatives can interfere with the ability to fall sleep and disrupt normal sleep cycles, reducing refreshment from sleep.

3. Changing behaviors to promote sleep can help decrease anxiety about sleeplessness.

4. A comfortable environment promotes sleep. A readily available source of light helps promote orientation should the client awaken suddenly from a nightmare.

5. These techniques can produce mental and physical relaxation, promoting sleep and providing a means of control over nightmares.

Outcome criteria

As treatment progresses, the health care professional should be able to:
• verbalize a reduction in feelings of anxiety or fear when intrusive thoughts emerge
• demonstrate the ability to manage emotional reactions effectively
• use individual clinical supervision to manage countertransference issues and to obtain support
• participate in group clinical supervision with peers
• identify feelings and effective methods to cope with them
• participate in decision to seek psychotherapy
• express a sense of control and mastery over the present situation and its outcome
• identify and use safe, effective measures to promote sleep.

Selected references

Allanrach, E.J. (1988). Perceived supportive behaviors and nursing occupational stress: An evolution of consciousness. *Advances in Nursing,* 10(7), 73-82.

Armstrong, K., O'Callahan, W., and Marmar, C.R. (1991). Debriefing Red Cross disaster personnel: The multiple stressor debriefing model. *Journal of Traumatic Stress,* 4(4), 581-93.

Bonnivier-Fest, J. (1992). A peer supervision group: Put countertransference to work. *Journal of Psychological Nursing,* 30(2), 5-8.

Dansky, B.S., Roth, S., and Kroenberger, W.G. (1990). The trauma constellation identification scale: A measure of the psychological impact of a stressful life event. *Journal of Traumatic Stress,* 3(4), 557-72.

Driedger, S.M., and Cox, D. (1991). Burnout in nurses who care for PWAs: The impact of social support. *AIDS Patient Care,* 5(4), 197-203.

Edelwich, J., and Brodsky, P. (1980). *Burnout: The stages of disillusionment in the helping professions.* New York: Human Sciences Press.

Flach, F. (1988). *Resilience: Discovering a new strength at times of stress.* New York: Fawcett Columbine.

Flach, F. (1989). *Stress and its management.* New York: Norton.

Genest, M., Levine, J., Ramsden, V., and Swanson, R. (1990). The impact of providing help: Emergency workers and cardiopulmonary resuscitation attempts. *Journal of Traumatic Stress*, 3(2), 305-13.

Lyons, J.A. (1991). Strategies for assessing the potential for positive adjustment following trauma. *Journal of Traumatic Stress*, 4(1), 93111.

McCammon, S., Dunham, T.W., Allison, E.J., and Williamson, J.E. (1988). Emergency workers' cognitive appraisal and coping with traumatic events. *Journal of Traumatic Stress*, 1(3), 353-72.

McCann, I.L., and Pearlman, L.A. (1990). Vicarious traumatization: A framework for understanding the psychological effects of working with victims. *Journal of Traumatic Stress*, 3(1), 131-49.

Schroder, P.J. (1985). Recognizing transference and countertransference. *Journal of Psychological Nursing and Mental Health Services*, 23(2), 21-26.

Scott, C.D., and Hawk, J. (1986). *Heal thyself: The health of healthcare professionals*. New York: Brunner-Mazel.

Talbot, A. (1990). The importance of parallel process in debriefing crisis counselors. *Journal of Traumatic Stress*, 3, 265-78.

Talbot, A., Manton, M., and Dunn, P.J. (1992). Debriefing the debriefers: An intervention strategy to assist psychologists after a crisis. *Journal of Traumatic Stress*, 5(1), 45-63.

Tanaka, K. (1988). Development of a tool for assessing post-trauma response. *Archives of Psychiatric Nursing*, 2(6), 350-56.

Section III: Assessment Tools

Assessment of Extrapyramidal Effects

Regular evaluation for extrapyramidal side effects is extremely important to the care of a client receiving psychotropic medications. However, maintaining consistency in assessment from one health care professional to another can be difficult. An assessment tool can reduce variation between examiners, as well as the influence of subjective observation. Two such tools are presented here: the Simpson Neurological Rating Scale and the Abnormal Involuntary Movement Scale (AIMS).

The Simpson Neurological Scale examines ten distinct areas of neuromuscular function, assessing the degree of rigidity, resistance, tremor, salivation, and general restlessness. The Abnormal Involuntary Movement Scale (AIMS) helps identify movements that result from specific psychotropic medications; it examines facial and oral movements, extremity movements, trunk movements, and global judgments. The AIMS can be especially helpful in assessing a client's response to medication given to reduce extrapyramidal side effects.

SIMPSON NEUROLOGICAL RATING SCALE

Conduct the examination in a room where the subject can walk a sufficient distance to get into a natural rhythm (at least 15 paces).

Examine each side of the body; if one side shows more pronounced pathology than the other, record more severe pathology.

Cogwheel rigidity may be palpated when the examination is carried out for items 3, 4, 5, and 6. It is not rated separately and is merely another way to detect rigidity. Cogwheel rigidity requires a minimum score of 2.

1. **GAIT:** The subject is examined walking into the examining room—gait, swing of the arms, and general posture form the basis for an overall score for this item.
1 = Normal
2 = Mild diminution in swing while the subject is walking
3 = Obvious diminution in swing suggesting shoulder rigidity
4 = Stiff gait with little or no armswing noticeable
5 = Rigid gait with arms slightly pronated or stooped, shuffling gait with propulsion and repropulsion
9 = Not ratable

2. **ARM DROPPING:** The subject and the examiner both raise their arms to shoulder height and let them fall to their sides. In a normal subject, a stout slap is heard as the arms hit the sides. In the subject with extreme Parkinson's syndrome, the arms fall very slowly.
1 = Normal, free fall with loud slap and rebound
2 = Fall slowed slightly with less audible contact and little rebound
3 = Fall slowed, no rebound
4 = Marked slowing, no slap at all
5 = Arms fall as though against resistance or as though through glue
9 = Not ratable

3. **SHOULDER SHAKING:** The subject's arms are bent at a right angle at the elbow and are taken one at a time by the examiner, who grasps one hand and also clasps the other around the subject's elbow. The subject's upper arm is pushed to and fro and the humerus is externally rotated. The degree of resistance from normal to extreme rigidity is scored as detailed. The procedure is repeated with one hand palpating the shoulder cuff while rotation takes place.
1 = Normal
2 = Slight stiffness and resistance
3 = Moderate stiffness and resistance
4 = Marked rigidity with difficulty in passive movement
5 = Extreme stiffness and rigidity with almost a frozen joint
9 = Not ratable

4. **ELBOW RIGIDITY:** The elbow joints are bent separately at right angles and passively extended and flexed, with the subject's biceps observed and simultaneously palpated. The resistance to this procedure is rated.
1 = Normal
2 = Slight stiffness and resistance
3 = Moderate stiffness and resistance
4 = Marked rigidity with difficulty in passive movement
5 = Extreme stiffness and rigidity with almost a frozen joint
9 = Not ratable

5. **WRIST RIGIDITY:** The wrist is held in one hand and the fingers held by the examiner's other hand, with the wrist moved to extension, flexion, and ulnar and radial deviation; or the extended wrist is allowed to fall under its own weight; or the arm can be grasped above the wrist and shaken to and fro. A score of 1 would be a hand that extends easily, falls loosely, or flaps easily upwards and downwards.
1 = Normal
2 = Slight stiffness and resistance
3 = Moderate stiffness and resistance
4 = Marked rigidity with difficulty in passive movement
5 = Extreme stiffness and rigidity with almost a frozen wrist
9 = Not ratable

6. **HEAD ROTATION:** The subject sits or stands and is told that the examiner is going to move the subject's head from side to side, that it will not hurt, and to relax. (Questions about pain in the cervical area or difficulty in moving the head should be obtained to avoid causing any pain.) Clasp the subject's head between the two hands with the fingers on the back of the neck. Gently rotate the head in a circular motion three times and evaluate the muscular resistance to this movement.
1 = Loose, no resistance
2 = Slight resistance to movement although the time to rotate may be normal
3 = Resistance is apparent and the time of rotation is shortened
4 = Resistance is obvious and rotation is slowed
5 = Head appears stiff and rotation is difficult to carry out
9 = Not ratable

7. **GLABELLAR TAP:** Subject is told to open eyes wide and not to blink. The glabellar region is tapped at a steady, rapid speed. Note number of times subject blinks in succession. Take care to stand behind the subject so that the movement of the tapping finger is not observable. A full blink need not be observed; there may be contraction of the infraorbital muscle producing a twitch each time a stimulus is delivered. Vary the speed of tapping to ensure that muscle contraction is related to the tap.
1 = 0 to 5 blinks
2 = 0 to 10 blinks
3 = 11 to 15 blinks
4 = 16 to 20 blinks
5 = 21 or more blinks
9 = Not ratable

8. **TREMOR:** Subject is observed walking into examining room and then is reexamined for this item with arms extended at right angles to the body and the fingers spread out as far as possible.
1 = Normal
2 = Mild finger tremor, obvious to sight and touch
3 = Tremor of hand or arm occurring spasmodically
4 = Persistent tremor of one or more limbs
5 = Whole body tremor
9 = Not ratable

continued

Simpson Neurological Rating Scale *(continued)*

9. **SALIVATION:** The subject is observed while talking and then asked to open the mouth and elevate the tongue.

1 = Normal
2 = Excess salivation so that pooling takes place if mouth is open and tongue raised
3 = Excess salivation is present and might occasionally result in difficulty in speaking
4 = Speaking with difficulty because of excess salivation
5 = Frank drooling
9 = Not ratable

10. **AKATHISIA:** The subject is observed for restlessness. If restlessness is noted, ask: "Do you feel restless or jittery inside? Is it difficult to sit still?" A response is not necessary for scoring, but the subject's report can help make the assessment.

1 = No restlessness reported or observed
2 = Mild restlessness observed, such as occasional jiggling of the foot when the subject is seated
3 = Moderate restlessness observed: for example, jiggles foot, crosses and uncrosses legs, or twists a body part on several occasions
4 = Restlessness is observed frequently: for example, the foot or legs move most of the time
5 = Restlessness persistently observed: for example, subject cannot sit still, may get up and walk
9 = Not ratable

ABNORMAL INVOLUNTARY MOVEMENT SCALE (AIMS)

INSTRUCTIONS: Complete Examination Procedure
MOVEMENT RATINGS: Rate highest severity observed. Rate movements that occur upon activation one point less than those observed spontaneously.

Code: 0 = None
1 = Minimal, may be extreme normal
2 = Mild
3 = Moderate
4 = Severe

EXAMINATION PROCEDURE

Either before or after completing the Examination Procedure, observe the client unobtrusively at rest (such as in the waiting room). The chair used in this examination should be a hard, firm one without arms.

1. Ask the client to remove shoes and socks.
2. Ask the client whether there is anything in the mouth (such as gum or candy) and if there is, to remove it.
3. Ask about the current condition of the client's teeth. Ask if the client wears dentures. Do teeth or dentures bother client now?
4. Ask whether the client notices any movements in the mouth, face, hands, or feet. If yes, ask for a description and to what extent they currently bother the client or interfere with activities.
5. Have the client sit in chair with hands on knees, legs slightly apart, and feet flat on the floor. Look at the entire body for movements while in this position.
6. Ask the client to sit with hands hanging unsupported: if male, between the legs; if female and wearing a dress, hanging over the knees. Observe the hands and other body areas.
7. Ask the client to open the mouth. Observe the tongue at rest within the mouth. Do this twice.

8. Ask the client to protrude the tongue. Observe abnormalities of tongue movement.
9. Ask client to tap the thumb with each finger as rapidly as possible for 10 to 15 seconds, first with the right hand, then with left hand. Observe facial and leg movements.
10. Flex and extend the client's left and right arms, one at a time. Note any rigidity.
11. Ask the client to stand up. Observe in profile. Observe all body areas again, hips included.
12. Ask the client to extend both arms outstretched in front with palms down. Observe the trunk, legs, and mouth.
13. Have the client walk a few paces, turn, and walk back to chair. Observe the hands and gait. Do this twice.

FACIAL AND ORAL MOVEMENTS
(Circle One)

1. Muscles of facial expression (such as movements of forehead, eyebrows, periorbital area, and cheeks; include frowning, blinking, smiling, and grimacing) 0 1 2 3 4

2. Lips and perioral area (such as puckering, pouting, and smacking) 0 1 2 3 4

3. Jaw (such as biting, clenching, chewing, mouth opening, and lateral movement) 0 1 2 3 4

4. Tongue (rate only increase in movement both in and out of mouth, *not* inability to sustain movement) 0 1 2 3 4

EXTREMITY MOVEMENTS

5. Upper: arms, wrists, hand, fingers (include choreic movements, such as rapid, objectively purposeless, irregular, or spontaneous, and athetoid movements, such as slow, irregular, complex, or serpentine) 0 1 2 3 4

6. Lower: legs, knees, ankles, toes (such as lateral knee movement, foot tapping, heel dropping, foot squirming, or inversion and eversion of foot) 0 1 2 3 4

Abnormal Involuntary Movement Scale (AIMS) *(continued)*

TRUNK MOVEMENTS
7. Neck, shoulders, and hips (such as rocking, twisting, squirming,   0 1 2 3 4
   or pelvic gyrations)

GLOBAL JUDGMENTS
8. Severity of abnormal movements

0 None, normal
1 Minimal
2 Mild
3 Moderate
4 Severe

9. Incapacitation resulting from abnormal movements

0 None, normal
1 Minimal
2 Mild
3 Moderate
4 Severe

10. Client's awareness of abnormal movements (rate only client's report)

0 No awareness
1 Aware, no distress
2 Aware, mild distress
3 Aware, moderate distress
4 Aware, severe distress

DENTAL STATUS
11. Current problems with teeth or dentures

1 No
2 Yes

12. Does client usually wear dentures?

1 No
2 Yes

Simpson Neurological Rating Scale used courtesy of Dr. George Simpson, Medical College of Pennsylvania, Philadelphia.

Barry Psychosocial Assessment

This comprehensive assessment tool uses Gordon's functional health patterns to facilitate the data-gathering process and promote the identification of corresponding nursing diagnoses.

The assessment categories include the following patterns:
- Health perception–health management
- Nutritional-metabolic
- Elimination
- Activity-exercise
- Sleep-rest
- Cognitive-perceptual
- Self-perception–self-concept
- Role-relationship
- Sexuality-reproductive
- Coping–stress tolerance
- Value-belief

These categories help the nurse focus on specific aspects of the assessment and identify problem areas. Problem areas are then clarified through a focused assessment.

Assess all boxed questions subjectively, rather than asking the client directly. Bold italic statements advise the nurse how to proceed.

Admitting Information

Name _____ Age _____ Date of admission _____

Marital status   S_____   M_____   W_____   D_____   How long? _____

Occupation _____ Years of education completed _____

Date of assessment _____ Admitting diagnosis _____

HEALTH PERCEPTION–HEALTH MANAGEMENT

Patient's Perception of Illness

What was the original problem that caused you to come to the hospital? _____

On what date did you first become ill? _____

What caused this illness? _____

How do you feel about being in a hospital? _____

How can the physicians and nurses help you most? _____

How will this illness affect you when you are out of the hospital? _____

Do you think it will cause any changes in your life? _____

How will it affect your family? _____

Potential for noncompliance?   Yes _____   No _____   Possible _____

Related to: _____ Anxiety

_____ Negative side effects
of prescribed treatment

_____ Unsatisfactory relationship with caregiving environment or caregivers

_____ Other

Explain:

Potential for injury?   Yes _____   No _____   Possible _____

Explain:

Barry Psychosocial Assessment *(continued)*

NUTRITIONAL-METABOLIC

How does your current appetite compare with your normal appetite?

Same _____   Increased _____   Decreased _____

How long has it been different? _____

Has your weight fluctuated by more than 5 lb in the last several weeks?

Yes _____   No _____   How many pounds? _____

What is your normal fluid intake per day? ml* _____   Your current intake? ml _____

Nurse can substitute estimate of milliliters for client's reported fluid intake.

Aspects of client's illness or condition that could contribute to organic mental disorder?   No _____   Yes _____

Delirium type _____   Dementia type _____

Possible cause:

_____ Metabolic

_____ Electrolytes

_____ Other metabolic or
            endocrine condition

_____ Arterial disease

_____ Mechanical disease

_____ Electrical disorder

_____ Infectious disease

_____ Neoplastic disease

_____ Nutritional disease

_____ Degenerative (chronic)
            brain disease

_____ Drug toxicity

ELIMINATION

What is your current pattern of bowel movements?

Constipated _____   Diarrhea _____   Incontinent _____

How does this compare to normal?

Same _____   Different _____

Explain:

What is your current pattern of urination? _____

How does this compare to normal?

Same _____   Different _____

Explain:

Possibility that emotional distress may be contributing to any change?

High _____   Moderate _____   Low _____

ACTIVITY-EXERCISE

What is your normal energy level?

High _____   Moderate _____   Low _____

Has it changed in the past 6 months?   Yes _____   No _____

To what do you attribute the cause? _____

How would you describe your normal activity level?

High _____   Moderate _____   Low _____

How may it change following this hospitalization? _____

What types of activities do you normally pursue outside the home? _____

What recreational activities do you enjoy? _____

Do you anticipate your ability to manage your home will be changed following your hospitalization? _____

Explain:

continued

Barry Psychosocial Assessment *(continued)*

ACTIVITY-EXERCISE *(continued)*

Current self-care deficits?

Feeding _____   Bathing _____   Dressing _____   Toileting _____

Anticipated deficits following hospitalization? _____

Current impairment in mobility? _____

Anticipated immobility following hospitalization? _____

Alterations in the following?

Airway clearance How? _____

Breathing patterns How? _____

Cardiac output How? _____

Respiratory function How? _____

Potential for altered tissue perfusion as manifested by altered cognitive-perceptual patterns?

SLEEP-REST

Normal sleeping pattern

How many hours do you normally sleep per night?   From what hour to what hour? _____ to _____

Changes in normal sleeping pattern

Do you have difficulty falling asleep? _____

Do you awaken in the middle of night? _____

Do you awaken early in the morning? _____

Are you sleeping more or fewer hours than normal? _____   How many? _____

COGNITIVE-PERCEPTUAL

Are you feeling pain now? _____   How severe? _____   How often? _____   What relieves the pain? _____

What information does this client need to know to manage this illness or health state?

Ability to comprehend this information?

Good _____   Moderate _____   Poor _____

If poor, explain:

Mental Status Exam

Level of awareness and orientation _____

Appearance and behavior _____

Speech and communication _____

Affect (mood) _____

Thinking process _____

Related to: Inability to evaluate reality _____   Aging _____   Other _____

Explain:

Barry Psychosocial Assessment *(continued)*

COGNITIVE-PERCEPTUAL *(continued)*

If there is a distortion of the thought process, a focused assessment is indicated.

Perception _____

Abstract thinking _____

Social judgment _____

Memory _____

Impairment in short-term memory _____   Long-term _____

Is there evidence of unilateral neglect?   Yes _____   No _____   Does not apply _____

Self-perception

Does the client describe feelings of anxiety or uneasiness? _____

Is he able to identify a cause?   Yes _____ No _____

Cause? _____

If the client feels anxious but cannot identify a cause, assess for the major coping risks of physical illness below.

Is there anything you are frightened of during this hospitalization or illness?

Yes _____   No _____   What is it? _____

How will this illness affect your future plans? _____

Normally, do you believe that you control what happens to you (internal locus of control) or do you believe that other people or events control what happens (external locus of control)?

Internal locus of control _____
External locus of control _____

Will this illness affect the way you feel about yourself? _____

How? _____   About your body? _____

Psychosocial Risks of Illness

What are the major issues of this illness for this client? _____

For this family? _____

Use the following space to record client and family comments illustrating how they are coping with these issues.

Trust   Client _____
                    Family _____

Self-esteem   Client _____
                    Family _____

Body image   Client _____
                    Family _____

Control   Client _____
                    Family _____

Loss   Client _____
                    Family _____

continued

Barry Psychosocial Assessment *(continued)*

Psychosocial Risks of Illness *(continued)*

Guilt

Client _____

Family _____

Intimacy

Client _____

Family _____

Could one or more of these issues be contributing to feelings of anxiety, hopelessness, powerlessness, or disturbance in self-concept?

Yes _____   No _____   Possible _____

If so, explain which ones and proceed with a focused assessment.

ROLE-RELATIONSHIP

What is your occupation? _____

How many years have you been in this occupation? _____

Do you anticipate that this illness will have an effect on your ability to work?   Yes _____   No _____   How? _____

With whom do you live? _____ Are they supportive? _____

Who are the most important people in your life? _____

Do you ever feel socially isolated?   Yes _____   No _____

Explain:

Is there any indication in this history of social isolation or impaired social interaction?   Yes _____   No _____
Explain:

Ability to communicate

Within normal limits _____   Impaired _____

Describe:

FAMILY HISTORY

Who are the members of your immediate family? What are their ages and how are they related to you? Please include deceased members and when they died.

Name of family member _____ Relationship to you _____ Age _____ Date of death _____

    _____   _____   _____   _____

    _____   _____   _____   _____

    _____   _____   _____   _____

    _____   _____   _____   _____

What is your position in relation to your brothers and sisters? For example, are you the second oldest, the youngest...? _____

How often do you see your immediate family members? _____

What goes on in your family when something bad happens? _____

What do most of the members do? _____

Barry Psychosocial Assessment *(continued)*

FAMILY HISTORY *(continued)*

Have any of your relationships within your immediate and extended family changed recently? _____

Which ones? _____

How have they changed? _____

Is there any change in the way you parent your children?   Yes _____   No _____

If so, to what do you attribute the cause?

_____ New baby

_____ Death of other family member

_____ Illness in other family member

_____ Change in residence (describe reason for change)

_____ Other (describe)

What is your normal role within your family? _____

What role do the significant other people in your family play? _____

Potential for disruption of these roles by this illness?   High _____   Moderate _____   Low _____

Explain:

While the client is describing the family, is there any indication of uncontrolled anger or rage?   Yes _____   No _____

Related to a specific issue or person?

Explain:

Open (trusting) or closed (untrusting) communication style in family? (Can be initially determined by statements and emotional

expression of client.) _____

Developmental stage of family

_____ Early married

_____ Married with no children

_____ Active childbearing

_____ Pre-school or school age children

_____ Adolescent children and children leaving home

_____ Middle-aged children no longer at home

_____ Elderly, well-functioning

_____ Elderly, infirm

Is there any other aspect of your family or the way your family normally operates that you think should be added here? What is it?

If any item discussed in this section appears to be a current stressor for this client or family, it can be assessed using a focused approach with the other items under coping–stress tolerance pattern.

Interpersonal style

_____ Dependent

_____ Controlled

_____ Dramatizing

_____ Suspicious

_____ Self-sacrificing

_____ Superior

_____ Uninvolved

_____ Mixed (usually two styles predominate)

_____ No predominant personality style

Write a brief sentence explaining your choice.

Response to you as the interviewer.   Guarded? _____   Open? _____

Is the client able to maintain good eye contact?

continued

Barry Psychosocial Assessment *(continued)*

SEXUALITY-REPRODUCTIVE

Have you experienced any recent change in your sexual functioning? Yes _____ No _____

How? _____ For how long? _____

Do you associate your change in sexual functioning with some event in your life? _____

Do you think this illness could change your normal pattern of sexual functioning? _____

How? _____

Is this change in sexuality patterns related to:

_____ Ineffective coping

_____ Change or loss of body part

_____ Prenatal or postpartum changes

Changes in neurovegetative functioning related to depression

Explain:

Use focus assessment if necessary.

COPING–STRESS TOLERANCE

Level of Stress During Year Before Admission

How long have you been out of work with this illness? _____

Have you experienced any recent change in your job? _____

Have you been under any unusual job stress during the past year? _____

What was the cause?

_____ Retirement

_____ Fired

_____ Other. Explain:

_____ Same job, but new boss or working relationship

_____ Promotion or demotion

Do you expect the stress will be present when you return to work? _____

The preceding questions should be adapted for students to a school situation.

Have there been changes in your family during the last 2 years?

Which family members are involved? Include dates.

Death _____

Was this someone you were close to? _____

Divorce _____

Child leaving home _____

Cause? _____

Other _____

Has there been any other unusual stress during the last year that is still affecting you?

Describe:

Any unusual stress in your family?

Describe:

Barry Psychosocial Assessment *(continued)*

COPING–STRESS TOLERANCE *(continued)*

Normal Coping Ability

When you go through a very difficult time, how do you handle it?

_____ Talk it out with someone

_____ Drink

_____ Ignore it

_____ Become anxious

_____ Withdraw from others

_____ Become depressed

_____ Get angry and yell

_____ Get angry and clam up

_____ Get angry and hit or throw something

_____ Other (explain)

How often do you experience feelings of depression? _____

In the past, what is the longest period of time this feeling has lasted? _____

Have you felt depressed during the past few weeks?   Yes _____   No _____

To what do you attribute the cause? _____

If rape trauma is the cause of this admission do not explore the psychological reaction with the client until reading the report of the rape crisis counselor, who should have met with the client within an hour of arrival at the emergency department. Either follow the recommendations on the report for ongoing assessment or proceed with gentle questioning about current feelings.

What is the most serious trauma you have experienced? _____

What was the most difficult time you have experienced in your life? _____

How long did it take you to get over it? _____

What did you do to cope with it? _____

Potential for Self-Harm

This part of the assessment should be included if moderate to severe depression is present.

Have you ever thought of committing suicide?   Yes _____   No _____

If yes, continue on.

What would you do to end your life?   No plan _____   Plan _____

Describe:

What would prevent you from committing suicide? _____

Substances That May Be Used as Stress-Relievers

Smoking history

Do you smoke? _____   How long have you been smoking? _____ How many packs per day? _____

Alcohol use history

Do you drink? _____   How often? _____   How much? _____

Is there a history of alcoholism in your family? _____   Who? _____

Drug use

What prescribed medications are you currently using?

Name of medications _____

Dose or schedule _____ Prescribing physician _____

Are you currently using any other drugs?   Yes _____   No _____

What are they? _____

How long have you been using them? _____

What is the usual amount? _____ How often? _____

Have you ever been treated for substance abuse? _____

continued

Barry Psychosocial Assessment *(continued)*

VALUE-BELIEF

What is your religious affiliation? _____

Do you consider yourself active or inactive in practicing your religion? Active _____   Inactive _____

Is your religious leader a supportive person?   Yes _____   No _____

Explain:

What does this illness mean to you? _____

Are you experiencing spiritual distress?   Yes _____   No _____

Explain:

What would you consider to be the primary cause of this spiritual distress (actual, possible, or potential)?

_____ Inability to practice spiritual rituals   _____ Crisis of illness, suffering, or death

_____ Conflict between religious, spiritual, or cultural beliefs and   _____ Other (explain)
prescribed health regimen

Do you expect there will be any disparity in your caregivers' approach that could present a problem to you? _____

Any problems in the areas of

_____ Spiritual rituals   _____ Communication

_____ Cause of illness   _____ Problem solving

_____ Perception of illness and sick role   _____ Nutrition

_____ Health maintenance   _____ Family response

Explain:

How has this illness affected your relationship with God or the supreme being of your religion?

Explain:

The 11 functional health patterns were named by Marjorie Gordon (1987) in *Nursing diagnosis: Process and application,* New York: McGraw-Hill.

From Barry, P.D. (1989). *Psychosocial nursing: Assessment and intervention.* (2nd ed.) Philadelphia: Lippincott. Used with permission.

Modified Overt Aggression Scale

The Modified Overt Aggression Scale (MOAS) is a psychometric tool for determining the severity of aggression. The MOAS can be used to describe the nature and prevalence of aggression in an inpatient psychiatric population. The MOAS assesses four categories of aggression, including verbal aggression, aggression against property, autoaggression, and physical aggression.

Scoring is based on a five-point rating system that represents increasing levels of severity. Each section has a weighted score that reflects the overall severity of aggression (the higher the score, the more severe the aggression). The total score is determined by multiplying the four individual scales by their specific weights and then adding the four weighted scores.

Client's name _____ Sex _____ Date _____

Rater _____ Unit _____ Shift _____ Hosp. no. _____

Period of observation _____

Directions: For each category of aggressive behavior, check the highest applicable rating point to describe the most serious act of aggression committed by the client during the specified observation period.

Verbal aggression
Verbal hostility, such as statements or invectives that seek to inflict psychological harm on another through devaluation or degradation, and threats of physical attack.

0–No verbal aggression
1–Shouts angrily, curses mildly, or makes personal insults
2–Curses viciously, is severely insulting, has temper outbursts
3–Impulsively threatens violence toward others or self
4–Threatens violence toward others or self repeatedly or deliberately (such as to gain money or sex)

Autoaggression
Physical injury toward oneself, such as self-mutilation or suicide attempt.

0–No autoaggression
1–Picks or scratches skin, pulls out hair, hits self (without injury)
2–Bangs head, hits fists into walls, throws self on floor
3–Inflicts minor cuts, bruises, burns, or welts on self
4–Inflicts major injury on self or makes a suicide attempt

Aggression against property
Wanton and reckless destruction of unit paraphernalia or others' possessions.

0–No aggression against property
1–Slams door angrily, rips clothing, urinates on floor
2–Throws objects down, kicks furniture, defaces walls
3–Breaks objects, smashes windows
4–Sets fires, throws objects dangerously

Physical aggression
Violent action intended to inflict pain, bodily harm, or death upon another.

0–No physical aggression
1–Makes menacing gestures, swings at people, grabs at clothing
2–Strikes, kicks, pushes, scratches, pulls hair of others (without injury)
3–Attacks others, causing mild injury (such as bruises, sprains, or welts)
4–Attacks others, causing serious injury (such as fracture, loss of teeth, deep cuts, or loss of consciousness)

RATING SUMMARY

Scale	Scaled Score		Weighted Score
Verbal aggression	_____	× 1 =	_____
Aggression against property	_____	× 2 =	_____
Autoaggression	_____	× 3 =	_____
Physical aggression	_____	× 4 =	_____
			_____ Total weighted score

From Kay, S.R., et al. (1988). Profiles of aggression among psychiatric patients. *The Journal of Nervous and Mental Disease.* 176(9), 539-46. Used with permission.

ASSESSMENT TOOLS

Suicide Risk Assessment Tool

The following assessment tool was developed by the Los Angeles Suicide Prevention Center to help identify clients at risk for suicide. Scores are given in each of several categories, then totaled and averaged based on the number of categories rated. An average score of 1 or 2 indicates that the client is at low risk for suicide; a score of 3 to 6, at medium risk; and a score of 8 or 9, at high risk.

Name _____ Age _____ Sex _____ Date _____

Rater _____ Evaluation _____

	Low	Medium	High
	1 2	3 4 5 6	7 8 9

SUICIDE POTENTIAL

Age and sex _____   Resources _____   Total _____
Symptoms _____   Prior suicidal behavior _____
Stress _____   Medical status _____   Number of categories related _____
Acute vs. chronic _____   Communication aspects _____
Suicidal plan _____   Reaction of significant other _____   Average _____

Rating for Category (left column) / **Rating for Category** (right column)

Age and sex (1-9)   _____

Male
    50 plus (7-9)   _____
    35-49 (4-6)   _____
    15-34 (1-3)   _____
Female
    50 plus (5-7)   _____
    35-49 (3-5)   _____
    15-34 (1-3)   _____

Symptoms (1-9)   _____

Severe depression: sleep disorder, anorexia, weight loss, withdrawal, despondent, loss of interest, apathy (7-9)   _____

Feelings of hopelessness, helplessness, exhaustion (7-9)   _____

Delusions, hallucination, loss of contact, disorientation (6-8)   _____

Compulsive gambler (6-8)   _____

Disorganization, confusion, chaos (5-7)   _____

Alcoholism, drug addiction, homosexuality (4-7)   _____

Agitation, tension, anxiety (4-6)   _____

Guilt, shame, embarrassment (4-6)   _____

Feelings of rage, anger, hostility, revenge (4-6)   _____

Poor impulse control, poor judgment (4-6)   _____

Frustrated dependency (4-6)   _____

Other (describe):   _____

Stress (1-9)   _____

Loss of loved person by death, divorce, separation (5-9)   _____

Loss of job, money, prestige, status (4-8)   _____

Sickness, serious illness, surgery, accident, loss of limb (3-7)   _____

Threat of prosecution, criminal involvement, exposure (4-6)   _____

Stress (continued)

Change(s) in life, environment, setting (4-6)   _____

Success, promotion, increased responsibilities (2-5)   _____

No significant stress (1-3)   _____

Other (describe):   _____

Acute versus chronic (1-9)   _____

Sharp, noticeable, and sudden onset of specific symptoms (1-9)   _____

Recurrent outbreak of similar symptoms (4-9)   _____

Recent increase in long-standing traits (4-7)   _____

No specific recent change (1-4)   _____

Other (describe):   _____

Suicidal plan (1-9)   _____

Lethality of proposed method—gun, jump, hanging, drowning, knife, poison, pills, aspirin (1-9)   _____

Availability of means in proposed method (1-9)   _____

Specific detail and clarity in organization of plan (1-9)   _____

Specificity in time planned (1-9)   _____

Bizarre plans (4-6)   _____

Rating of previous suicide attempts(s) (1-9)   _____

No plans (1-3)   _____

Other (describe):   _____

Resources (1-9)   _____

No sources of support (family, friends, agencies, employment) (7-9)   _____

Family and friends available, unwilling to help (4-7)   _____

Financial problem (4-7)   _____

Available professional help, agency, or therapist (2-4)   _____

Suicide Risk Assessment Tool *(continued)*

	Rating for Category *(continued)*		Rating for Category *(continued)*

Resources *(continued)*

Family or friends willing to help (1-3) _____

Stable life history (1-3) _____

Physician or clergy available (1-3) _____

Employed (1-3) _____

Finances no problem (1-3) _____

Other (describe): _____

Prior suicidal behavior (1-7) _____

One or more prior attempts of high lethality (6-7) _____

One or more prior attempts of low lethality (4-5) _____

History of repeated threats and depression (3-5) _____

No prior suicidal or depressed history (1-3) _____

Other (describe): _____

Medical status (1-7) _____

Chronic debilitating illness (5-7) _____

Pattern of failure in previous therapy (4-6) _____

Many repeated unsuccessful experiences with doctors (4-6) _____

Psychosomatic illness (such as asthma, ulcer) (2-4) _____

Chronic minor illness complaints, hypochondria (1-3) _____

No medical problems (1-2) _____

Other (describe): _____

Communication aspects (1-7) _____

Communication broken with rejection of efforts to reestablish by both client and others (5-7) _____

Communications have internalized goal (such as to cause guilt in others or to force behavior) (2-4) _____

Communications directed toward world and people in general (3-5) _____

Communications directed toward one or more specific persons (1-3) _____

Other (describe): _____

Reaction of significant other (1-7) _____

Defensive, paranoid, rejected, punishing attitude (5-7) _____

Denial of own or client's need for help (5-7) _____

No feelings of concern about the client; does not understand the client (4-6) _____

Indecisiveness, feelings of helplessness (3-5) _____

Alternation between feelings of anger and rejection and feelings of responsibility and desire to help (2-4) _____

Sympathy and concern plus admission of need for help (1-3) _____

Other (describe): _____

From Los Angeles Suicide Prevention Center. *Assessment of Suicidal Potentiality.* Los Angeles, The Center. Used with permission.

Appendices and Index

Appendix A: *DSM III-R* Classification— Axes I and II Categories and Codes

Disorders Usually First Evident in Infancy, Childhood, or Adolescence

DEVELOPMENTAL DISORDERS

Note: These are coded on Axis II.

Mental Retardation
317.00   Mild mental retardation
318.00   Moderate mental retardation
318.10   Severe mental retardation
318.20   Profound mental retardation
319.00   Unspecified mental retardation

Pervasive Developmental Disorders
299.00   Autistic disorder
      Specify if childhood onset
299.80   Pervasive developmental disorder not otherwise specified (NOS)

Specific Developmental Disorders
      Academic skills disorders
315.10   Developmental arithmetic disorder
315.80   Developmental expressive writing disorder
315.00   Developmental reading disorder
      Language and speech disorders
315.39   Developmental articulation disorder
315.31   Developmental expressive language disorder
315.31   Developmental receptive language disorder
      Motor skills disorder
315.40   Developmental coordination disorder
315.90   Specific developmental disorder NOS

Other Developmental Disorders
315.90   Developmental disorder NOS

Disruptive Behavior Disorders
314.01   Attention-deficit hyperactivity disorder
      Conduct disorder,
312.10   group type
312.00   solitary aggressive type
312.90   undifferentiated type
313.81   Oppositional defiant disorder

Anxiety Disorders of Childhood or Adolescence
309.21   Separation anxiety disorder
313.21   Avoidant disorder of childhood or adolescence
313.00   Overanxious disorder

Eating Disorders
307.10   Anorexia nervosa
307.51   Bulimia nervosa
307.52   Pica
307.53   Rumination disorder of infancy
307.50   Eating disorder NOS

Gender Identity Disorders
302.60   Gender identity disorder of childhood
302.50   Transsexualism
      Specify sexual history: asexual, homosexual, heterosexual, unspecified
302.85   Gender identity disorder of adolescence or adulthood, nontranssexual type
      Specify sexual history: asexual, homosexual, heterosexual, unspecified
302.85   Gender identity disorder NOS

Tic Disorders
307.23   Tourette's disorder
307.22   Chronic motor or vocal tic disorder
307.21   Transient tic disorder
      Specify: single episode or recurrent
307.20   Tic disorder NOS

Elimination Disorders
307.70   Functional encopresis
      Specify: primary or secondary type
307.60   Functional enuresis
      Specify: primary or secondary type
      Specify: nocturnal only, diurnal only, nocturnal and diurnal

Speech Disorders Not Elsewhere Classified
307.00   Cluttering
307.00   Stuttering

Other Disorders of Infancy, Childhood, or Adolescence
313.23   Elective mutism
313.82   Identity disorder
313.89   Reactive attachment disorder of infancy or early childhood
307.30   Stereotypy/habit disorder
314.00   Undifferentiated attention-deficit disorder

ORGANIC MENTAL DISORDERS

Dementias Arising in the Senium and Presenium
      Primary degenerative dementia of the Alzheimer type, senile onset,
290.30   with delirium
290.20   with delusions
290.21   with depression
290.00   uncomplicated
      (Note: code 331.00 Alzheimer's disease on Axis III)
Code in fifth digit: 1= with delirium, 2= with delusions, 3= with depression, 0= uncomplicated
290.1x   Primary degenerative dementia of the Alzheimer type, presenile onset, _____
      (Note: code 331.00 Alzheimer's disease on Axis III)
290.4x   Multi-infarct dementia, _____
290.00   Senile dementia NOS
      Specify etiology on Axis III if known
290.10   Presenile dementia NOS
      Specify etiology on Axis III if known (e.g., Pick's disease, Jakob-Creutzfeldt disease)

Psychoactive Substance-Induced Organic Mental Disorders
      Alcohol
303.00   intoxication
291.40   idiosyncratic intoxication
291.80   Uncomplicated alcohol withdrawal
291.00   withdrawal delirium
291.30   hallucinosis
291.10   amnestic disorder
291.20   Dementia associated with alcoholism

      Amphetamine or similarly acting sympathomimetic
305.70   intoxication
292.00   withdrawal
292.81   delirium
292.11   delusional disorder
      Caffeine
305.90   intoxication

continued

DSM III-R Classification—Axes I and II Categories and Codes *(continued)*

Cannabis
305.20	intoxication
292.11	delusional disorder

Cocaine
305.60	intoxication
292.00	withdrawal
292.81	delirium
292.11	delusional disorder

Hallucinogen
305.30	hallucinosis
292.11	delusional disorder
292.84	mood disorder
292.89	Posthallucinogen perception disorder

Inhalant
305.90	intoxication

Nicotine
292.00	withdrawal

Opioid
305.50	intoxication
292.00	withdrawal

Phencyclidine (PCP) or similarly acting arylcyclohexylamine
305.90	intoxication
292.81	delirium
292.11	delusional disorder
292.84	mood disorder
292.90	organic mental disorder NOS

Sedative, hypnotic, or anxiolytic
305.40	intoxication
292.00	Uncomplicated sedative, hypnotic, or anxiolytic withdrawal
292.00	withdrawal delirium
292.83	amnestic disorder

Other or unspecified psychoactive substance
305.90	intoxication
292.00	withdrawal
292.81	delirium
292.82	dementia
292.83	amnestic disorder
292.11	delusional disorder
292.12	hallucinosis
292.84	mood disorder
292.89	anxiety disorder
292.89	personality disorder
292.90	organic mental disorder NOS

Organic Mental Disorders associated with Axis III physical disorders or conditions, or whose etiology is unknown.

293.00	Delirium
294.10	Dementia
294.00	Amnestic disorder
293.81	Organic delusional disorder
293.82	Organic hallucinosis
293.83	Organic mood disorder
	Specify: manic, depressed, mixed
294.80	Organic anxiety disorder
310.10	Organic personality disorder
	Specify if explosive type
294.80	Organic mental disorder NOS

PSYCHOACTIVE SUBSTANCE USE DISORDERS

Alcohol
303.90	dependence
305.00	abuse

Amphetamine or similarly acting sympathomimetic
304.40	dependence
305.70	abuse

Cannabis
304.30	dependence
305.20	abuse

Cocaine
304.20	dependence
305.60	abuse

Hallucinogen
304.50	dependence
305.30	abuse

Inhalant
304.60	dependence
305.90	abuse

Nicotine
305.10	dependence

Opioid
304.00	dependence
305.50	abuse

Phencyclidine (PCP) or similarly acting arylcyclohexylamine
304.50	dependence
305.90	abuse
304.90	Polysubstance dependence
304.90	Psychoactive substance dependence NOS
305.90	Psychoactive substance abuse NOS

SCHIZOPHRENIA

Code in fifth digit: 1=subchronic, 2=chronic, 3=subchronic with acute exacerbation, 4=chronic with acute exacerbation, 5=in remission, 0=unspecified.

Schizophrenia,
295.2x	catatonic, _____
295.1x	disorganized, _____
295.3x	paranoid, _____
	Specify if stable type
295.9x	undifferentiated, _____
295.6x	residual, _____
	Specify if late onset

DELUSIONAL (PARANOID) DISORDER

297.10	Delusional (Paranoid) disorder
	Specify type: erotomanic, grandiose, jealous, persecutory, somatic, unspecified

PSYCHOTIC DISORDERS NOT ELSEWHERE CLASSIFIED

298.80	Brief reactive psychosis
295.40	Schizophreniform disorder
	Specify: without good prognostic features or with good prognostic features
295.70	Schizoaffective disorder
	Specify: bipolar type or depressive type
297.30	Induced psychotic disorder
298.90	Psychotic disorder NOS (Atypical psychosis)

DSM *III-R* Classification—Axes I and II Categories and Codes *(continued)*

MOOD DISORDERS

Code current state of Major Depression and Bipolar Disorder in fifth digit: 1 = mild, 2 = moderate, 3 = severe, without psychotic features, 4 = with psychotic features (specify mood-congruent or mood-incongruent), 5 = in partial remission, 6 = in full remission, 0 = unspecified

For major depressive episodes, specify if chronic and specify if melancholic type.

For Bipolar Disorder, Bipolar Disorder NOS, Recurrent Major Depression, and Depressive Disorder NOS, specify if seasonal pattern.

Bipolar Disorders

	Bipolar disorder,
296.6x	mixed, _____
296.4x	manic, _____
296.5x	depressed, _____
301.13	Cyclothymia
296.70	Bipolar disorder NOS

Depressive Disorders

	Major Depression,
296.2x	single episode, _____
296.3x	recurrent, _____
300.40	Dysthymia (or Depressive neurosis)
	Specify: primary or secondary type
	Specify: early or late onset
311.00	Depressive disorder NOS

ANXIETY DISORDERS (or Anxiety and Phobic Neuroses)

	Panic disorder
300.21	with agoraphobia
	Specify current severity of agoraphobic avoidance
	Specify current severity of panic attacks
300.01	without agoraphobia
	Specify current severity of panic attacks
300.22	Agoraphobia without history of panic disorder
	Specify with or without limited symptom attacks
300.23	Social phobia
	Specify if generalized type
300.29	Simple phobia
300.30	Obsessive compulsive disorder (or Obsessive compulsive neurosis)
309.89	Post-traumatic stress disorder
	Specify if delayed onset
300.02	Generalized anxiety disorder
300.00	Anxiety disorder NOS

SOMATOFORM DISORDERS

300.70	Body dysmorphic disorder
300.11	Conversion disorder (or Hysterical neurosis, conversion type)
	Specify: single episode or recurrent
300.70	Hypochondriasis (or Hypochondriacal neurosis)
300.81	Somatization disorder
307.80	Somatoform pain disorder
300.70	Undifferentiated somatoform disorder
300.70	Somatoform disorder NOS

DISSOCIATIVE DISORDERS (or Hysterical Neuroses, Dissociative Type)

300.14	Multiple personality disorder
300.13	Psychogenic fugue
300.12	Psychogenic amnesia
300.60	Depersonalization disorder (or Depersonalization neurosis)
300.15	Dissociative disorder NOS

SEXUAL DISORDERS

Paraphilias

302.40	Exhibitionism
302.81	Fetishism
302.89	Frotteurism
302.20	Pedophilia
	Specify: same sex, opposite sex, same and opposite sex
	Specify if limited to incest
	Specify: exclusive type or nonexclusive type
302.83	Sexual masochism
302.84	Sexual sadism
302.30	Transvestic fetishism
302.82	Voyeurism
302.90	Paraphilia NOS

Sexual Dysfunctions

Specify: psychogenic only, or psychogenic and biogenic (Note: If biogenic only, code on Axis III)
Specify: lifelong or acquired
Specify: generalized or situational

	Sexual desire disorders
302.71	Hypoactive sexual desire disorder
302.79	Sexual aversion disorder
	Sexual arousal disorders
302.72	Female sexual arousal disorder
302.72	Male erectile disorder
	Orgasm disorders
302.73	Inhibited female orgasm
302.74	Inhibited male orgasm
302.75	Premature ejaculation
	Sexual pain disorders
302.76	Dyspareunia
306.51	Vaginismus
302.70	Sexual dysfunction NOS

Other Sexual Disorders

302.90	Sexual disorder NOS

SLEEP DISORDERS

Dyssomnias

	Insomnia disorder
307.42	related to another mental disorder (nonorganic)
780.50	related to known organic factor
307.42	Primary insomnia
	Hypersomnia disorder
307.44	related to another mental disorder (nonorganic)
780.50	related to a known organic factor
780.54	Primary hypersomnia
307.45	Sleep-wake schedule disorder
	Specify: advanced or delayed phase type, disorganized type, frequently changing type
	Other dyssomnias
307.40	Dyssomnia NOS

Parasomnias

307.47	Dream anxiety disorder (Nightmare disorder)
307.46	Sleep terror disorder
307.46	Sleepwalking disorder
307.40	Parasomnia NOS

FACTITIOUS DISORDERS

	Factitious disorder
301.51	with physical symptoms
300.16	with psychological symptoms
300.19	Factitious disorder NOS

continued

DSM III-R Classification—Axes I and II Categories and Codes *(continued)*

IMPULSE CONTROL DISORDERS NOT ELSEWHERE CLASSIFIED

312.34	Intermittent explosive disorder
312.32	Kleptomania
312.31	Pathological gambling
312.33	Pyromania
312.39	Trichotillomania
312.39	Impulse control disorder NOS

ADJUSTMENT DISORDER

Adjustment disorder

309.24	with anxious mood
309.00	with depressed mood
309.30	with disturbance of conduct
309.40	with mixed disturbance of emotions and conduct
309.28	with mixed emotional features
309.82	with physical complaints
309.83	with withdrawal
309.23	with work (or academic) inhibition
309.90	Adjustment disorder NOS

PSYCHOLOGICAL FACTORS AFFECTING PHYSICAL CONDITION

316.00	Psychological factors affecting physical condition

Specify physical condition on Axis III

PERSONALITY DISORDERS

Note: These are coded on Axis II.

Cluster A

301.00	Paranoid
301.20	Schizoid
301.22	Schizotypal

Cluster B

301.70	Antisocial
301.83	Borderline
301.50	Histrionic
301.81	Narcissistic

Cluster C

301.82	Avoidant
301.60	Dependent
301.40	Obsessive compulsive
301.84	Passive aggressive
301.90	Personality disorder NOS

V CODES FOR CONDITIONS NOT ATTRIBUTABLE TO A MENTAL DISORDER THAT ARE A FOCUS OF ATTENTION OR TREATMENT

V62.30	Academic problem
V71.01	Adult antisocial behavior
F40.00	Borderline intellectual functioning (Note: This is coded on Axis II.)
V71.02	Childhood or adolescent antisocial behavior
V65.20	Malingering
V61.10	Marital problem
V15.81	Noncompliance with medical treatment
V62.20	Occupational problem
V61.20	Parent-child problem
V62.81	Other interpersonal problem
V61.80	Other specified family circumstances
V62.89	Phase of life problem or other life circumstance-problem
V62.82	Uncomplicated bereavement

ADDITIONAL CODES

300.90	Unspecified mental disorder (nonpsychotic)
V71.09	No diagnosis or condition on Axis I
799.90	Diagnosis or condition deferred on Axis I

Appendix B: NANDA Diagnostic Categories Arranged by Gordon's Functional Health Patterns

Below is a list of the North American Nursing Diagnosis Association's (NANDA) approved diagnostic categories arranged according to Gordon's functional health patterns.

Health-Perception–Health-Management Pattern
Altered health maintenance
Health-seeking behaviors (specify)
Ineffective management of therapeutic regimen (individual)*
Noncompliance (specify)
High risk for infection
High risk for injury
High risk for poisoning
High risk for trauma
High risk for aspiration
High risk for disuse syndrome
High risk for suffocation
Altered protection

Nutritional-Metabolic Pattern
Altered nutrition: high risk for more than body requirements
Altered nutrition: more than body requirements
Altered nutrition: less than body requirements
Ineffective breast-feeding
Interrupted breast-feeding*
Effective breast-feeding
Ineffective infant feeding pattern*
Impaired swallowing
High risk for aspiration
Altered oral mucous membrane
High risk for fluid volume deficit
Fluid volume deficit
Fluid volume excess
High risk for impaired skin integrity
Impaired skin integrity
Impaired tissue integrity
High risk for altered body temperature
Ineffective thermoregulation
Hyperthermia
Hypothermia

Elimination Pattern
Constipation
Colonic constipation
Perceived constipation
Diarrhea
Bowel incontinence
Altered urinary elimination pattern
Functional incontinence
Reflex incontinence
Stress incontinence
Urge incontinence
Total incontinence
Urinary retention

Activity-Exercise Pattern
High risk for activity intolerance
Activity intolerance (specify level)
Fatigue
Impaired physical mobility (specify level)
High risk for peripheral neurovascular dysfunction*
High risk for disuse syndrome
Total self-care deficit (specify level)
Bathing or hygiene self-care deficit (specify level)
Dressing or grooming self-care deficit (specify level)
Feeding self-care deficit (specify level)
Toileting self-care deficit (specify level)
Diversional activity deficit
Impaired home maintenance management
   (mild, moderate, severe, potential, chronic)
Ineffective airway clearance

Ineffective breathing pattern
Inability to sustain spontaneous ventilation*
Dysfunctional ventilatory weaning response*
Impaired gas exchange
Decreased cardiac output
Altered tissue perfusion (specify)
Dysreflexia
Altered growth and development

Sleep-Rest Pattern
Sleep-pattern disturbance

Cognitive-Perceptual Pattern
Pain
Chronic pain
Sensory or perceptual alterations (specify visual, auditory, kinesthetic, gustatory, tactile, olfactory)
Unilateral neglect
Knowledge deficit (specify)
Altered thought processes
Decisional conflict (specify)

Self-Perception–Self-Concept Pattern
Fear
Anxiety
Hopelessness
Powerlessness
Self-esteem disturbance
Chronic low self-esteem
Situational low self-esteem
Body-image disturbance
Personal identity disturbance

Role-Relationship Pattern
Anticipatory grieving
Dysfunctional grieving
Altered role performance
Social isolation
Impaired social interaction
Altered family processes
High risk for altered parenting
Altered parenting
Parental role conflict
Impaired verbal communication
High risk for violence: self-directed or directed at others
Caregiver role strain*
High risk for caregiver role strain*

Sexuality-Reproductive Pattern
Sexual dysfunction
Altered sexuality patterns
Rape-trauma syndrome
Rape-trauma syndrome: compound reaction
Rape-trauma syndrome: silent reaction

Coping–Stress-Tolerance Pattern
Ineffective individual coping
Defensive coping
Ineffective denial
Impaired adjustment
Relocation stress syndrome*
High risk for self-mutilation*
Post-trauma response
Family coping: potential for growth
Ineffective family coping: compromised
Ineffective family coping: disabling

Value-Belief Pattern
Spiritual distress (distress of human spirit)

*Adopted summer 1992

Adapted from Gordon, M. (1991). *Manual of Nursing Diagnosis: 1991-1992*. St. Louis: Mosby-Year Book. Used with permission.

Appendix C: Psychiatric Nursing Taxonomy

The following classification is based on the work of the Phenomenon Task Force and the Advisory Panel on Classifications for Nursing Practice of the American Nurses' Association. The psychiatric nursing diagnostic categories listed here are among those diagnoses proposed for review by the North American Nursing Diagnosis Association in April 1992.

01. Human Response Patterns in Activity Processes

01.01 Altered motor behavior
  01.01.01 Bizarre motor behavior
  01.01.02 Catatonia
  01.01.03 Impaired coordination
  01.01.04 Hyperactivity
  01.01.05 Hypoactivity
  01.01.06 Muscular rigidity
  01.01.07 Psychomotor retardation

01.02 Altered recreation patterns
  01.02.01 Inadequate diversional activity

01.03 Altered self-care
  01.03.01 Altered eating
  *01.03.02 Altered grooming
  01.03.03 Altered health maintenance
  *01.03.04 Altered hygiene
  01.03.05 Altered participation in health care
  *01.03.06 Altered toileting

01.04 Altered sleep/arousal patterns
  01.04.01 Difficult transition to and from sleep
  01.04.02 Hypersomnia
  01.04.03 Insomnia
  01.04.04 Nightmares
  01.04.05 Somnolence

01.97 Undeveloped activity processes

01.98 Altered activity processes not otherwise specified

01.99 Potential for altered activity processes

02. Human Response Patterns in Cognition Processes

02.01 Altered decision making

02.02 Altered judgment

*02.03 Altered knowledge processes
  02.03.01 Agnosia
  02.03.02 Altered intellectual functioning
  *02.03.03 Knowledge deficit

02.04 Altered learning processes

02.05 Altered memory
  02.05.01 Amnesia
  02.05.02 Distorted memory
  02.05.03 Long-term memory loss
  02.05.04 Short-term memory loss

02.06 Altered orientation
  02.06.01 Confusion
  02.06.02 Delirium
  02.06.03 Disorientation

02.07 Altered thought content
  02.07.01 Delusions
  02.07.02 Ideas of reference
  02.07.03 Magical thinking
  02.07.04 Obsessions

*02.08 Altered thought processes
  02.08.01 Altered abstract thinking
  02.08.02 Altered concentration
  02.08.03 Altered problem solving
  02.08.04 Thought insertion

02.97 Undeveloped cognition processes

02.98 Altered cognition processes not otherwise specified

02.99 Potential for altered cognition processes

03. Human Response Patterns in Ecological Processes

03.01 Altered community maintenance
  03.01.01 Community safety hazards
  03.01.02 Community sanitation hazards

03.02 Altered environmental integrity

*03.03 Altered home maintenance
  03.03.01 Home safety hazards
  03.03.02 Home sanitation hazards

04. Human Response Patterns in Emotional Processes

04.01 Abuse response patterns
  *04.01.01 Rape-trauma syndrome
04.02 Altered feeling patterns
  04.02.01 Anger
  *04.02.02 Anxiety
  04.02.03 Elation
  04.02.04 Envy
  *04.02.05 Fear
  *04.02.06 Grief
  04.02.07 Guilt
  04.02.08 Sadness
  04.02.09 Shame

04.03 Undifferentiated feeling pattern

04.97 Undeveloped emotional responses

04.98 Altered emotional processes not otherwise specified

04.99 Potential for altered emotional processes

05. Human Response Patterns in Interpersonal Processes

*05.01 Altered communication processes
  05.01.01 Altered nonverbal communication
  *05.01.02 Altered verbal communication

05.02 Altered conduct/impulse processes
  05.02.01 Aggressive/violent behaviors
    05.02.01.01 Aggressive/violent behaviors toward environment
    05.02.01.02 Aggressive/violent behaviors toward others
    05.02.01.03 Aggressive/violent behaviors toward self
  05.02.02 Dysfunctional behaviors
    05.02.02.01 Age-inappropriate behaviors
    05.02.02.02 Bizarre behaviors
    05.02.02.03 Compulsive behaviors
    05.02.02.04 Disorganized behaviors
    05.02.02.05 Unpredictable behaviors

05.03 Altered role performance
  05.03.01 Altered family role
  05.03.02 Altered leisure role
  *05.03.03 Altered parenting role
  05.03.04 Altered play role
  05.03.05 Altered student role
  05.03.06 Altered work role

05.04 Altered sexuality processes

05.05 Altered social interaction
  05.05.01 Social intrusiveness
  *05.05.02 Social isolation/withdrawal

05.97 Undeveloped interpersonal processes

05.98 Altered interpersonal processes not otherwise specified

05.99 Potential for altered interpersonal processes
  *05.99.01 Potential for violence

Psychiatric Nursing Taxonomy *(continued)*

06. Human Response Patterns in Perception Processes

06.01 Altered attention
  06.01.01 Distractibility
  06.01.02 Hyperalertness
  06.01.03 Inattention
  06.01.04 Selective attention

*06.02 Altered comfort patterns
  06.02.01 Discomfort
  06.02.02 Distress
  *06.02.03 Pain

06.03 Altered self-concept
  *06.03.01 Altered body image
  06.03.02 Altered gender identity
  *06.03.03 Altered personal identity
  *06.03.04 Altered self-esteem
  06.03.05 Altered social identity
  06.03.06 Undeveloped self-concept

06.04 Altered sensory perception
  *06.04.01 Auditory
  *06.04.02 Gustatory
  06.04.03 Hallucinations
  06.04.04 Illusions
  *06.04.05 Kinesthetic
  *06.04.06 Olfactory
  *06.04.07 Tactile
  *06.04.08 Visual

06.97 Undeveloped perception processes

06.98 Altered perception processes not otherwise specified

06.99 Potential for altered perception processes

07. Human Response Patterns in Physiological Processes

07.01 Altered circulation processes
  07.01.01 Altered vascular circulation
    *07.01.01.01 Tissue perfusion
    *07.01.01.02 Altered fluid volume
  07.01.02 Altered cardiac circulation

07.02 Altered elimination processes
  *07.02.01 Altered bowel elimination
    *07.02.01.01 Constipation
    *07.02.01.02 Diarrhea
    *07.02.01.03 Incontinence
    07.02.01.04 Encopresis
  *07.02.02 Altered urinary elimination
    *07.02.02.01 Incontinence
    *07.02.02.02 Retention
    07.02.02.03 Enuresis
  07.02.03 Altered skin elimination

07.03 Altered endocrine/metabolic processes
  07.03.01 Altered growth
  07.03.02 Altered hormone regulation
    07.03.02.01 Premenstrual stress syndrome

07.04 Altered gastrointestinal processes
  07.04.01 Altered absorption
  07.04.02 Altered digestion

07.05 Altered neuro/sensory processes
  07.05.01 Altered levels of consciousness
  07.05.02 Altered sensory acuity
  07.05.03 Altered sensory processing
  07.05.04 Altered sensory integration
    07.05.04.01 Learning disabilities

07.06 Altered nutrition processes
  07.06.01 Altered cellular processes
  07.06.02 Altered systemic processes
    *07.06.02.01 More than body requirements
    *07.06.02.02 Less than body requirements
  07.06.03 Altered eating processes
    07.06.03.01 Anorexia
    07.06.03.02 Pica

07.07 Altered oxygenation processes
  07.07.01 Altered respiration
    07.07.01.01 Altered gas exchange
    *07.07.01.02 Ineffective airway clearance
    *07.07.01.03 Ineffective breathing pattern

07.08 Altered physical integrity processes
  *07.08.01 Altered skin integrity
  *07.08.02 Altered tissue integrity

07.09 Altered physical regulation processes
  07.09.01 Altered immune responses
    07.09.01.01 Infection

07.10 Altered body temperature
  *07.10.01 Hypothermia
  *07.10.02 Hyperthermia
  *07.10.03 Ineffective thermoregulation

07.97 Undeveloped physiological processes

07.98 Altered physiological processes not otherwise specified

07.99 Potential for altered physiological processes

08. Human Response Patterns in Valuation Processes

*08.01 Altered meaningfulness
  *08.01.01 Hopelessness
  08.01.02 Helplessness
  08.01.03 Loneliness
  *08.01.04 Powerlessness

08.02 Altered spirituality
  *08.02.01 Spiritual distress
  08.02.02 Spiritual despair

08.03 Altered values
  08.03.01 Conflict with social order
  08.03.02 Inability to internalize values
  08.03.03 Unclarified values

08.97 Undeveloped valuation processes

08.98 Altered valuation processes not otherwise specified

08.99 Potential for altered valuation processes

---

* NANDA-approved diagnostic category

Adapted from Loomis, M., O'Toole, A.O., Pothier, P., West, P., Wilson, H., and the American Nurses' Association Phenomenon Task Force. (1987). *Classification of human responses of concern for psychiatric-mental health nursing practice.* Used with permission.

Appendix D: Recommended Laboratory Tests in Long-term Drug Therapy

Long-term use of drugs can cause physiologic abnormalities best detected by laboratory tests. This chart lists recommended laboratory tests during therapy with selected psychotropic drugs. The drugs are grouped according to primary therapeutic use.

Drug	Laboratory tests	Rationale	Special considerations
Anticonvulsants			
carbamazepine (Tegretol)	CBC, platelet count	To detect aplastic anemia or agranulocytosis	Establish baseline and monitor routinely; incidence of aplastic anemia is low. Transient decreases in platelet and leukocyte counts are common and usually don't signal an impending problem.
	Liver function tests	To detect hepatotoxicity	Establish baseline and repeat periodically. Hepatotoxicity may occur after prolonged use.
	Urinalysis, blood urea nitrogen (BUN)	To detect nephrotoxicity	Establish baseline and repeat periodically.
	Ophthalmologic examinations (fundoscopy, slit-lamp, and tonometry)	To detect adverse ophthalmologic effects, including glaucoma	Drug has mild anticholinergic effects and may elevate intraocular pressure.
clonazepam (Klonopin)	Liver function tests	To detect hepatotoxicity	Transient elevations of serum aminotransferase and alkaline phosphatase may occur.
	Ophthalmologic tests	To detect glaucoma	Contraindicated in acute angle-closure glaucoma; establish baseline screening to identify undiagnosed glaucoma.
	Renal function tests	To detect nephrotoxicity	Renal problems are relatively rare with prolonged use.
	Blood counts	To detect blood dyscrasias	A few cases of leukopenia and aplastic anemia reported with other benzodiazepines.
clorazepate (Tranxene)	CBC, platelet count	To detect blood dyscrasias	Relatively rare; establish baseline and repeat periodically.
	Liver function tests	To detect hepatotoxicity	Establish baseline and repeat periodically; elevated aspartate aminotransferase (AST), alanine aminotransferase (ALT), lactate dehydrogenase, and total and direct bilirubin has occurred with benzodiazepines.
	Kidney function tests	To detect nephrotoxicity	Establish baseline and repeat periodically.
ethosuximide (Zarontin)	CBC, platelet count	To detect blood dyscrasias	May produce direct positive Coomb's test or systemic lupus erythematosus.
	Urinalysis	To detect nephrotoxicity	Establish baseline and repeat periodically.
	Liver function tests	To detect hepatotoxicity	Establish baseline and repeat periodically. Hepatotoxicity may occur after prolonged use.

Recommended Laboratory Tests in Long-term Drug Therapy *(continued)*

Drug	Laboratory tests	Rationale	Special considerations
Anticonvulsants *(continued)*			
ethotoin (Peganone)	CBC, platelet count	To detect blood dyscrasias	Reversible lymphadenopathy has been reported.
	Liver function tests	To detect hepatotoxicity	Establish baseline and repeat periodically. Hepatotoxicity may occur after prolonged use.
mephenytoin (Mesantoin)	CBC, platelet count	To detect blood dyscrasias	Higher incidence than some other anticonvulsants; establish baseline, repeat after 2 weeks of initial therapy, then after 2 weeks of maintainance. Repeat monthly for first year then at 3-month intervals.
	Liver function tests	To detect hepatotoxicity	Establish baseline and repeat periodically. Hepatotoxicity may occur after prolonged use.
mephobarbital (Mebaral)	CBC, platelet count	To detect blood dyscrasias	Establish baseline and repeat periodically.
methsuximide (Celontin)	CBC, platelet count	To detect blood dyscrasias	Establish baseline and repeat periodically.
	Liver function tests	To detect hepatotoxicity	Establish baseline and repeat periodically. Hepatotoxicity may occur after prolonged use.
	Urinalysis	To detect nephrotoxicity	Establish baseline and repeat periodically.
paramethadione (Paradione)	CBC, platelet count	To detect blood dyscrasias	Higher incidence of blood dyscrasias than some other anticonvulsants; establish baseline and repeat monthly for the first year.
	Urinalysis	To detect nephrotoxicity	Establish baseline and repeat monthly for the first year.
	Liver function tests	To detect hepatotoxicity	Establish baseline and repeat monthly for the first year.
phenacemide (Phenurone)	CBC, platelet count	To detect blood dyscrasias	Establish baseline then repeat monthly for first year; reduce frequency if no problems detected after 1 year.
	Urinalysis	To detect nephrotoxicity	Establish baseline and repeat periodically.
	Liver function tests	To detect hepatotoxicity	Establish baseline and repeat monthly.
phenobarbital (Barbita)	CBC, platelet count	To detect blood dyscrasias	Establish baseline and repeat periodically.
phensuximide (Milontin)	CBC, platelet count	To detect blood dyscrasias	Establish baseline and repeat periodically.
	Urinalysis	To detect nephrotoxicity	Establish baseline and repeat periodically.
	Liver function tests	To detect hepatotoxicity	Establish baseline and repeat periodically. Hepatotoxicity may occur after prolonged use.

continued

Recommended Laboratory Tests in Long-term Drug Therapy *(continued)*

Drug	Laboratory tests	Rationale	Special considerations
Anticonvulsants *(continued)*			
phenytoin (Dilantin)	CBC, platelet count	To detect blood dyscrasias	Macrocytosis and megaloblastic anemia may respond to folic acid therapy. May be associated with lymphoma.
	Liver function tests	To detect hepatotoxicity	Establish baseline and repeat periodically. Hepatotoxicity may occur after prolonged use.
	Renal function studies	To prevent toxicity	Higher incidence of glycosuria and hyperglycemia in clients with renal impairment.
primidone (Mysoline)	CBC, platelet count	To detect blood dyscrasias	Establish CBC and SMA 12 every 6 months.
	Liver function tests	To detect hepatotoxicity	Establish baseline and repeat periodically. Hepatotoxicity may occur after prolonged use.
trimethadione (Tridione)	CBC, platelet count	To detect blood dyscrasias	Higher incidence than some other anticonvulsants; establish baseline and repeat monthly for the first year.
	Urinalysis	To detect nephrotoxicity	Establish baseline and repeat monthly for the first year.
	Liver function tests	To detect hepatotoxicity	Establish baseline and repeat monthly for the first year.
	Ophthalmologic examinations	To detect hemeralopia or other visual disturbances	Discontinue if scotomata is detected.
valproic acid (Depakene)	Liver function tests	To detect hepatotoxicity	Establish baseline and repeat frequently, especially during first 6 months. May be dose-related. Higher incidence of fatal hepatotoxicity in children under age 2. Hepatotoxic effects not always preceded by abnormal liver function tests.
	Platelet count, bleeding time, coagulation studies	To detect clotting abnormalities	Some clinicians recommend thromboelastography as the most reliable assessment of drug effects on coagulation.
	Liver function tests	To detect hepatotoxicity	Establish baseline and repeat periodically. Hepatotoxicity may occur after prolonged use.
Antidepressants			
amitriptyline (Elavil)	Liver function tests	To detect hepatotoxicity	Establish baseline and repeat periodically.
	Blood counts	To detect blood dyscrasias	Establish baseline and repeat periodically, especially in symptomatic clients.
	Electrocardiogram (ECG)	To detect cardiotoxicity	Establish baseline and repeat periodically, especially in clients receiving high doses.
	Ophthalmologic examinations, including tonometry	To detect glaucoma	Anticholinergic effects may exacerbate glaucoma.

Recommended Laboratory Tests in Long-term Drug Therapy *(continued)*

Drug	Laboratory tests	Rationale	Special considerations
Antidepressants *(continued)*			
amoxapine (Asendin)	Liver function tests	To detect hepatotoxicity	Establish baseline and repeat periodically; asymptomatic elevations of transaminase and alkaline phosphatase levels, which can progress to signs of hepatic failure, have occurred in clients receiving TCAs.
	Blood counts	To detect blood dyscrasias	Establish baseline and repeat periodically, especially in symptomatic clients.
	ECG	To detect cardiotoxicity	Establish baseline and repeat periodically, especially in clients receiving high doses.
	Ophthalmologic examinations, including tonometry	To detect glaucoma	Anticholinergic effects may exacerbate glaucoma.
bupropion (Wellbutrin)	Blood counts	To detect blood dyscrasias	Establish baseline and repeat periodically, especially in symptomatic clients.
	ECG	To detect cardiotoxicity	Establish baseline and repeat periodically; bupropion has minimal effects on ECG.
	Body weight	To detect excessive weight loss	Anorectic action noted with short-term use.
clomipramine (Anafranil)	Liver function tests	To detect hepatotoxicity	Establish baseline and repeat periodically; asymptomatic elevations of transaminase and alkaline phosphatase levels, which can progress to signs of hepatic failure, have occurred in clients receiving TCAs.
	Blood counts	To detect blood dyscrasias	Establish baseline and repeat periodically, especially in symptomatic clients.
	ECG	To detect cardiotoxicity	Establish baseline and repeat periodically, especially in clients receiving high doses.
	Ophthalmologic examinations, including tonometry	To detect glaucoma	Anticholinergic effects may exacerbate glaucoma.
desipramine (Norpramin)	Liver function tests	To detect hepatotoxicity	Establish baseline and repeat periodically; asymptomatic elevations of transaminase and alkaline phosphatase levels, which can progress to signs of hepatic failure, have occurred in clients receiving TCAs.
	Blood counts	To detect blood dyscrasias	Establish baseline and repeat periodically, especially in symptomatic clients.
	ECG	To detect cardiotoxicity	Establish baseline and repeat periodically, especially in clients receiving high doses.
	Ophthalmologic examinations, including tonometry	To detect glaucoma	Anticholinergic effects may exacerbate glaucoma.

continued

Recommended Laboratory Tests in Long-term Drug Therapy *(continued)*

Drug	Laboratory tests	Rationale	Special considerations
Antidepressants *(continued)*			
doxepin (Sinequan)	Liver function tests	To detect hepatotoxicity	Establish baseline and repeat periodically; asymptomatic elevations of transaminase and alkaline phosphatase levels, which can progress to signs of hepatic failure, have occurred in clients receiving TCAs.
	Blood counts	To detect blood dyscrasias	Establish baseline and repeat periodically, especially in symptomatic clients.
	ECG	To detect cardiotoxicity	Establish baseline and repeat periodically, especially in clients receiving high doses.
	Ophthalmologic examinations, including tonometry	To detect glaucoma	Anticholinergic effects may exacerbate glaucoma.
fluoxetine (Prozac)	Blood counts	To detect blood dyscrasias	Establish baseline and repeat periodically, especially in symptomatic clients.
	ECG	To detect cardiotoxicity	Establish baseline and repeat periodically; fluoxetine has minimal effects on ECG
	Ophthalmologic examinations, including tonometry	To detect glaucoma	Anticholinergic effects may exacerbate glaucoma.
	Body weight	To detect excessive weight loss	Anorectic action noted with short-term use.
imipramine (Tofranil)	Liver function tests	To detect hepatotoxicity	Establish baseline and repeat periodically; asymptomatic elevations of transaminase and alkaline phosphatase levels, which can progress to signs of hepatic failure, have occurred in clients receiving TCAs.
	Blood counts	To detect blood dyscrasias	Establish baseline and repeat periodically, especially in symptomatic clients.
	ECG	To detect cardiotoxicity	Establish baseline and repeat periodically, especially in clients receiving high doses.
	Ophthalmologic examinations, including tonometry	To detect glaucoma	Anticholinergic effects may exacerbate glaucoma.
isocarboxazid (Marplan)	Blood pressure	To detect toxicity	May cause orthostatic hypotension, especially in hypertensive clients.
	Ophthamologic examinations	To detect toxicity	Prolonged use may be associated rarely with amblyopia, visual disturbances, or glaucoma.
	Blood counts	To detect blood dyscrasias	Establish baseline and repeat periodically; normocytic and normochromic anemia, leukocytosis, agranulocytosis, and thrombocytopenia have been reported with monoamine oxidase (MAO) inhibitors.
	Liver function studies	To detect hepatotoxicity	Prevalent in clients on prolonged, high-dose therapy.

Recommended Laboratory Tests in Long-term Drug Therapy *(continued)*

Drug	Laboratory tests	Rationale	Special considerations
Antidepressants *(continued)*			
maprotiline (Ludiomil)	Liver function tests	To detect hepatotoxicity	Establish baseline and repeat periodically; asymptomatic elevations of transaminase and alkaline phosphatase levels, which can progress to signs of hepatic failure, have occurred in clients receiving TCAs.
	Blood counts	To detect blood dyscrasias	Establish baseline and repeat periodically, especially in symptomatic clients.
	ECG	To detect cardiotoxicity	Establish baseline and repeat periodically, especially in clients receiving high doses.
	Ophthalmologic examinations, including tonometry	To detect glaucoma	Anticholinergic effects may exacerbate glaucoma.
nortriptyline (Aventyl)	Liver function tests	To detect hepatotoxicity	Establish baseline and repeat periodically; asymptomatic elevations of transaminase and alkaline phosphatase levels, which can progress to signs of hepatic failure, have occurred in clients receiving TCAs.
	Blood counts	To detect blood dyscrasias	Establish baseline and repeat periodically, especially in symptomatic clients.
	ECG	To detect cardiotoxicity	Establish baseline and repeat periodically, especially in clients receiving high doses.
	Ophthalmologic examinations, including tonometry	To detect glaucoma	Anticholinergic effects may exacerbate glaucoma.
phenelzine (Nardil)	Blood pressure	To detect toxicity	May cause orthostatic hypotension, especially in hypertensive clients.
	Ophthamologic examinations	To detect toxicity	Prolonged use may be associated rarely with amblyopia, visual disturbances, or glaucoma.
	Blood counts	To detect blood dyscrasias	Establish baseline and repeat periodically; normocytic and normochromic anemia, leukocytosis, agranulocytosis, and thrombocytopenia have been reported with MAO inhibitors.
	Liver function studies	To detect hepatotoxicity	Prevalent in clients on prolonged, high-dose therapy.
protriptyline (Vivactil)	Liver function tests	To detect hepatotoxicity	Establish baseline and repeat periodically; asymptomatic elevations of transaminase and alkaline phosphatase levels, which can progress to signs of hepatic failure, have occurred in clients receiving TCAs.
	Blood counts	To detect blood dyscrasias	Establish baseline and repeat periodically, especially in symptomatic clients.

continued

Recommended Laboratory Tests in Long-term Drug Therapy *(continued)*

Drug	Laboratory tests	Rationale	Special considerations
Antidepressants *(continued)*			
protriptyline *(continued)*	ECG	To detect cardiotoxicity	Establish baseline and repeat periodically, especially in clients receiving high doses.
	Ophthalmologic examinations, including tonometry	To detect glaucoma	Anticholinergic effects may exacerbate glaucoma.
tranylcypromine (Parnate)	Blood pressure	To detect toxicity	May cause orthostatic hypotension, especially in hypertensive clients.
	Ophthalmologic examinations	To detect toxicity	Prolonged use may be associated rarely with amblyopia, visual disturbances, or glaucoma.
	Blood counts	To detect blood dyscrasias	Establish baseline and repeat periodically; normocytic and normochromic anemia, leukocytosis, agranulocytosis, and thrombocytopenia have been reported with MAO inhibitors.
	Liver function studies	To detect hepatotoxicity	Prevalent in clients on prolonged, high-dose therapy
trazodone (Trazon)	Blood counts	To detect blood dyscrasias	Establish baseline and repeat periodically, especially in symptomatic clients.
	ECG	To detect cardiotoxicity	Establish baseline and repeat periodically, especially in clients receiving high doses.
trimipramine (Surmontil)	Liver function tests	To detect hepatotoxicity	Establish baseline and repeat periodically; asymptomatic elevations of transaminase and alkaline phosphatase levels, which can progress to signs of hepatic failure, have occurred in clients receiving TCAs.
	Blood counts	To detect blood dyscrasias	Establish baseline and check periodically, especially in symptomatic clients.
	ECG	To detect cardiotoxicity	Establish baseline and repeat periodically, especially in clients receiving high doses.
	Ophthalmologic examinations, including tonometry	To detect glaucoma	Anticholinergic effects may exacerbate glaucoma.
Antiparkinsonian agents			
amantadine (Symmetrel)	Liver function studies	To detect toxicity	Establish baseline and repeat periodically; reversible elevations in liver enzymes seen occasionally.
benztropine (Cogentin)	Ophthalmologic examinations, especially tonometry	To detect toxic effect	Anticholinergic effect may unmask glaucoma in predisposed clients.
biperiden (Akineton)	Ophthalmologic examinations, especially tonometry	To detect toxic effect	Anticholinergic effect may unmask glaucoma in predisposed clients.

Recommended Laboratory Tests in Long-term Drug Therapy *(continued)*

Drug	Laboratory tests	Rationale	Special considerations
Antiparkinsonian agents *(continued)*			
bromocriptine (Parlodel)	Blood pressure	To detect hypotension	Orthostatic hypotension is common when therapy is initiated; however, a persistent hypotensive effect usually accompanies therapy.
	Hematologic studies	To detect chronic toxicity	Recommended by most clinicians for clients on prolonged therapy; establish baseline and repeat periodically.
	Liver function studies	To detect and prevent toxicity	Transient elevations of AST, ALT, creatine phosphokinase, and alkaline phosphatase levels and of some transaminases have been noted.
	Renal function studies	To detect and prevent toxicity	Transient elevations of BUN and uric acid levels have been noted.
carbidopa-levodopa (Sinemet)	Liver function studies	To detect toxic effects	Establish baseline and repeat periodically.
	Hematologic tests	To detect toxic effects	Establish baseline and repeat periodically; check clotting studies before any surgical procedures.
	Cardiovascular studies (ECG, blood pressure)	To detect toxicity	Establish baseline and repeat periodically; orthostatic hypotension is common, especially at initiation of therapy and during dosage increases.
	Renal function	To detect toxicity	Establish baseline and repeat periodically.
diphenhydramine (Benadryl)	Blood counts	To detect toxicity	Establish baseline and repeat periodically; pancytopenia, agranulocytosis, and thrombocytopenia reported rarely with prolonged use.
levodopa (Dopar)	Liver function studies	To detect toxic effects	Establish baseline and repeat periodically.
	Hematologic tests	To detect toxic effects	Establish baseline and repeat periodically; check clotting studies before any surgical procedures.
	Cardiovascular studies (ECG, blood pressure)	To detect toxicity	Check baseline and repeat periodically; orthostatic hypotension is common, especially at initiation of therapy and during dosage increases.
	Renal function	To detect toxicity	Establish baseline and repeat periodically.
orphenadrine (Orphenate)	Ophthalmologic examinations, especially tonometry	To detect toxic effect	Anticholinergic effect may unmask glaucoma in predisposed clients.
pergolide (Permax)	Ophthalmologic examinations, especially tonometry	To detect toxic effect	Anticholinergic effect may unmask glaucoma in predisposed clients.
procyclidine (Kemadrin)	Ophthalmologic examinations, especially tonometry	To detect toxic effect	Anticholinergic effect may unmask glaucoma in predisposed clients.
trihexyphenidyl (Artane)	Ophthalmologic examinations, especially tonometry	To detect toxic effect	Anticholinergic effect may unmask glaucoma in predisposed clients.

continued

Recommended Laboratory Tests in Long-term Drug Therapy *(continued)*

Drug	Laboratory tests	Rationale	Special considerations
Antimanic agent			
lithium (Lithane)	Blood counts	To detect blood dyscrasias	Establish baseline and repeat periodically.
	Serum electrolytes (particularly sodium)	To prevent toxicity	Sodium depletion can decrease lithium clearance and increase risk of toxicity.
	Serum lithium levels	To prevent toxicity	Toxic effects associated with levels above 1.5 mEq/liter.
	Thyroid function studies	To evaluate decreased thyroid function	About 5% of all clients develop goiters; evaluate triiodothyronine, thyroxine, and thyroid-stimulating hormone concentrations.
	Kidney function tests	To detect nephron atrophy	Establish baseline renal function (serum creatinine, urinalysis) every 1 to 2 months for the first 6 months then every 6 months thereafter.
	Urine specific gravity	To detect diabetes insipidus	Specific gravity should be above 1.015.
Antipsychotic agents			
acetophenazine (Tindal)	Blood counts	To detect blood dyscrasias	Phenothiazines can cause mild leukopenia; agranulocytosis is more frequently seen in females after 4 to 10 weeks of therapy. Incidence of blood dyscrasias is low but mortality is high; check blood studies promptly in symptomatic clients.
	Ophthalmologic examinations	To detect adverse drug effect	Corneal opacities and retinopathy have been reported after prolonged, high-dose therapy.
	ECG	To detect toxicity	Establish baseline and check periodically.
chlorpromazine (Thorazine)	Blood counts	To detect blood dyscrasias	Phenothiazines can cause mild leukopenia; agranulocytosis is more frequently seen in females after 4 to 10 weeks of therapy. Incidence of blood dyscrasias is low but mortality is high. Check blood studies promptly in symptomatic clients.
	Ophthalmologic examinations	To detect adverse drug effect	Corneal opacities and retinopathy have been reported after prolonged, high-dose therapy.
	ECG	To detect toxicity	Establish baseline and check periodically.
chlorprothixene (Taractan)	Blood counts	To detect blood dyscrasias	Drug can cause mild leukopenia or agranulocytosis. Incidence of blood dyscrasias is low. Check blood studies promptly in symptomatic clients.
	Ophthalmologic examinations	To detect adverse drug effect	Corneal opacities and retinopathy may occur after prolonged, high-dose therapy.
	ECG	To detect toxicity	Establish baseline and repeat periodically.

Recommended Laboratory Tests in Long-term Drug Therapy *(continued)*

Drug	Laboratory tests	Rationale	Special considerations
Antipsychotic agents *(continued)*			
clozapine (Clozaril)	Blood counts	To detect adverse drug effects	Drug can cause granulocytopenia or fatal agranulocytosis; baseline WBC count and differential required before therapy, and weekly WBC and granulocyte counts are mandatory during therapy and for at least 4 weeks after drug is discontinued.
fluphenazine (Prolixin)	Blood counts	To detect blood dyscrasias	Phenothiazines can cause mild leukopenia; agranulocytosis is more frequently seen in females after 4 to 10 weeks of therapy. Incidence of blood dyscrasias is low but mortality is high. Check blood studies promptly in symptomatic clients.
	Ophthalmologic examinations	To detect adverse drug effects	Corneal opacities and retinopathy have been reported after prolonged, high-dose therapy.
	ECG	To detect toxicity	Establish baseline and repeat periodically.
	Blood pressure	To detect adverse drug effects	Orthostatic hypotension may be problematic at initiation of therapy.
haloperidol (Haldol)	Blood counts	To detect blood dyscrasias	Drug can cause mild leukopenia or agranulocytosis (only when combined with other drugs). Incidence of blood dyscrasias is low. Check blood studies promptly in symptomatic clients.
	ECG	To detect toxicity	Establish baseline and check periodically
	Blood pressure	To detect adverse drug effects	Orthostatic hypotension may be problematic at initiation of therapy; hypertension can occur with prolonged use.
loxapine (Loxitane)	Blood counts	To detect blood dyscrasias	Drug can cause mild leukopenia or agranulocytosis. Incidence of blood dyscrasias is low. Check blood studies promptly in symptomatic clients.
	Ophthalmologic examinations	To detect adverse drug effectd	Corneal opacities and retinopathy may occur after prolonged, high-dose therapy. Anticholinergic effects may aggravate glaucoma.
	ECG	To detect toxicity	Establish baseline and repeat periodically.
	Blood pressure	To detect adverse drug effects	Tachycardia or orthostatic hypotension may be problematic, especially at initiation of therapy.

continued

Recommended Laboratory Tests in Long-term Drug Therapy *(continued)*

Drug	Laboratory tests	Rationale	Special considerations
Antipsychotic agents *(continued)*			
mesoridazine (Serentil)	Blood counts	To detect blood dyscrasias	Phenothiazines can cause mild leukopenia; agranulocytosis is more frequently seen in females after 4 to 10 weeks of therapy. Incidence of blood dyscrasias is low but mortality is high. Check blood studies promptly in symptomatic clients.
	Ophthalmologic examinations	To detect adverse drug effects.	Corneal opacities and retinopathy have been reported after prolonged, high-dose therapy.
	ECG	To detect toxicity	Establish baseline and repeat periodically.
molindone (Moban)	Blood counts	To detect blood dyscrasias	Drug can cause mild leukopenia or agranulocytosis. Incidence of blood dyscrasias is low. Check blood studies promptly in symptomatic clients.
	Ophthalmologic examinations	To detect adverse drug effects	Corneal opacities and retinopathy may occur after prolonged, high-dose therapy. Anticholinergic effects may aggravate glaucoma.
	ECG	To detect toxicity	Establish baseline and repeat periodically.
perphenazine (Trilafon)	Blood counts	To detect blood dyscrasias	Phenothiazines can cause mild leukopenia; agranulocytosis is more frequently seen in females after 4 to 10 weeks of therapy. Incidence of blood dyscrasias is low but mortality is high. Check blood studies promptly in symptomatic clients.
	Ophthalmologic examinations	To detect adverse drug effects	Corneal opacities and retinopathy have been reported after prolonged, high-dose therapy.
	ECG	To detect toxicity	Establish baseline and repeat periodically.
prochlorperazine (Compazine)	Blood counts	To detect blood dyscrasias	Phenothiazines can cause mild leukopenia; agranulocytosis is more frequently seen in females after 4 to 10 weeks of therapy. Incidence of blood dyscrasias is low but mortality is high. Check blood studies promptly in symptomatic clients.
	Ophthalmologic examinations	To detect adverse drug effects	Corneal opacities and retinopathy have been reported after prolonged, high-dose therapy.
	ECG	To detect toxicity	Establish baseline and repeat periodically.

Recommended Laboratory Tests in Long-term Drug Therapy *(continued)*

Drug	Laboratory tests	Rationale	Special considerations
Antipsychotic agents *(continued)*			
promazine (Sparine)	Blood counts	To detect blood dyscrasias	Phenothiazines can cause mild leukopenia; agranulocytosis is more frequently seen in females after 4 to 10 weeks of therapy. Incidence of blood dyscrasias is low but mortality is high. Check blood studies promptly in symptomatic clients.
	Ophthalmologic examinations	To detect adverse drug effects	Corneal opacities and retinopathy have been reported after prolonged, high-dose therapy.
	ECG	To detect toxicity	Establish baseline and repeat periodically.
	Blood pressure	To detect adverse drug effects	Orthostatic hypotension may be problematic at initiation of therapy.
thioridazine (Mellaril)	Blood counts	To detect blood dyscrasias	Phenothiazines can cause mild leukopenia; agranulocytosis is more frequently seen in females after 4 to 10 weeks of therapy. Incidence of blood dyscrasias is low but mortality is high. Check blood studies promptly in symptomatic clients.
	Ophthalmologic examinations	To detect adverse drug effect	Corneal opacities and retinopathy have been reported after prolonged, high-dose therapy.
	ECG	To detect toxicity	Establish baseline and repeat periodically
	Blood pressure	To detect adverse drug effects	Orthostatic hypotension may be problematic at initiation of therapy.
thiothixene (Navane)	Blood counts	To detect blood dyscrasias	Drug can cause mild leukopenia or agranulocytosis. Incidence of blood dyscrasias is low. Check blood studies promptly in symptomatic clients.
	Ophthalmologic examinations	To detect adverse drug effects	Corneal opacities and retinopathy may occur after prolonged, high-dose therapy.
	ECG	To detect toxicity	Establish baseline and repeat periodically
	Blood pressure	To detect adverse drug effects	Orthostatic hypotension may be problematic at initiation of therapy.
trifluoperazine (Stelazine)	Blood counts	To detect blood dyscrasias	Phenothiazines can cause mild leukopenia; agranulocytosis is more frequently seen in females after 4 to 10 weeks of therapy. Incidence of blood dyscrasias is low but mortality is high. Check blood studies promptly in symptomatic clients.
	Ophthalmologic examinations	To detect adverse drug effects	Corneal opacities and retinopathy have been reported after prolonged, high-dose therapy.
	ECG	To detect toxicity	Establish baseline and repeat periodically.
	Blood pressure	To detect adverse drug effects	Orthostatic hypotension may be problematic at initiation of therapy.

continued

Recommended Laboratory Tests in Long-term Drug Therapy *(continued)*

Drug	Laboratory tests	Rationale	Special considerations
Anxiolytics			
alprazolam (Xanax)	Blood counts	To detect blood dyscrasias	Establish baseline and repeat periodically during prolonged therapy.
	Liver function tests	To detect hepatotoxicity	Elevated liver function tests reported after prolonged benzodiazepine use.
	Renal function tests	To detect nephrotoxicity	Decreased renal function may occur after prolonged benzodiazepine use.
chlordiazepoxide (Librium)	Blood counts	To detect blood dyscrasias	Establish baseline and repeat periodically during prolonged therapy.
	Liver function tests	To detect hepatotoxicity	Elevated liver function tests reported after prolonged benzodiazepine use.
	Renal function tests	To detect nephrotoxicity	Decreased renal function may occur after prolonged benzodiazepine use.
diazepam (Valium)	Blood counts	To detect blood dyscrasias	Relatively rare; establish baseline and repeat periodically during prolonged therapy.
	Plasma testolactone levels	To detect chronic toxicity	Decreases reported in males with prolonged therapy.
	Liver function tests	To detect hepatotoxicity	Elevated AST, ALT, lactate dehydrogenase, alkaline phosphatase, and total and direct bilirubin reported occasionally with chronic use.
	Renal function studies	To detect nephrotoxicity	May occur with prolonged use; also transient decreased renal function after parenteral diazepam has been reported.
halazepam (Paxipam)	Blood counts	To detect blood dyscrasias	Establish baseline and repeat periodically during prolonged therapy.
	Liver function tests	To detect hepatotoxicity	Elevated liver function tests reported after prolonged benzodiazepine use.
	Renal function tests	To detect nephrotoxicity	Decreased renal function may occur after prolonged benzodiazepine use.
lorazepam (Ativan)	Liver function tests	To detect hepatotoxicity	Elevated liver enzymes reported after prolonged benzodiazepine use.
	Blood counts	To detect blood dyscrasias	Establish baseline and repeat periodically during prolonged use.
	Renal function tests	To detect nephrotoxicity	Nephrotoxicity may occur after prolonged use.
meprobamate (Miltown)	Blood counts	To detect blood dyscrasias	Establish baseline and repeat periodically; blood dyscrasias has been reported rarely.
oxazepam (Serax)	Blood counts	To detect blood dyscrasias	Establish baseline and repeat periodically.
	Kidney function tests	To detect nephrotoxicity	May occur after prolonged benzodiazepine use.
	Liver function tests	To detect hepatotoxicity	May occur after prolonged benzodiazepine use.

Recommended Laboratory Tests in Long-term Drug Therapy (continued)

Drug	Laboratory tests	Rationale	Special considerations
Anxiolytics (continued)			
prazepam (Centrax)	Blood counts	To detect blood dyscrasias	Establish baseline and repeat periodically.
	Kidney function tests	To detect nephrotoxicity	May occur after prolonged benzodiazepine use.
	Liver function tests	To detect hepatotoxicity	May occur after prolonged benzodiazepine use.
Sedative-hypnotics			
amobarbital (Amytal)	CBC, platelet count	To detect blood dyscrasias	Establish baseline and repeat periodically.
aprobarbital (Alurate)	CBC, platelet count	To detect blood dyscrasias	Establish baseline and repeat periodically.
butabarbital (Butisol)	CBC, platelet count	To detect blood dyscrasias	Establish baseline and repeat periodically.
chloral hydrate (Noctec)	Blood counts	To detect blood dyscrasias	Leukopenia and eosinophilia reported rarely with prolonged use.
flurazepam (Dalmane)	Blood counts	To detect blood dyscrasias	Establish baseline and repeat periodically.
	Liver function tests	To detect hepatotoxicity	Reported with prolonged benzodiazepine use.
	Kidney function tests	To detect nephrotoxicity	Reported with prolonged benzodiazepine use.
glutethimide (Doriden)	Blood counts	To detect blood dyscrasias	May be symptom of an acute hypersensitivity reaction.
pentobarbital (Nembutal)	CBC, platelet count	To detect blood dyscrasias	Establish baseline and repeat periodically.
quazepam (Doral)	Blood counts	To detect blood dyscrasias	Establish baseline and repeat periodically.
	Kidney function tests	To detect nephrotoxicity	Reported with prolonged use of benzodiazepines.
	Liver function tests	To detect hepatotoxicity	Reported with prolonged benzodiazepine use.
secobarbital (Seconal)	CBC, platelet count	To detect blood dyscrasias	Establish baseline and repeat periodically.
temazepam (Restoril)	Blood counts	To detect blood dyscrasias	Establish baseline and repeat periodically.
	Liver function tests	To detect hepatotoxicity	Reported with prolonged benzodiazepine use.
	Kidney function tests	To detect nephrotoxicity	Reported with prolonged benzodiazepine use.
triazolam (Halcion)	Blood counts	To detect blood dyscrasias	Establish baseline and repeat periodically.
	Liver function tests	To detect hepatotoxicity	Reported with prolonged benzodiazepine use.
	Kidney function tests	To detect nephrotoxicity	Reported with prolonged benzodiazepine use.

From *Handbook of psychotropic drugs.* Springhouse, PA: Springhouse Corp., 1992.

Appendix E: Psychiatric Drug Reactions

The following list reports generic drugs and pharmacologic classes that have been associated with psychiatric symptoms or disorders. If unspecified, reported incidence for individual drugs is less than 1%.

Symptom	Generic name	Trade name	Incidence
Agitation	alprazolam	Xanax	
	antidepressants		
	atropine		
	bromocriptine	Parlodel	
	clonidine	Catapres	3%
	diazepam	Valium	
	diphenhydramine	Benadryl	
	ephedrine		
	fluoxetine	Prozac	
	indapamide	Lozol	5%
	isoniazid (INH)		
	MAO inhibitors		
	methadone		
	morphine sulfate		
Akathisia	alprazolam	Xanax	
	chlorprothixene	Taractan	common
	phenothiazines		
Amnesia	alprazolam	Xanax	>1%
	benzodiazepines		
	triazolam	Halcion	
Anxiety	amantadine	Symmetrel	1% to 5%
	CNS stimulants		
	diazoxide	Proglycem	frequent
	dronabinol	Marinol	16%
	epinephrine	Adrenalin	
	indapamide	Lozol	5%
	indomethacin	Indocin	
	leuprolide acetate	Lupron	>3%
	maprotiline	Ludiomil	3%
	naltrexone	Trexan	>10%
	oxymetazoline		
	pindolol	Visken	4%
	ritodrine	Yutopar	5% to 6% (I.V.)
	sympathomimetics		
	theophylline		
Apathy	CNS depressants		
	digitalis glycosides		
	halazepam	Paxipam	9%
Behavioral changes	clonazepam	Klonopin	25%
	meperidine	Demerol	
Catatonia	atenolol	Tenormin	
	butyrophenones		
	chlorprothixine	Taractan	
	fluphenazine hydrochloride	Permitil Hydrochloride	
	labetalol	Trandate	
	methdilazine hydrochloride	Tacaryl	
	perphenazine	Trilafon	
	perphenazine and amitriptyline	Etrafon, Triavil	

Symptom	Generic name	Trade name	Incidence
Catatonia (continued)	phenothiazines		
	prochlorperazine	Compazine	
	promethazine	Phenergan	
	propranolol	Inderal	
	propranolol and hydrochlorothiazide	Inderide	
	thioxanthines		
	trifluoperazine	Stelazine	
	trimeprazine	Temaril	
Choreoathetotic movements	chlorprothixene	Taractan	
	levodopa	Larodopa	
	lithium	Cibalith, Eskalith	
	loxapine hydrochloride	Loxitane C	
	methyldopa	Aldomet	
	methyldopa and chlorothiazide	Aldoclor	
	methyldopa and hydrochlorothiazide	Aldoril	
Clonic movements	lithium	Eskalith, Lithane	
Clonus	doxapram	Dopram	
Confusion	alprazolam	Xanax	9.9%
	amantadine	Symmetrel	1% to 5%
	baclofen	Lioresal	1% to 11%
	benzodiazepines		
	carbamazepine	Mazepine, Tegretol	
	clonidine	Catapres	
	CNS depressants		
	cyclosporine	Sandimmune	2%
	diazepam	Valium	
	esmolol	Brevibloc	2%
	guanadrel sulfate	Hylorel	14.8%
	halazepam	Paxipam	9%
	interferon alfa-2a, recombinant	Roferon-A	10%
	isocarboxazid	Marplan	most common
	levodopa	Larodopa	
	MAO inhibitors		
	meperidine	Demerol	
	metoclopramide	Octamide	>10%
	mexiletine	Mexitil	2.6%
	penicillin		
	pentazocine	Fortral, Talwin	30%
	phenobarbital		
	phenytoin	Dilantin	most common
	temazepam	Restoril	2% to 3%
	tocainide	Tonocard	>1%
	valproic acid	Depakene	

Psychiatric Drug Reactions *(continued)*

Symptom	Generic name	Trade name	Incidence
Delirium	acyclovir	Zovirax	
	amantadine	Symmetrel	
	amphetamines		
	anticholinergics		
	atropine		
	baclofen	Lioresal	
	chloramphenicol	Chloromy-cetin	
	cimetidine	Tagamet	
	clonidine	Catapres	
	corticosteroids		
	digitalis glyco-sides		
	ephedrine		
	famotidine	Pepcid	
	fentanyl citrate with droperidol	Innovar	
	indomethacin	Indocin	
	lithium	Eskalith, Lithane	
	lorazepam	Ativan	
	meperidine	Demerol	
	methohexital sodium	Brevital Sodium	
	methoxyflurane	Penthrane	
	methyldopa	Aldomet	
	mexiletine	Mexitil	
	nizatidine	Axid	
	opium alkaloids	Pentopon	
	pentazocine	Talwin	
	phenelzine	Nardil	
	phenylephrine		
	phenylpropanolamine		
	phenytoin	Dilantin	
	propranolol	Inderal	
	quinidine gluconate	Duraquin	
	ranitidine	Zantac	
	sympathomimetics		
	thiamylal	Surital	
Delusions	amitriptyline	Elavil	
	carbidopa-levodopa	Sinemet	
	chlordiazepoxide hydrochloride	Limbitrol	
	desipramine	Pertofrane	
	imipramine	Tofranil	
	levodopa	Larodopa	frequent
	nortriptyline	Pamelor	
	perphenazine and amitriptyline	Etrafon, Triavil	
	protriptyline	Vivactil	
	trimipramine	Surmontil	
Dementia	carbidopa-levodopa	Sinemet	
	levodopa	Larodopa	
	methotrexate	Mexate	
	quinidine sulfate	Quinidex Extentabs	

Symptom	Generic name	Trade name	Incidence
Depression	alprazolam	Xanax	
	amantadine	Symmetrel	1% to 5%
	atenolol	Tenormin	12%
	atenolol and chlorthalidone	Tenoretic	12%
	baclofen	Lioresal	
	clonidine	Catapres	
	digitalis glyco-sides		
	dronabinol	Marinol	7%
	flecainide	Tambocor	1% to 3%
	flunisolide	Aerobid Inhaler	1% to 3%
	guanabenz	Wytensin	3%
	guanadrel	Hylorel	1.9%
	halazepam	Paxipam	9%
	indapamide	Lozol	5%
	indomethacin	Indocin	1% to 3%
	metoclopramide	Octamide	<10%
	metoprolol	Lopressor	5%
	mexiletine	Mexitil	2.4%
	naltrexone	Trexan	<10%
	NSAIDs		
	reserpine	Serpasil	
	tolmetin	Tolectin	<3%
Disorientation	benzodiazepines		
	cimetidine	Tagamet	
	CNS depressants		
	famotidine	Pepcid	
	halazepam	Paxipam	9%
	lidocaine	Xylocaine	
	methadone		
	metronidazole	Flagyl	
	morphine		
	nizatidine	Axid	
	NSAIDs		
	penicillin		
	pentazocine	Talwin	30%
	ranitidine	Zantac	
Emotional disturbances	imipramine	Tofranil	
	primidone	Mysoline	
	ritodrine	Yutopar	5 to 6%
	valproic acid	Depakene	
Euphoria	antidepressants		
	atropine		
	baclofen	Lioresal	
	levodopa	Larodopa	
	methadone		
	morphine sulfate		
	pentazocine	Talwin	
Hallucinations	acyclovir	Zovirax	
	amantadine	Symmetrel	1% to 5%
	atropine		
	baclofen	Lioresal	
	beta-adrenergic blockers		
	bromocriptine	Parlodel	
	carbidopa-levodopa	Sinemet	
	cimetidine	Tagamet	

continued

Psychiatric Drug Reactions *(continued)*

Symptom	Generic name	Trade name	Incidence
Hallucinations *(continued)*	corticosteroids		
	diazepam	Valium	
	digitalis glyco-sides		
	diphenhydramine	Benadryl	
	dronabinol	Marinol	5%
	ephedrine		
	famotidine	Pepcid	
	levodopa	Larodopa	
	lidocaine	Xylocaine	
	methyldopa	Aldomet	
	metronidazole	Flagyl	
	nizatidine	Axid	
	oxymetazoline		
	penicillin		
	pentazocine	Talwin	
	phenylephrine		
	propranolol	Inderal	
	ranitidine	Zantac	
Hysteria	azatidine	Optimine	
	clemastine	Tavist	
	clonazepam	Klonopin	
	codeine and bromodiphen-hydramine	Ambenyl	
	cyproheptadine	Periactin	
	dexchlorpheni-ramine, pseu-doephedrine, and guaifene-sin	Polaramine	
	ethchlorvynol	Placidyl	
	methdilazine hy-drochloride	Tacaryl	
	phenylpropa-nolamine and chlorphenir-amine	Ornade, Tria-minic	
	promethazine	Phenergan	
	pseudoephedrine		
	trimeprazine	Temaril	
	tripelennamine	PBZ	
	triprolidine, pseudoephed-rine, and co-deine phosphate	Actifed with codeine	
Insomnia	acebutolol	Sectral	3%
	albuterol	Proventil, Ventolin	2%
	alprazolam	Xanax	>8%
	amantadine	Symmetrel	5% to 10%
	amphetamines		
	antidepressants		
	baclofen	Lioresal	2% to 7%
	clomiphene	Serophene	1.9%
	estramustine	Emcyt	3% to 4%
	fluoxetine	Prozac	
	guanfacine	Tenex	4%
	indapamide	Lozol	<5%
	interferon alfa-2b, recombi-nant	Intron	5%

Symptom	Generic name	Trade name	Incidence
Insomnia *(continued)*	isocarboxazid	Marplan	most frequent
	ketoprofen	Orudis	>3%
	leuprolide ace-tate	Lupron	<3%
	MAO inhibitors		
	maprotiline	Ludiomil	2%
	metoclopramide	Octamide	10%
	pentoxifylline	Trental	2.3%
	phenylpropa-nolamine		
	pindolol	Visken	19%
	sympathomi-metics		
	theophylline		
Jitteriness	acyclovir	Zovirax	
	amitriptyline	Elavil	
	amphetamines		
	chlorpromazine	Thorazine	
	diethylpropion	Tenuate	
	isocarboxazid	Marplan	most frequent
	metoclopramide	Octamide	
	nifedipine	Adalat, Pro-cardia	2%
	phenelzine	Nardil	
	prochlorperazine	Compazine	
	ritodrine	Yutopar	5% to 8%
	sympathomi-metics		
	trifluoperazine	Stelazine	
Lethargy	atenolol	Tenormin	3%
	atenolol and chlorthalidone	Tenoretic	3%
	butalbital, aspi-rin, caffeine and codeine phosphate	Fiorinal with codeine	most com-mon
	butorphanol	Stadol	2%
	clonidine	Catapres	3%
	estramustine	Emcyt	3% to 4%
	etretinate	Tegison	1% to 10%
	immune globulin	RhoGam	25%
	indapamide	Lozol	5%
	interferon alfa-2a, recombi-nant	Roferon-A	3%
	leuprolide ace-tate	Lupron	3%
	metoprolol	Lopressor	10%
	pindolol	Visken	3%
	temazepam	Restoril	3%
Manic symptoms	alprazolam	Xanax	
	antidepressants		20% to 30%
	baclofen	Lioresal	
	bromocriptine	Parlodel	
	corticosteroids		
	levodopa	Larodopa	
	metoclopramide	Octamide	
	propranolol	Inderal	
	triazolam	Halcion	

Psychiatric Drug Reactions *(continued)*

Symptom	Generic name	Trade name	Incidence
Memory impairment	acebutolol	Sectral	
	alprazolam	Xanax	>1%
	atenolol	Tenormin	
	atenolol and chlorthalidone	Tenoretic	
	benztropine	Cogentin	
	carbamazepine	Tegretol	
	clonazepam	Klonopin	
	diphenhydramine	Benadryl	
	glutethimide	Doriden	
	isocarboxazid	Marplan	most frequent
	isoniazid (INH)		
	labetalol	Trandate	
	leuprolide acetate	Lupron	<3%
	lithium	Eskalith	
	MAO inhibitors		
	maprotiline	Ludiomil	
	metoprolol	Lopressor	
	oxazepam	Serax	
	phenobarbital		
	phenytoin	Dilantin	
	propranolol and hydrochlorothiazide	Inderide	
	timolol	Blocadren, Timoptic	
	tocainide	Tonocard	
	trazodone	Desyrel	>1%
	triazolam	Halcion	
	valproic acid	Depakene	
Memory loss, short term	benzodiazepines		
	mexilitine	Mexitil	
	propranolol	Inderal	
Mood changes	carbidopa-levodopa	Sinemet	
	fenfluramine	Pondimin	
	flunisolide	AeroBid Inhaler	1% to 3%
	hydrocodone and acetaminophen	Co-Gesic, Vicodin, Zydone	
	hydrocodone, aspirin, and caffeine	Damason P	
	hydrocodone and chlorpheniramine	Hycomine	
	hydromorphone	Dilaudid	
	nifedipine	Adalat, Procardia	
	phenelzine	Nardil	
	piroxicam	Feldene	
	tocainide	Tonocard	>1%
Nervousness	albuterol	Proventil, Ventolin	4% to 20%
	alprazolam	Xanax	4.1%
	bitolterol	Tornalate	5%
	dicyclomine	Bentyl	6%
	flunisolide	AeroBid Inhaler	3% to 9%
	indapamide	Lozol	>5%

Symptom	Generic name	Trade name	Incidence
Nervousness *(continued)*	isoetharine hydrochloride	Arm-a-Med Isoetharine	
	ketoprofen	Orudis	>3%
	maprotiline	Ludiomil	6%
	metaproterenol	Alupent	
	mexiletine	Mexitil	5%
	naltrexone	Trexan	>10%
	nifedipine	Adalat, Procardia	7%
	pindolol	Visken	11%
	ritodrine	Yutopar	5% to 6%
	triazolam	Halcion	5.2%
	trihexyphenidyl	Artane	30% to 50%
Neuromuscular reactions, extrapyramidal	butyrophenones		frequent
	chlorpromazine	Thorazine	frequent
	haloperidol	Haldol	frequent
	phenothiazines		frequent
	pimozide	Orap	frequent
	prochlorperazine	Compazine	frequent
	thioxanthines		
	trifluoperazine	Stelazine	frequent
	vincristine	Vincasar PFS	frequent
Nightmares	amantadine	Symmetrel	
	amoxapine	Asendin	>1%
	atropine		
	baclofen	Lioresal	
	beta-adrenergic blockers		
	bromocriptine	Parlodel	
	levodopa	Larodopa	frequent
	propranolol	Inderal	
Night terrors	ethosuximide	Zarontin	
	penicillin		
Paradoxical anxiety	hydrochlorothiazide and deserpidine	Oreticyl	
	methyclothiazide	Enduron	
	perphenazine	Trilafon	
Paranoia	alprazolam	Xanax	
	amphetamines		
	bromocriptine	Parlodel	
	carbidopa-levodopa	Sinemet	
	dronabinol	Marinol	2%
	ephedrine		
	fluphenazine hydrochloride	Permitil Hydrochloride	
	indomethacin	Indocin	
	lidocaine		
	meperidine	Demerol	
	naltrexone	Trexan	
	NSAIDs		
	perphenazine	Trilafon	
	perphenazine and amitriptyline	Etrafon, Triavil	
	phenylephrine		
	sympathomimetics		
	triazolam	Halcion	

continued

Psychiatric Drug Reactions (continued)

Symptom	Generic name	Trade name	Incidence
Parkinson-like symptoms	asparaginase	Elspar	
	chlorothiazide and reserpine	Diupres	
	chlorprothixene	Taractan	common
	chlorthalidone and reserpine	Demi-Regroton	
	fluphenazine hydrochloride	Permitil Hydrochloride, Prolixin Hydrochloride	
	haloperidol	Haldol	
	hydrochlorothiazide and reserpine	Hydropres-25	
	hydroflumethiazide	Saluron	
	indomethacin	Indocin	
	mesoridazine	Serentil	
	methychlothiazide and reserpine	Diutensen-R	
	methyldopa	Aldomet	
	methyldopa and chlorothiazide	Aldoclor	
	methyldopa and hydrochlorothiazide	Aldoril	
	metoclopramide	Octamide	
	metyrosine	Demser	
	perphenazine	Trilafon	
	perphenazine and amitriptyline	Etrafon, Triavil	
	pimozide	Orap	
	polythiazide	Renese	
	prochlorperazine	Compazine	
	rauwolfia serpentina	Raudixin	
	reserpine	Ser-Ap-Es, Serpasil	
	thiothixene	Navane	
	trichlormethiazide and reserpine	Metatensin	
	trifluoperazine	Stelazine	
	trimethobenzamide	Tigan	
Psychiatric disturbances	guanadrel	Hylorel	3.8%
	phenacemide	Phenurone	17%
Psychosis	amantadine	Symmetrel	
	bromocriptine	Parlodel	
	chlorprothixene	Taractan	
	cimetidine	Tagamet	
	clonazepam	Klonopin	
	cycloserine	Seromycin	
	dapsone	Avlosulfon	
	digoxin	Lanoxicaps, Lanoxin	1% to 4%
	divalproex sodium	Depakote	
	ethionamide	Trecator-SC	

Symptom	Generic name	Trade name	Incidence
Psychosis (continued)	Iohexol	Omnipaque	
	methadone (I.V.)		
	methyldopa	Aldomet	
	metrizamide	Amipaque	
	morphine sulfate	Duramorph	
	perphenazine	Trilafon	
	phendimetrazine	Plegine	
	phentermine	Adipex-P	
	prednisolone sodium phosphate	Hydeltrasol	
	procainamide	Pronestyl	
	sulfisoxazole and phenazopyridine	Azo Gantrisin	
	valproic acid	Depakene	
	vidarabine	Vira-A	
Psychosis, activation	bromocriptine	Parlodel	
	desipramine	Pertofrane	
	fluphenazine hydrochloride	Prolixin Hydrochloride	
	perphenazine and amitriptyline	Etrafon, Triavil	
	prochlorperazine	Compazine	
Psychosis, exacerbation	desipramine	Norpramin	
	fluphenazine hydrochloride	Permetil Hydrochloride, Prolixin Hydrochloride	
	imipramine	Tofranil	
	nortriptyline	Pamelor	
	protriptyline	Vivactil	
	thiethylperazine	Torecan	
	thioridazine	Mellaril	
	trimipramine	Surmontil	
Psychosis, toxic	isoniazid (INH)		
	methylphenidate	Ritalin	
	morphine sulfate	Duramorph	
Rage reactions	indomethacin	Indocin	
	sulindac	Clinoril	
Seizures	alprazolam	Xanax	2 to 3 days (after abrupt discontinuation)
	bromocriptine	Parlodel	
	chloroquine	Aralen	
	chlorpromazine	Thorazine	
	cyclosporine	Sandimmune	>3%
	desipramine	Pertofrane	
	esmolol	Brevibloc	
	fluphenazine	Permitil	
	lidocaine	Xylocaine	
	lithium	Eskalith	
	methdilazine hydrochloride	Tacaryl	
	methocarbamol	Robaxin	
	metoclopramide	Reglan	
	metrizamide	Amipaque	
	metronidazole	Flagyl	

Psychiatric Drug Reactions *(continued)*

Symptom	Generic name	Trade name	Incidence
Seizures *(continued)*	mezlocillin	Mezlin	
	paramethadione	Paradione	
	pemoline	Cylert	
	penicillin		
	perphenazine	Etrafon, Triavil	
	perphenazine and amitriptyline	Etrafon Trianil	
	promethazine	Phenergan	
	ticarcillin/clavulanate	Timentin	
	tocainide	Tonocard	
	trimeprazine	Temaril	
	trimethadione	Tridione	
Sensorium, clouded	atenolol	Tenormin	
	CNS depressants		
	labetalol	Trandate	
	labetalol and hydrochlorothiazine	Normozide	
	mepivacaine	Carbocaine	
	nadolol and bendroflumethiazide	Corzide	
	propranolol	Inderal	
	propranolol and hydrochlorothiazide	Inderide	
	timolol	Blocadren, Timoptic	
Sleep disturbances	bromocriptine	Parlodel	
	diazepam	Valium	
	diphenidol	Vontrol	
	ethosuximide	Zarontin	
	guanabenz	Wytensin	3%
	guanadrel	Hylorel	2.1%
	imipramine	Tofranil	
	metoprolol	Lopressor	
	mexiletine	Mexitil	7.1%
	naltrexone	Trexan	>10%
	nifedipine	Adalat, Procardia	2%
Suicidal ideation	amitriptyline	Elavil	
	carbidopa-levodopa	Sinemet	
	chlorthalidone and reserpine	Demi-Regroton, Regroton	
	clonazepam	Klonopin	
	desipramine	Pertofrane	
	meprobamate	Meprospan, Miltown	
	perphenazine	Trilafon	

Symptom	Generic name	Trade name	Incidence
Tardive dyskinesia	chlorpromazine	Thorazine	
	chlorprothixine	Taractan	
	fluphenazine hydrochloride	Permitil Hydrochloride, Prolixin Hydrochloride	
	haloperidol	Haldol	
	loxapine hydrochloride	Loxitane C	
	mesoridazine	Serentil	
	metoclopramide	Octamide, Reglan	
	molindone	Moban	
	perphenazine	Trilafon	
	perphenazine and amitriptyline	Etrafon, Triavil	
	pimozide	Orap	
	prochlorperazine	Compazine	
	thioridazine	Mellaril	
	thiothixine	Navane	
	trifluoperazine	Stelazine	
Tourette's syndrome	dextroamphetamine	Dexedrine	
	methamphetamine	Desoxyn	
	pemoline	Cylert	

From *Handbook of psychotropic drugs.* Springhouse, PA: Springhouse Corp., 1992.

Appendix F: Managing Medication Adverse Reactions

The list below covers some of the most common adverse reactions to pharmacologic therapy and what to tell clients to minimize or prevent those reactions.

Coping with Dry Mouth

- Brush teeth using a fluoridated toothpaste after each meal.
- Use a fluoride rinse and floss daily.
- Drink lots of fluids between meals and with meals (unless your physician restricts your fluid intake).
- Avoid acidic beverages, such as citrus juices, because they may irritate sore tissues.
- Limit consumption of alcohol and caffeinated drinks because they are dehydrating.
- Stop smoking—it irritates the mouth.
- Avoid dry, coarse, or very spicy foods.
- Moisten foods with water, juices, dressings, or by dipping them into sauce or soup.
- Suck on sugarless lemon drops to stimulate saliva. Ask your doctor for a saliva substitute (such as Xero-lube).
- Sip cool liquids and suck on ice chips or sugarless candy.

Coping with Dizziness

- When getting out of bed, stand up slowly.
- Sit on the edge of the bed for a minute and dangle your legs before arising.
- When getting up from a chair, stand up slowly and do not move quickly.
- Do not drive or operate machinery if you feel dizzy or unsteady.
- When walking up or down stairs, take one step at a time; use the handrail to keep your balance.

Coping with Constipation

- Try to eat such foods as bran cereal and raw leafy vegetables and fruits; these foods add bulk and help soften stool.
- Eat dried fruits, such as prunes, dates, and raisins, for their laxative effect.
- Ask your doctor about using over-the-counter artificial bulk laxatives, such as Metamucuil or Citrucel, and stool softeners, such as Colace.
- Drink lots of fluids (unless your physician restricts your fluid intake).
- Maintain activity level, exercising in moderation.
- Allow adequate time for bowel movements.

Coping with Sleep Disturbances

- Sleep as much as you need to feel refreshed and alert during the day.
- Go to bed at the same time each night.
- Avoid napping during the day because it may make it harder for you to fall asleep at night.
- Exercise daily to promote deep sleep. However, do not exercise 3 to 4 hours before bedtime; it disturbs sleep.
- Keep the bedroom at a comfortable temperature; avoid temperature extremes.
- Avoid alcohol and caffeine.
- Eat a light snack before bedtime to avoid nighttime hunger.
- Engage in a relaxing activity, such as reading, listening to soft music, or taking a warm bath.
- If you cannot fall asleep, turn on a light, get out of bed, and do something relaxing until you feel sleepy.
- Avoid regular use of sleeping pills; they may make you drowsy the next day, and may even make the insomnia worse.
- If your insomnia lasts for 3 weeks or more, or if you are sleepy during the day and fall asleep suddenly in situations where you used to remain awake, talk to your physician immediately.

Appendix G: Managing Acute Substance Abuse

Substance	Signs and symptoms	Interventions
Alcohol (ethanol) • beer and wine • distilled spirits • other preparations, such as cough syrup or mouthwash	• Ataxia • Seizures • Coma • Hypothermia • Alcohol breath odor • Respiratory depression • Bradycardia • Hypotension • Nausea and vomiting	• Induce vomiting or perform gastric lavage if ingestion occurred within the past 4 hours. Give activated charcoal and a saline cathartic. • Start I.V. fluid replacement and administer dextrose, thiamine, B-complex vitamins, and Vitamin C, to prevent dehydration and hypoglycemia and to correct nutritional deficiencies. • The client may need padded bed rails and cloth restraints for protection from injury. • Control seizures with an anticonvulsant such as diazepam (Valium). • Monitor for hallucinations and alcohol withdrawal syndrome. If these occur, treat with chlordiazepoxide (Librium), chloral hydrate, or paraldehyde. • Monitor for crackles or rhonchi, possibly indicating aspiration pneumonia. Treat with antibiotics, as appropriate. • Clearly monitor neurologic status and vital signs until the client is stable. Consider dialysis if the client's vital functions are severely depressed.
Amphetamines • amphetamine sulfate (Benzedrine)—bennies, greenies, cartwheels • dextroamphetamine sulfate (Dexedrine)—dexies, hearts, oranges • methamphetamine—speed, meth, crystal	• Dilated reactive pupils • Altered mental status (from confusion to paranoia) • Hallucinations • Tremor and seizure activity • Hyperactive deep tendon reflexes • Exhaustion • Coma • Dry mouth • Shallow respirations • Tachycardia • Hypertension • Hyperthermia • Diaphoresis	• If the drug was taken orally, induce vomiting or perform gastric lavage; give activated charcoal and a sodium or magnesium sulfate cathartic. • Acidify the client's urine by adding ammonium chloride or ascorbic acid to I.V. solution to lower pH to 5. • Force diuresis with mannitol. • Use short-acting barbiturate, such as pentobarbital, to control stimulant-induced seizures. • Restrain the paranoid or hallucinating client to prevent injury. • Treat agitation or assaultive behavior with haloperidol (Haldol) I.M. • Treat hypertension with an alpha-adrenergic blocking agent, such as phentolamine (Regitine). • Monitor for cardiac arrhythmias. Treat tachyarrhythmias or ventricular arrhythmias with propranolol or lidocaine. • Treat hyperthermia with tepid sponge baths or a hypothermia blanket. • Provide a quiet environment to avoid overstimulation. • Monitor for signs and symptoms of withdrawal, such as abdominal tenderness, muscle aches, and prolonged periods of sleep. • Observe suicide precautions, especially if the client shows signs of withdrawal.
Antipsychotics • haloperidol (Haldol) • phenothiazines such as chlorpromazine (Thorazine) or thioridazine (Mellaril)	• Constricted pupils • Photosensitivity • Extrapyramidal (dyskinesia, opisthotonos, muscle rigidity, ocular deviation) • Dry mouth • Decreased level of consciousness • Decreased deep tendon reflexes • Seizures • Hypothermia or hyperthermia • Dysphagia • Respiratory depression • Hypotension • Tachycardia	• Perform gastric lavage if the client ingested the drug within the past 6 hours. (Don't administer ipecac, because phenothiazines have an antiemetic effect.) Give activated charcoal and a cathartic. • Treat extrapyramidal adverse reactions with diphenhydramine (Benadryl) or benztropine (Cogentin). • Give physostigmine salicylate (Antilirium) to reverse the drug's anticholinergic effects in severe cases. • Replace fluids I.V. to correct hypotension; monitor vital signs. • Monitor respiratory rate and provide supplemental oxygen to treat respiratory depression. • Control seizures with an anticonvulsant, such as diazepam, or a short-acting barbiturate, such as pentobarbital sodium (Nembutal). • Keep the client's room dark to avoid exacerbating his photosensitivity.

continued

Managing Acute Substance Abuse (continued)

Substance	Signs and symptoms	Interventions
Anxiolytic sedative-hypnotics • benzodiazepines such as chlordiazepoxide hydrochloride (Librium) and diazepam (Valium)	• Confusion • Drowsiness • Stupor • Decreased reflexes • Seizures • Coma • Shallow respirations • Hypotension	• Induce vomiting or perform gastric lavage; give activated charcoal and a cathartic. • Provide supplemental oxygen to correct hypoxia-induced seizures. • Administer fluids I.V. to correct hypotension; monitor the client's vital signs frequently. • In severe toxicity, give physostigmine salicylate (Antilirium) to reverse respiratory and CNS depression.
Barbiturate sedative-hypnotics • amobarbital sodium (Amytal Sodium) — blue angels, blue devils, blue birds • phenobarbital (Luminal) — phennies, purple hearts, goofballs • secobarbital sodium (Seconal) — reds, red devils, seccy	• Poor pupil reaction to light • Nystagmus • Depressed level of consciousness (from confusion to coma) • Flaccid muscles and absent reflexes • Hyperthermia or hypothermia • Cyanosis • Respiratory depression • Hypotension • Blisters or bullous lesions	• Induce vomiting or perform gastric lavage if the client ingested the drug within the past 4 hours; give activated charcoal and a saline cathartic. • Maintain blood pressure with I.V. fluid challenges and vasopressors. • After phenobarbital overdose, give sodium bicarbonate I.V. to alkalinize urine and speed the drug's elimination. • Provide a hyperthermia or hypothermia blanket to help return the client's temperature to normal. • Consider hemodialysis or hemoperfusion if toxicity is severe. • Closely monitor neurologic status and vital signs. • Monitor for respiratory distress or pulmonary edema and signs of withdrawal, such as hyperreflexia, generalized tonic-clonic seizures, and hallucinations. • Provide symptomatic relief of withdrawal symptoms, as appropriate.
Cocaine • cocaine hydrochloride • crack • "free-base"	• Dilated pupils • Confusion • Alternating euphoria and apprehension • Hyperexcitability • Visual, auditory, and olfactory hallucinations • Spasms and seizures • Coma • Tachypnea • Hyperpnea • Pallor or cyanosis • Respiratory arrest • Tachycardia • Hypertension or hypotension • Fever • Nausea and vomiting • Abdominal pain • Perforated nasal septum or oral sores	• If cocaine was ingested, induce vomiting or perform gastric lavage; give activated charcoal followed by a saline cathartic. • Administer an antipyretic to reduce fever. • Monitor blood pressure and heart rate and treat symptomatic tachycardia with propranolol. • Control seizures with an anticonvulsant, such as diazepam (Valium). • Scrape the inside of the client's nose to remove residual amounts of inhaled cocaine. • Monitor cardiac rate and rhythm — ventricular fibrillation and cardiac standstill can occur as a direct cardiotoxic result of cocaine. Defibrillate and initiate cardiopulmonary resuscitation, as indicated.
Glutethimide (Doriden) • blues • CD • cibas	• Small, reactive pupils • Nystagmus • Drowsiness • Irritability • Impaired thought processes (memory, judgment, attention span) • Slurred speech • Twitching, spasms, and seizures	• If the drug was taken orally, induce vomiting or perform gastric lavage; give activated charcoal and a cathartic. • Maintain the client's blood pressure with I.V. fluid challenges and vasopressors. • Consider hemodialysis or hemoperfusion if the client has hepatic or renal failure or prolonged coma. • Control seizures with an anticonvulsant, such as diazepam (Valium). • Closely monitor neurologic status. Coma may recur because of the drug's slow release from fat deposits.

Managing Acute Substance Abuse *(continued)*

Substance	Signs and symptoms	Interventions
Glutethimide (Doriden) *(continued)*	• Hypothermia • CNS depression (unresponsive to deep coma) • Apnea • Respiratory depression • Hypotension • Paralytic ileus • Poor bladder control	• Monitor for signs of increased intracranial pressure, such as decreasing level of consciousness and widening pulse pressure. Give mannitol I.V. as indicated. • Watch for signs of withdrawal, such as hyperreflexia, generalized tonic-clonic seizures, and hallucinations. • Provide symptomatic relief of withdrawal symptoms.
Hallucinogens • lysergic acid diethylamide (LSD) — hawk, acid, sunshine • mescaline (peyote) — mese, cactus, big chief	• Dilated pupils • Intensified perceptions • Agitation and anxiety • Synesthesia • Impaired judgment • Hyperactive movement • Flashback experiences • Hallucinations • Depersonalization • Moderately increased blood pressure • Increased heart rate • Fever	• Impose safety precautions to protect the client from injury. • If the drug was taken orally, induce vomiting or perform gastric lavage; give activated charcoal and a cathartic. • Control seizures with diazepam (Valium) I.V.
Narcotics • codeine • heroin — smack, H, junk, snow • hydromorphone (Dilaudid) — D, lords • morphine — mort, monkey, M, Miss Emma	• Constricted pupils • Depressed level of consciousness (but the client is usually responsive to persistent verbal or tactile stimuli) • Seizures • Hypothermia • Slow, deep respirations • Hypotension • Bradycardia • Skin changes (pruritus, urticaria, and flushed skin)	• Repeat naloxone (Narcan) administration until the drug's CNS depressant effects are reversed. • Replace fluids I.V. to increase circulatory volume. • Correct hypothermia as indicated. • Auscultate frequently for crackles, possibly indicating pulmonary edema. (Onset may be delayed.) • Provide oxygen via nasal cannula, mask, or mechanical ventilation to correct hypoxemia from hypoventilation. • Monitor cardiac rate and rhythm, being alert for atrial fibrillation. (This should resolve spontaneously when hypoxemia is corrected.) • Monitor for signs of withdrawal, such as piloerection (goose flesh), diaphoresis, and hyperactive bowel sounds.
Nonbarbiturate sedative-hypnotics • methaqualone (Quaaludes) — ludes, soapers, love drug	• Dilated pupils • Nystagmus • Disorientation • Slurred speech • Hypertonicity • Ataxia • Twitching and seizures • Coma • Dry mouth • Anorexia • Nausea, vomiting, or diarrhea	• Induce vomiting or perform gastric lavage if the client ingested the drug within the past 2 to 4 hours. Give activated charcoal and a cathartic. • Maintain blood pressure with I.V. fluids and vasopressors. • Consider hemodialysis or hemoperfusion for severe toxicity. • Initially treat hypertonicity with diazepam (Valium). If hypertonicity doesn't improve, the client may require treatment with curare and mechanical ventilation. • Control seizures with diazepam, phenytoin (Dilantin), or phenobarbital (Luminal). • Monitor for crackles, rhonchi, or decreased breath sounds, possibly indicating aspiration pneumonia. Provide supplemental oxygen and antibiotics, as indicated. • Monitor for signs of withdrawal, such as hyperreflexia, generalized tonic-clonic seizures, and hallucinations. • Treat withdrawal signs and symptoms with pentobarbital or phenobarbital, as indicated.

continued

Managing Acute Substance Abuse *(continued)*

Substance	Signs and symptoms	Interventions
Phencyclidine (PCP) • angel dust • hog • peace pill	• Blank staring • Nystagmus • Amnesia • Decreased awareness of surroundings • Recurrent coma • Violent behavior • Hyperactivity • Seizures • Gait ataxia • Muscle rigidity • Drooling • Hyperthermia • Hypertensive crisis • Cardiac arrest	• If the drug was taken orally, induce vomiting or perform gastric lavage; instill and remove activated charcoal repeatedly. • Force acidic diuresis by acidifying the client's urine with ascorbic acid to increase excretion of the drug. Continue to acidify urine for 2 weeks, because toxic symptoms may recur when fat cells release their stores of PCP. • Control agitation or psychotic behavior with diazepam (Valium) and haloperidol (Haldol). • Control seizures with diazepam. • Treat hypertension and tachycardia with propranolol or, if the client's hypertension is severe, nitroprusside. • Closely monitor urine output and serial renal function tests—rhabdomyolysis, myoglobinuria, and renal failure may occur in severe intoxication. • If the client develops renal failure, perform hemodialysis.
Tricyclic antidepressants • amitriptyline (Elavil) • imipramine (Tofranil)	• Dilated pupils • Blurred vision • Altered mental status (from agitation to hallucinations) • Loss of deep tendon reflexes • Seizures • Coma • Anticholinergic effects (dry mucous membranes, diminished secretions) • Tachycardia • Hypotension • Nausea and vomiting • Urine retention	• Induce vomiting or perform gastric lavage if the client ingested the drug within the past 24 hours. (Anticholinergic effects of these drugs decrease gastric emptying.) Give activated charcoal and a magnesium sulfate cathartic. • Replace fluids I.V. to correct hypotension. • Give hypertonic sodium bicarbonate I.V. to correct hypotension and arrhythmias; if bifascicular or complete heart block occurs, a temporary transvenous pacemaker may be required. • Treat seizures with diazepam (Valium) or phenobarbital I.V. • Some clinicians administer physostigmine salicylate (Antilirium) to reverse central anticholinergic effects.

From *Handbook of psychotropic drugs.* Springhouse, PA: Springhouse Corp., 1992.

Appendix H: Resources for Clients and Families

ADDICTIONS

Alcoholism

Adult Children of Alcoholics
P.O. Box 3216
2522 W. Sepulueda Blvd.
Suite 200
Torrance, CA 90505
1-213-534-1815

Al-Anon Family Group Headquarters
P.O. Box 862
Midtown Station
New York, NY 10018-0862
1-212-302-7240

Alcoholics Anonymous World Services, Inc.
P.O. Box 459
Grand Central Station
New York, NY 10163
1-212-686-1100

California Hispanic Commission on Alcohol and Drug Abuse
2400 O Street
Sacramento, CA 95816
1-916-443-5473

Catholic Alcoholics — Calix Society
7601 Wayzata Blvd.
Minneapolis, MN 55426
1-612-546-0544

Children of Alcoholics Foundation
P.O. Box 4185
Dept. R.C.
Grand Central Station
New York, NY 10163
1-212-754-0656

Institute on Black Chemical Abuse
2614 Nicollet Avenue South
Minneapolis, MN 55408
1-612-871-7878

International Conference of Young People in AA Advisory Council
Box 19312
Eastgate Station
Indianapolis, IN 46219

Jewish Alcoholics, Chemically Dependent Persons and
    Significant Others
197 Broadway
Room M-7
New York, NY 10002
1-212-473-4747

National Asian Pacific Families Against Substance Abuse
6303 Friendship Court
Bethesda, MD 20817
1-301-530-0945

National Association for Children of Alcoholics
31582 Coast Highway
Suite B
South Laguna, CA 92677-3044
1-714-499-3889

National Association of Lesbian and Gay Alcoholism
    Professionals
204 West 20th Street
New York, NY 10011
1-212-713-5074

National Association of Native American Children of Alcoholics
c/o Seattle Indian Health Board
P.O. Box 3364
Seattle, WA 98114

Substance and Alcohol Intervention Services for the Deaf
50 W. Main Street
Room 215
Rochester, NY 14614
1-716-475-4978 (Voice)
1-716-475-4979 (TTY)

Women for Sobriety, Inc.
P.O. Box 618
Quakertown, PA 18951
1-215-536-8026

Drug Abuse

Action on Smoking and Health
2013 H Street N.W.
Washington, DC 20006
1-202-659-4310

American Lung Association
National Headquarters
1740 Broadway
New York, NY 10019-4374

Cocaine Anonymous
6125 Washington Blvd.
Suite 202
Los Angeles, CA 90230
1-213-559-5833
1-800-347-8998

Cocanon Family Groups
P.O. Box 64742-66
Los Angeles, CA 90064
1-213-859-2206

Nar-Anon Family Groups
P.O. Box 2562
Palos Verdes, CA 90274
1-213-547-5800

Narcotics Anonymous World Service Office
P.O. Box 9999
Van Nuys, CA 91409
1-818-780-3951

Pill Addicts Anonymous
General Service Board
P.O. Box 278
Reading, PA 19603
1-215-372-1128

Eating Disorders

American Anorexia and Bulimia Association, Inc.
418 E. 76th Street
New York, NY 10021
1-201-734-1114

Anorexics and Bulimics Anonymous
P.O. Box 112214
San Diego, CA 92111

National Anorexic Aid Society, Inc.
1925 E. Dublin Granville Road
Columbus, OH 43229
1-614-436-1112

National Association to Aid Fat Americans, Inc.
P.O. Box 43
Bellerose, NY 11426
1-516-352-3120

Overeater's Anonymous World Service Office
P.O. Box 92870
Los Angeles, CA 90009
1-310-657-6252

continued

Resources for Clients and Families *(continued)*

AGING AND ALZHEIMER'S DISEASE

Alzheimer's Association
919 N. Michigan Avenue
Suite 1000
Chicago, IL 60611-1676

American Association of Retired Persons
601 E Street N.W.
Washington, DC 20049
1-202-434-2277

Gerontological Society of America
1275 K Street, N.W.
Suite 350
Washington, DC 20005
1-202-842-1275

National Council on the Aging, Inc.
409 3rd Street, N.W.
Suite 200
Washington, DC 20024
1-202-479-1200

AIDS, ARC, and HIV+

AIDS Project Los Angeles, Inc.
7362 Santa Monica Blvd.
West Hollywood, CA 90046
1-213-876-8951

HIVIES
c/o the Illinois Alcoholism & Drug
   Dependence Association
500 W. Monroe
Springfield, IL 62704
1-217-528-7335

New Life
P.O. Box 851
19-21 Belmont Avenue
Kids Center for Hope
Hope House
Dover, NJ 07801
1-201-361-5555

Positives Anonymous World Services Office
25 Saint Marks Place
New York, NY 10003
1-212-732-6879

ANXIETY DISORDERS

Anxiety Disorders

Agoraphobics in Motion
605 West Eleven Mile Road
Royal Oak, MI 48067
1-313-547-0400

Anxiety Disorders Association of America
6000 Executive Blvd., Suite 200
Rockville, MD 20852
1-301-231-9350

Emotions Anonymous
P.O. Box 4245
Saint Paul, MN 55104
1-612-647-9712

Obsessive-Compulsive Disorder Foundation
Box 60
Vernon, CT 06066

Panic and Phobic Disorders

Phobia Society of America
133 Rollins Avenue
Suite 4B
Rockville, MD 20852

CHILD AND DOMESTIC ABUSE

American Association for Protecting Children
American Humane
63 Inverness Drive East
Englewood, CO 80012
1-303-695-0811
1-800-227-5242

Batterers Anonymous
8485 Tamarind
Suite D
Fontana, CA 92335
1-714-355-1100

National Coalition Against Domestic Violence
P.O. Box 34103
Washington, DC 20043-4103
1-202-638-6388

National Organization for Victims
   Assistance (NOVA)
1757 Park Road, N.W.
Washington, DC 20010
1-202-393-6682

FAMILY SUPPORT GROUPS

Codependents Anonymous
P.O. Box 33577
Phoenix, AZ 85067-3577
1-602-277-7991

Codependents of Sex Addicts
Twin Cities COSA
P.O. Box 14537
Minneapolis, MN 55414
1-612-537-6904

Families Anonymous, Inc.
14553 Delano Street
Van Nuys, CA 91411
1-818-989-7841

Gam-Anon International Service Office (for families of
   compulsive gamblers)
P.O. Box 157
Whitestone
New York, NY 11357
1-212-903-4200

National Alliance for the Mentally Ill
2101 Wilson Blvd
Suite 302
Arlington, VA 22201
1-703-524-7600

Parents Anonymous
520 S. Lafayette Park
Suite 316
Los Angeles, CA 90057
1-800-421-0353

Parents Without Partners, Inc.
8807 Colesville Road
Silver Spring, MD 20910
1-301-588-9354

Resources for Clients and Families (continued)

FAMILY SUPPORT GROUPS (continued)

Step Family Foundation, Inc.
333 West End Avenue
New York, NY 10023
1-212-877-3244

Tough Love
P.O. Box 1069
Doylestown, PA 18901
1-215-348-7090 or
1-800-333-1069

GENERAL INFORMATION RESOURCE

National Self-Help Clearinghouse
Graduate School University Center
City University of New York
33 W. 42nd Street
New York, NY 10036

MOOD DISORDERS

Depressive and Manic Depressive Association
222 S. Riverside Plaza
Suite 2812
Chicago, IL 60606
1-312-993-0066

Manic and Depressive Support Group, Inc.
P.O. Box 1747
Madison Square Station
New York, NY 10159
1-212-533-MDSG

PERSONALITY DISORDERS

International Society for the Study of Multiple Personality and
    Dissociation
5700 Old Orchard Road
1st Floor
Skokie, IL 60077-1024

Multiple Personality Clinic
Department of Psychiatry
Rush University
600 S. Paulina
Chicago, IL 60612

SCHIZOPHRENIA AND CHRONIC MENTAL ILLNESS

GROW, Inc.
2403 W. Springfield
Box 3667
Champaign, IL 61826
1-217-352-6989

National Alliance for the Mentally Ill
2101 Wilson Blvd
Suite 302
Arlington, VA 22201
1-703-524-7600

National Crisis Prevention Institute
3315 K N 124th Street
Brookfield, WI 53005
1-800-558-8976 or 1-414-783-5787

National Mental Health Association
1021 Prince Street
Alexandria, VA 22314-2971
1-703-684-7722

Recovery, Inc: The Association of Nervous and Former Mental
    Patients
802 Dearborn Street
Chicago, IL 60610
1-312-337-5661

SEXUAL DISORDERS, SEXUAL ABUSE, AND VIOLENCE

Impotence Information Center
P.O. Box 9
Minneapolis, MN 55440
1-800-843-4315

Impotents Anonymous
119 S. Ruth Street
Maryville, TN 37801
1-615-983-6064

Incest Survivors Anonymous
P.O. Box 5613
Long Beach, CA 90805-0613
1-213-428-5599

J2CP Information Service (Sex Change Surgery and
    Transsexualism)
P.O. Box 184
San Juan Capistrano, CA 92693
1-714-496-J2CP

Parents United (incest)
P.O. Box 952
San Jose, CA 95108
1-408-280-5055

Resolve, Inc. (problems of infertility)
1310 Broadway
Somerville, MA 02144
1-617-623-0744

Sex and Love Addicts Anonymous (SLAA)
Augustine Fellowship
P.O. Box 119
Newtown Branch
Boston, MA 02258
1-617-332-1845

Sex Information and Education Council of the United States
New York University
130 West 42nd Street
Suite 2500
New York, NY 10036
1-212-819-9770

Survivors of Incest Anonymous
World Service Office
P.O. Box 21817
Baltimore, MD 21222-6817
1-301-282-3400

Index

t refers to a table.

t refers to a table.

t refers to a table.

t refers to a table.

S

Sadism, sexual, 239
Sadistic personality disorder, 126, 127t
Schizoaffective disorder, 108
Schizoid personality disorder, 113
Schizophrenic disorders. 92-102
 altered oral mucous membrane in, 101
 altered thought processes in, 93-94
 assessment guidelines for, 92-93
 assessment in hospital, 96t
 catatonic type, 92
 complications of, 93
 discharge criteria for, 101
 disorganized type, 92
 etiology of, 92
 neuroleptics, guidelines for use, 95t
 outcome criteria for, 101
 physical findings for, 93
 potential activity intolerance in, 99
 potential anxiety in, 100-101
 potential for violence in, 97-99
 residual type, 92
 resources for clients and families with, 305
 self-care assessment for, 100t
 undifferentiated type, 92
 visual alterations in, 94, 96-97
Schizophreniform disorder, 108
Schizotypal personality disorder, 113
Secobarbital, 27t, 179t, 291
Sedatives, 27-29t, 29, 291
Seizures, 296-297
Self-care deficit, 222
Self-defeating personality disorder, 126, 127t
Self-destructive behavior, 208
Self-esteem disturbance, 49, 69-70, 80, 147-148, 152, 192, 205
Selye, H., 31
Sensorium, clouded, 297
Serotonin, 208
Sexual disorders, 239-241. See also Gender identity disorder.
 altered sexuality patterns in, 241
 assessment guidelines for, 240
 complications of, 241
 discharge criteria for, 241
 etiology of, 239
 outcome criteria for, 241
 paraphilias, 239, 239t
 physical findings for, 240
 sexual dysfunctions and, 239
Sexual dysfunctions, 239
Sexual history, elements of, 234-235t
Sexual response variations, 233, 239
Simpson Neurological Rating Scale, 255-256
Skinner, B.F., 9
Sleep disorders, 226-232
 assessment guidelines for, 226-227
 complications of, 228
 discharge criteria for, 231
 dyssomnias, 226
 etiology of, 226
 hypersomnias, 226
 outcome criteria for, 231
 parasomnias, 226
 physical findings for, 227-228
 psychiatric and medical disorders as cause of, 229t
 sleep history assessment for, 230t
 sleep pattern disturbance, 228-229, 231
 sleep-promoting techniques and, 231t
 sleep stages, 227t
 sleep-wake schedule disorder, 226

Sleep disturbance, 226, 297
Sleep-wake schedule disorder, 226
Social isolation, 49-50, 131, 163-164, 223
Social model, 10
Social readjustment rating scale, 31, 32t
Sociocultural influences, 208
Somatization disorder, 217
Somatoform pain disorder, 217
Somatotype, 233
Spiritual distress, 71, 193
Splitting in personality disorders, 119
Stimulant dependence, 187-195
 altered health maintenance in, 189
 altered nutrition (less than body requirements) in, 190
 assessment guidelines for, 187-188
 cocaine effects and, 188t
 complications of, 189
 decreased cardiac output in, 191
 discharge criteria for, 194
 dressing or grooming self-care deficit in, 191
 etiology of, 187
 fear in, 192
 impaired social interactions in, 193
 ineffective family coping in, 194
 knowledge deficit in, 194
 outcome criteria for, 194
 physical findings for, 188-189
 potential altered body temperature in, 190
 potential for violence in, 193
 potential impaired skin integrity in, 190
 self-esteem disturbance in, 192
 sensory-perceptual alteration in, 192
 sleep pattern disturbance in, 191
 spiritual distress in, 193
Stress, 31, 34
 general adaptation syndrome stages, 33t
 social readjustment rating scale, 32t
Stressors, 217
Substance abuse, 169, 178, 187, 196, 202
 acute, managing, 299-302
Suicidal ideation, 297
Suicide Risk Assessment Tool, 268-269
Sullivan, Harry Stack, 9, 42
Support groups for clients and families, 304-305
Symbiosis, 119
Szasz, Thomas, 10

T

Tardive dyskinesia, 297
Temazepam, 28t, 178, 291
Theory
 behavioral, 119-120, 187, 196, 217, 233
 biogenetic, 208
 cognitive, 31, 120
 family, 113, 120, 126, 187, 196, 208
 goal attainment, 13
 interpersonal, 34
 intrapersonal, 217
 of nursing, general, 12
 object-relations, 73-74, 113, 126
 psychoanalytic, 113, 233
 psychodynamic, 113, 119, 187, 196, 208
Therapy
 behavioral, 16-17
 biological, 16-17
 family, 16
 group, 16
 milieu, 16
 short-term medication, 46t

Thioridazine, 26t, 289
Thiothixene, 26t, 289
Thioxanthene, 26t
Tourette's syndrome, 297
Transsexualism, 233
Transvestism, 239
Tranylcypromine, 21t, 284
Traumatization, vicarious, 249-253
 assessment guidelines for, 249-250
 burnout and, 249
 complications of, 250
 countertransference in, 249
 etiology of, 249
 outcome criteria for, 252
 physical findings for, 250
 post-trauma response and, 251
 powerlessness in, 251
 sleep pattern disturbance in, 252
Trazodone, 22t, 284
Treatment modalities
 behavioral therapy, 16-17
 biological therapies, 17
 crisis intervention, 15-16
 family therapy, 16
 group therapy, 16
 milieu therapy, 16
 psychopharmacology, 17, 18-29t, 29
 psychotherapy, 15
Triazolam, 28t, 178, 291
Tricyclic antidepressants, 17, 22-24t, 302
 client-family guidelines for, 88t
Trifluoperazine, 26t, 289
Trihexyphenidyl, 285
Trimethadione, 280
Trimipramine, 24t, 284

UV

Unitary human model, 13
Valproic acid, 280
Violence, 242
 assessing victims of, 243t
 disorders associated with
  rape-trauma syndrome, 242-247
  vicarious traumatization, 249-252
 resources for victims of, 304
Voyeurism, 239

WXYZ

Wolpe, J., 9
Zoophilia, 239

t refers to a table.